MW01142898

TRANSFORMED

TRANSFORMED

How Oregon's Public Health University Won Independence and Healed Itself

William Graves

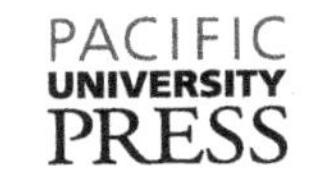

FOREST GROVE, OREGON

PACIFIC UNIVERSITY PRESS
2043 College Way
Forest Grove, Oregon 97116

Cover design by Alex Bell

ISBN (hbk) 978-1-945398-98-8
ISBN (pbk) 978-0-9884827-9-1
ISBN (epub) 978-1-945398-94-0
ISBN (PDF) 978-1-945398-97-1

Published in the United States of America

I know of no other academic health center or major public research university that ever made a change as radical as OHSU made in 1995: It left the state and the state system of higher education to operate largely on its own as a private corporation with a public mission.

The architect of this change was Dr. Peter Kohler along with his leadership team, whose story unfolds in this excellent book, a worthwhile read for anyone with connections to academia or government.

Phil Knight, Chairman Emeritus, Nike Inc.

Table of Contents

List of Figures

Acknowledgements

I am indebted to the scores of people who helped me in so many ways to write this book. Dr. Peter Kohler, who proposed the project to me, provided continuous and thoughtful support and insight at every turn from beginning to end. Similarly, members of his former leadership team at Oregon Health & Science University and key players in this story—Lesley Hallick, Janet Billups, Lois Davis, Timothy Goldfarb, and James Walker—each were readily available repeatedly for interviews and questions.

Isaac Gilman, library director and director of Pacific University Press, proved indispensible in publishing this book with his steady hand, skilled editing, and thoughtful and patient guidance. Former library director Marita Kunkel helped in the early stages to get the project rolling.

I am also indebted to the OHSU Foundation and OHSU staff, including the former and present faculty, administrators and community supporters who granted me their time for interviews. Special thanks to OHSU President Joseph Robertson for his support of this book and help providing me access to the campus and staff. Thanks also to OHSU employees Caryn Ruch, communications manager; Amy Johnson, office manager to the legal department; Mary Bianchini, executive assistant to the president; and the staff in the OHSU Historical Collections & Archives, Maija Anderson, head librarian; Max Johnson, archivist and assistant professor; and Meg Langford, public services coordinator.

Additionally, I'm grateful to Barbara Archer, professor of health care administration at Concordia University in Portland, and Dana Director, OHSU vice president for research operations and student affairs, for sharing their insights and doctoral theses on OHSU's conversion to a public corporation.

Many thanks also to my son, Mark Graves, for his help with photographs and graphics, and my niece, Dawn Rohrer, for her superior work transcribing many of my interviews.

And thanks to those who provided feedback on the manuscript, including author and friend Bill Geroux, and members of my writing group, called 546: Don Colburn, Sally Cheriel, Wendy Lawton, and Paige Parker. I'm also grateful for the support of my siblings, Jill Cain and Jack and Douglas Graves; and for friends who encouraged me throughout this project: Neal and Anita Perrine, John Sutton, Spencer Heinz, Chris and David Parent, Chris and Louise Brantley, Duane and Patricia Pellervo, John and JoAnn Ullstrom, Cynthia and Arnie Eriksen, Sherrie and Larry Wade, and Mary Kogen, my piano teacher.

Finally, my deepest gratitude to my wife, Karin Graves; my son, Max Graves; daughter and son-in-law, Emma and Kwame Harlin; our German son, Sebastian Franke; and my father, Earl Graves, for their patience, support, and encouragement through the more than two years I worked on this book.

Author's Note

Peter Kohler, the former president of Oregon Health & Science University, contacted me in the winter of 2014 to see if I might be interested in helping him and the five members of his former administrative team write a book. I had spent twenty-three years covering education and health care for *The Oregonian* in Portland, knew of Kohler, and had on a few occasions reported on OHSU when he was its president. He and his team wanted to tell the story of how they battled to free Oregon's sole academic health center from the bureaucratic trappings of the state and its university system by converting it into an independent and entrepreneurial public benefit corporation and of the remarkable transformation that followed. Kohler also wanted to show that OHSU's transformation could serve as a model for other public universities and academic health centers struggling with declining state support and revenue.

He and his team initially set out to write this story themselves as a kind of collective memoir. When I joined them, it became clear I would need to write this remarkable story with them as the key players and primary sources. They contributed money to the OHSU Foundation, which in turn provided me a salary while I researched hundreds of documents and newspaper stories and interviewed scores of current and former OHSU employees and state leaders involved in its transformation. Without this funding, I would have been unable to write the story of these people and their institution.

I have approached this project as a journalist, striving to find various and opposing views on the issues and to be as accurate as I can. I do, however, tell this story from the perspective of Kohler and his team. I relied on multiple interviews with all of them, worked closely with Kohler throughout, and I try to tell the story they wanted to tell. At no time did any of them interfere. All of them reviewed the manuscript, in some cases multiple times, all with the view of ensuring the story was accurate.

Introduction

A Singular Path to Change

On July 1, 1995, Oregon Health & Science University broke from the state's higher education system and plunged into the health care marketplace as an independent public corporation. While other public bodies in Oregon and elsewhere had mixed government and corporate qualities, no academic health center or major public research university had ever made such a radical change—to break from the state and its university system and chart its fate alone as a private corporation with a public mission.

OHSU's transformation—and the way its administrative team carried it out—offers a vivid case study in institutional change and leadership. It is an instructive story for the growing number of public academic health centers and universities facing the same disruptive forces that drove OHSU to convert to a public corporation. And beyond public institutions, it provides insights for any large organization willing to go through the cultural and structural changes necessary to truly transform into a high-performing operation.

LEADING CHANGE

As in all stories of organizational change, OHSU's transformation is a story about people. Dr. Peter Kohler—a trim, tall, forty-nine-year-old endocrinologist—arrived at OHSU in 1988 for his first attempt at running one of about 125 academic health centers across the nation at that time.

Like many of the researchers and faculty whom he would draw to OHSU, he was a rising star, most recently as dean of the medical school at the University of Texas Health Science Center in San Antonio. He had a strong track record of handling administrative duties at other academic health centers, and he had a solid research background, including a prominent role during his eight years at the National Institutes of Health.

"He was exactly the kind of president we needed," says Dr. Markus Grompe, genetic researcher and professor in the departments of Pediatrics and Molecular and Medical Genetics at OHSU. "He was someone who wanted research and had actually done it. He was a Howard Hughes [Medical Institute] investigator, which is the elite. He had a really good balance of knowing the research world and knowing the business world."[1]

Kohler's soft Virginian accent and genial, unassuming manner made him an instant hit among Oregon leaders. And he deftly picked the right people for the right jobs, assembling a young leadership team that developed a unique camaraderie over the years in their galvanizing struggle to win autonomy for OHSU. Lesley Hallick, a molecular biology professor and researcher, joined Kohler as vice president of academic affairs, the leader who would convince a skeptical faculty it should support conversion to a public corporation. Lois Davis, former chief of staff for Congressman Ron Wyden (Democrat from Oregon), led the charge in the legislature as the health center's chief lobbyist. Timothy Goldfarb, director of hospitals and clinics, showed how OHSU's clinical services could be a powerful economic engine for the health center if freed from state restrictions and allowed to compete as a business. James B. Walker, the university's vice president of finance and administration, had deep experience running the hospital business in the face of state bureaucratic rules. He built a compelling financial argument for making OHSU a public corporation even as he worried through sleepless nights whether it could ever really happen. The state assigned Janet Billups to OHSU as a young assistant attorney general, but she soon became the university's lawyer, charged with the monumental job of combing Oregon's statutes and nearly single-handedly writing Senate Bill 2, which would define OHSU's powers and obligations as a public corporation.

It wasn't long after Kohler arrived at OHSU that he and his leadership team concluded transformational change offered the best, and possibly the only, path to a stable future. State funding had been declining for decades. The university's other major source of money, its small teaching hospital, served largely indigent patients: it was a money loser that legislators more than once proposed closing. It was widely viewed as a hospital of last resort, even by OHSU employees, who went elsewhere for care. Rusty water poured from its taps. Its maternity ward put as many as four mothers to a room and was so limited in space that OHSU had to send some of its pregnant patients to other hospitals or into the hallway to deliver their babies. Scuffed, worn, and cramped classrooms, research labs, and offices across the campus needed repairs and remodeling.

After Kohler's team led OHSU's conversion into a public corporation, state regulatory barriers fell like the Berlin Wall, releasing pent-up entrepreneurial talent that produced explosive growth. The expansion lifted the university into the top research echelon of American academic health centers. It quickly upgraded and expanded its hospital, which has become the preferred choice for Oregonians and one of the top ten hospitals in the nation for handling the most complex medical cases. Most of OHSU's new laboratories, clinics, surgery centers, and research institutes emerged after it became a public corporation. It is impossible to say precisely how much of the university's dramatic growth can be attributed to its becoming a public corporation, but research, business, and education leaders both inside and outside the university agree that the change played a major role.

Steve Stadum, a lawyer and former chief operating officer for OHSU's Knight Cancer Institute, argues the university could not have grown so much if it had remained a state agency and part of the state university system. "We would have never had a board," he says. "We would have never been able to issue debt, and we would not have ever been able to take risks, be entrepreneurial and opportunistic."[2]

Current President Joseph Robertson says OHSU would be half its size today if it had not become a public corporation,[3] which he says was "a foundational change" instrumental in its success. "OHSU is a much larger yet leaner, more entrepreneurial institution," he writes, "with widespread excellence: nationally ranked education programs and world-class research and patient-care programs."[4]

Dr. Eric Orwoll, who directs OHSU's clinical research program, says "everything changed over a very short period of time" after the university became a public corporation. Research expanded rapidly on campus, says Orwoll, a world expert on bone biology and osteoporosis in men. "There were new collaborations, new people, new opportunities for me as a young faculty member," he says. "It was a really fortuitous time to be here."

Orwoll arrived at OHSU in 1977 before the conversion and initially worked in "small, old, dark" laboratories in the old Veterans Administration Hospital on campus. Now he works on the top floor of the fourteen-story Hatfield Research Center, which opened in 1998. The laboratories are modern, well-equipped, "state of the art," he says, not only in the Hatfield Center, but also in the rebuilt VA Hospital and in OHSU's remodeled labs and towering new research buildings.[5]

RISE OF ACADEMIC HEALTH CENTERS

OHSU's identity as an academic health center underscores the significance of its transformation. The challenges of transforming any organization rise with complexity, and there are few enterprises more complex than academic health centers, which employ and enroll high concentrations of society's most intelligent people. Neither students nor faculty can retreat into the groves of academe because they are daily immersed in the practical demands and drama of helping people who are injured, sick, and sometimes dying, says Dr. Steven Wartman, president of the Association of Academic Health Centers (AAHC). University medical centers "are unique hybrids of business and academics. That, paradoxically, makes them the hardest institutions in the world to manage."[6]

Medical education, research, and health care programs coalesced into academic health centers in the 1950s, 1960s, and 1970s as federal research support and state funding increased. The federal government also offered states financial incentives to enlarge their medical schools because health leaders warned of a looming doctor shortage. Academic health centers refined their professional and accreditation standards, writes Dr. Roger Bulger, former president of the AAHC, and soon the university hospital rose as the "clinical court of last resort for the most complex medical problems."[7]

More recently, academic health centers have evolved into what might better be described as systems or networks, says Wartman. They encompass a growing geographic range of health and educational facilities with a host of services, he says, and each "can be viewed as an organization without boundaries."[8] Though they share the same three central missions—education, health care, and research—they differ widely in size, structure, and areas of focus and expertise. About two-thirds are part of a comprehensive undergraduate university, such as the University of Washington Medical Center; 19 percent are part of a university system; and 21 percent are freestanding health science universities like OHSU.[9] About a third are public, though the gap between public and private academic medical centers has narrowed, says Wartman.

"The economic realities and political realities have made the public act more like the private," he says. "They had to become more entrepreneurial."[10]

Although academic health centers play a critical national role in training most health professionals, save lives in the most complex medical cases, provide health care for the poor, and conduct advanced medical research, their collective force on the American health care landscape is not clearly documented. While the AAHC does not provide a current number of academic health centers, a recent publication estimates it to be about 140.[11] These centers command a significant share of the $3.1 trillion annual health care spending in the United States, but neither the AAHC nor the Association of American Medical Colleges can say precisely what that portion is. A 2014 report on the nation's academic health centers says the more than "110" academic health centers earned more than $175 billion a year from patient services and $14 billion in National Institutes of Health research funding. The report estimated that US academic health centers collectively employ about 1.2 million people.[12]

In addition, reports by the AAHC say the medical centers collectively enroll more than 325,000 health profession and graduate students and spend $19 billion on research and more than $6 billion on uncompensated patient care each year.[13]

"They are (major) economic engines in the communities in which they are embedded," says Wartman. "Many serve as safety nets as well."[14]

DECLINING PUBLIC SUPPORT FOR PUBLIC HIGHER EDUCATION

By the time Kohler arrived at OHSU in 1988, the academic health center boom of the 1950s through the 1970s had subsided, giving way to rising health education costs and waning state support. The hospital struggled financially in a market that was becoming increasingly competitive as the health insurance industry moved away from fee-for-service to managed care. The latter model limits customer choices in doctors and hospitals and pays providers on a flat per patient basis, all to control costs. OHSU, like all academic health centers, had a disadvantage in the managed care market because of the higher costs of its more complex services. What's more, Oregon voters in 1990 passed a property tax limitation measure that almost guaranteed OHSU its state revenue would plummet rather than rise.

When he was hired, Kohler had been told to expect state funding to soon climb to about 30 percent of the health center's budget. But instead, it remained flat, and the tax limit pushed it lower. This dramatic decrease in state funding, more than any other force, drove Kohler to seek more independence for OHSU. The university needed to fix buildings, upgrade its clinics, and expand its research capacity if it was to draw paying patients and first-rate faculty. So Kohler had to either succumb to the decline and bury his dream of making OHSU a great academic health center or find another way. When the medical center transformed to a public corporation and split from the state and its higher education system, it was collecting about a fifth of its operating budget from Oregon's general fund, down from two-fifths twenty years earlier. The decline in state support continued over the following two decades, during which OHSU's budget grew fivefold to $2.5 billion a year, less than 2 percent of which came from the state.

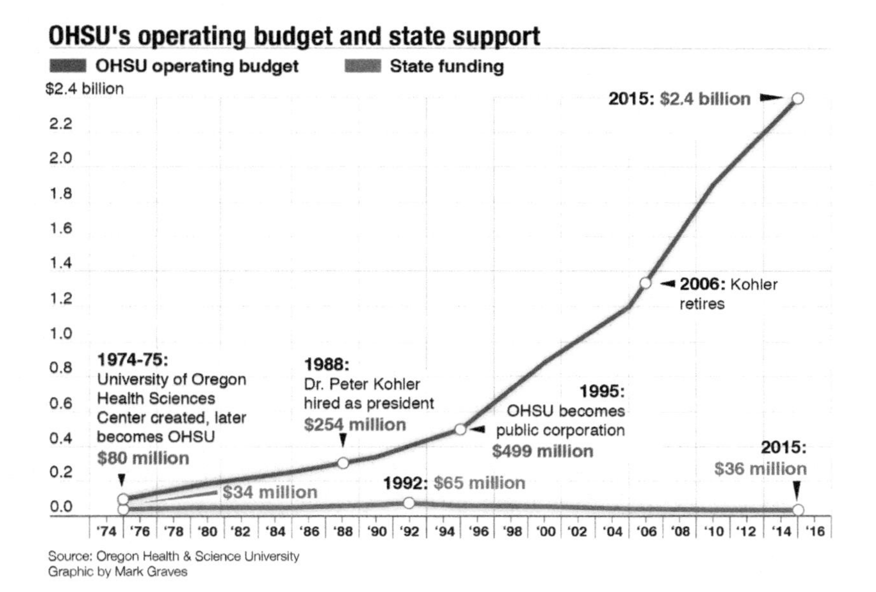

Today, public universities across the country face similar irreversible declines in state support. In early 2016, the University of California at Berkeley launched a "strategic planning process" aimed at helping it adjust to what Chancellor Nicholas Dirks called the "new normal" of decreasing state support. The prestigious public research university once depended on the state for half of its support, but that had plunged to only 13 percent of its $2.6 billion budget. With state limits on tuition increases and rapidly rising pension and health care costs, the university was operating with an annual deficit of about 6 percent or $150 million.[15]

At about the same time, public universities in Illinois were faced with layoffs and other drastic measures because a legislative budget fight had blocked their state money for seven months. Eastern Illinois University prepared to lay off 198 civil service workers and possibly close early.[16] Chicago State University had exhausted its reserves, could not meet its next month's payroll, and declared financial exigency, which, among other cuts, would allow it to fire tenured professors.[17] The City College of New York—a system of twenty-four colleges, including eleven four-year schools, serving 274,000 students—had a 17 percent drop in state funding over the eight preceding years, while tuition climbed by $300 per year in a system that was tuition-free in 1976.[18] In Louisiana, faced with a $900 million deficit in its state budget, the state higher education system braced for at least $70 million in cuts on top of $684 million in cuts since 2008.[19] Former US Secretary of Education Margaret Spellings had just taken office as the new president of the University of North Carolina system and was greeted by faculty and student protests after years of budget cuts, pay freezes, and fears the system was losing its national stature.[20] In Kansas, Governor Sam Brownback ordered a $17 million cut in spending on the state's public colleges over the next four months to close a revenue gap.[21] Dirks concluded the American public university was under siege. "What we are engaged in here is a fundamental defense of the concept of the public university," he says, "a concept that we must reinvent in order to preserve."[22]

Despite modest increases in state support for public institutions four, five, and six years after the Great Recession, most observers do not expect those increases to be permanent nor to reverse a long-term trend of decline. State funding for higher education, including community colleges, collectively climbed 5.7 percent nationwide in the 2013–14 year to $86.3 billion, but still fell below annual levels for 2008 through 2011. Between the Great Recession and fiscal year 2014, state support dropped 19 percent nationwide in per student spending, from $8,081 per student to $6,552 (in constant-adjusted 2014 dollars). Changes varied widely among states. Funding shot up 50 percent in Illinois, 38 percent in North Dakota and 6 percent in Alaska during this period. But it dropped in every other state. Allocations plunged 41 percent in Louisiana, 39 percent in Alabama, and 37 percent in Pennsylvania, and fell by a more modest 5 percent in Wyoming, New York, Montana, and Nebraska.[23]

Over the long run, state funding can be expected to continue to decline, says Thomas G. Mortenson, a higher education policy analyst. Based on trends since 1980, Mortenson figures, "average state support for higher education will reach zero by 2059."[24]

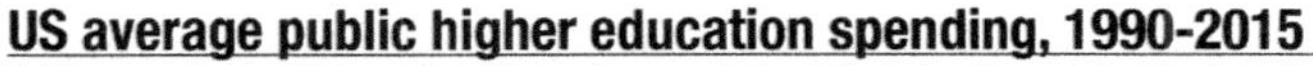

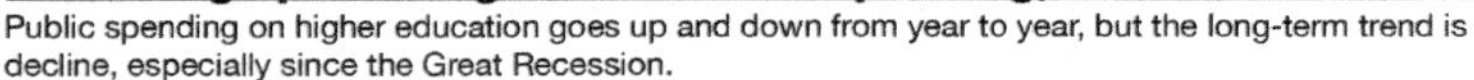

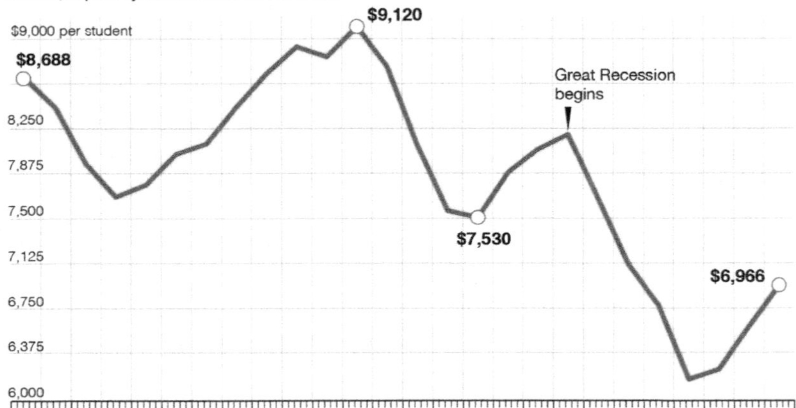

Note: Numbers are average annual spending per full-time student.

Source: State Higher Educaton Executive Officers from report, State Higher Education Finance: FY 2015.
Graphic by Mark Graves

Public universities have turned to tuition to make up for lost state support. Over the two decades between 1995 and 2015, on average tuition and fees more than doubled from $4,399 to $9,410 in 2015 dollars.[25] Tuition and fees have climbed so high they threaten to squeeze out middle-class students, let alone those more economically disadvantaged. Federal student financial aid through loans and grants, which totaled about $134 billion in the 2013–14 school year, has helped replace lost state revenues, but university leaders believe that, too, is finite.[26] The federal government may start requiring states to demonstrate a certain level of support before it will provide financial aid to their students, says Portland State University President Wim Wiewel. He says he does not see how public universities can sustain their quality without more state support.

"We'll continue to raise class sizes because we are going to continue to increase the number of non-tenured track faculty," he said. "We will do whatever it takes to make a cheap education possible. And clearly there are pressures to make that happen. Because we have reached a limit to what we can do through tuition. We can't keep raising tuition without seriously reducing the number of students we get, and then you get into a downward spiral."[27]

Universities have other sources of money, including research grants, investment earnings, dormitory and dining hall fees, event ticket sales, and parking receipts. Yet while their collective income from all sources continues to outpace inflation, it is not enough. Public universities in recent years have frozen salaries, cut staff, allowed class sizes to grow, deferred maintenance on their buildings, and reduced programs, slipping into a vicious cycle of decline.

"Even while their tuition charges are soaring, revenue-starved public campuses are in a long-term state of decline that shows no sign of reversing," writes James Garland, former president of Miami University in Ohio, an alarm echoed by many other authors.[28]

As a result of this trend, universities have had to cut into the heart of their enterprise—the quality of their faculty. They are replacing full-time professors with lower-cost lecturers, instructors, and part-time adjuncts. The proportion of full-time faculty in all public and private universities has plunged from 78 percent in 1970 to 51 percent in 2013,[29] and not all of those full-time professors are tenured or on tenure tracks. About 70 percent of US higher education's professors are contingent—adjuncts and non-tenure track lecturers and instructors.[30] Universities also are skimping on deferred maintenance to balance their budgets, creating growing backlogs of buildings in need of repair. The deferred maintenance price tag for Arizona's three public universities, for example, stood at over a half a billion dollars in the 2014–15 school year. The state gave the universities $3 million for maintenance that year after seven years of no money at all.[31] A 2015 survey of Schools of Agriculture at ninety-one universities found a total $8.4 billion in deferred maintenance that reduced the asset value of more than 15,000 buildings by nearly a third, according to a report by Sightlines, a firm that helps universities manage their facilities, and the Association of Public and Land-grant Universities.[32] The *New York Times* described how declining state support played out at City College of New York, where on its "handsome Gothic campus, leaking ceilings have turned hallways into obstacle courses of buckets. The bathrooms sometimes run out of toilet paper. The lectures are becoming uncomfortably overcrowded, and course selections are dwindling, because of steep budget cuts."[33]

PUBLIC DEFUNDING OF ACADEMIC HEALTH CENTERS

The trend of eroding state funding for public higher education in general is no less significant for academic health centers. Over the quarter century between 1987 and 2012, the declines in state support are stark and nearly universal. The portion of total revenue coming from the state dropped from 68 percent to 20 percent at the University of Arkansas for Medical Sciences in Little Rock, from 65 percent to 35 percent at Georgia Health

Sciences University, from 64 percent to 39 percent at the University of Oklahoma Health Sciences Center, from 46 percent to 29 percent at the University of Texas Health Science Center at Houston, and from 32 percent to 17 percent at the University of California at San Francisco.[34]

Academic health centers cannot count on much money from tuition since they enroll relatively few students, but they are slightly better positioned than other public universities to deal with declining state revenue: they can generate income through their hospital and clinical services. Those services also bring some indirect government support. The federal government pays for Medicare patients, and the federal and state governments share the costs of Medicaid patients. In addition, Medicare recognizes the benefits to society of training doctors by giving academic health centers $3 billion a year. Medicare also gives teaching hospitals about $6.5 million a year to compensate for the added costs of caring for more severe cases.[35] But depending on clinical revenues and Medicaid and Medicare payments has limits. At OHSU, for example, Medicare and Medicaid account for 55 percent of the payer mix and so about half or less of its patient revenue.[36] The realities of declining government support have brought other academic health centers to the same place OHSU was two decades ago, when it faced a growing deferred maintenance backlog, staff cuts, legislative threats to close its hospital, and declining quality.

INSTITUTION, HEAL THYSELF: THE OHSU MODEL

At OHSU, Kohler's solution to declining state support was to win the university enough autonomy to take charge of its fate. By becoming a public corporation, OHSU was freed of state regulations that hampered its ability to grow and compete in the health care marketplace. Once on its own as a public corporation, it could borrow its own money on Wall Street to improve its research and clinical facilities, attract top-quality researchers and faculty, and reposition itself on an upward trajectory. Not all academic health centers and public universities need to become public corporations, but they need to find more independence and more ways to sustain themselves with less government help, say many experts. John Woodward, a health finance specialist who helped OHSU during its transition, says other public universities and academic health centers need to prepare for that day when state tax money dries up.

OHSU "is the model," he says. "You have to be able to stand on your own."[37]

Other higher education leaders are reaching the same conclusion. For example, James Garland, the former Miami University president, says the traditional business model of public universities, with its heavy reliance on state subsidies and tuition, is failing. He proposes a different business model that resembles the OHSU public corporation. He argues that instead of giving money directly to their public universities, states should give it to students in the form of scholarships. This would create market incentives among universities to compete for students and their money by offering better education at better prices. To compete effectively, Garland says, the universities should be freed from state systems and bureaucracies to become "semiautonomous, publicly owned but independently governed, tax exempt corporations." Each university would have its own governing board and the power to set tuition and salaries, award contracts, accept gifts, and make changes in admission and graduation standards.[38]

Most academic health centers and universities are fervently seeking options to stay solvent, even as they draw more heavily on hospital and clinical revenue, tuition, alumni contributions, philanthropy, endowments, and investments to cover their bottom lines. Because Oregon was among the first states to see state funding on an inexorable descent, it was the first to release an entire academic health center from its state university system. Other venerated public institutions over the last two decades have shown an interest in seeking more autonomy, but their legislatures and political barriers have limited their success. State funding had slipped to 14 percent of the total budget for the University of Virginia and 22 percent at Virginia's College of William & Mary when, in 2005, both won some independence from the state system in exchange for meeting certain performance goals. In recent years, the University of Oregon, University of Wisconsin at Madison, Medical University of South Carolina, University of California at San Francisco, and others have sought to win legislative approval to part with their state systems and become independent universities.

Many of these efforts failed because of political blowback. Richard Lariviere, for example, was fired as president of the University of Oregon (UO) in 2011 after he defied the State Board of Higher Education in a hard-charging push to pry UO away from the Oregon University System and create its own board. In the same year, Chancellor Carolyn A. "Biddy" Martin tried to broker a deal with Governor Scott Walker to sever Madison, the flagship, from the University of Wisconsin system. After facing nearly a year of political turmoil and protests over that plan, Martin moved on to lead Amherst College in Massachusetts, and Madison remained in the university system.

In contrast, Kohler and his team were fortunate to encounter a favorable political climate in Oregon, which contributed to their success in winning support for OHSU's conversion to a public corporation. Republicans, who controlled both houses of the Oregon Legislature, had long preached that government should operate like a business, and now here was a government enterprise proposing to do exactly that. State leaders and voters were in the mood for big changes. The legislature had just passed a sweeping public school reform plan, and voters had approved the property tax limit that made it harder for the state to pay for its universities. OHSU's proposed change had the support of newly-elected Democratic Governor John Kitzhaber, an emergency room physician who trained at its medical school. And state leaders knew the university's hospital was struggling to make money and could become a serious economic drain on the state if something didn't change. Still, the university had proposed a radical move. Not everyone was ready to turn the state's only academic health center loose. Some university leaders still saw OHSU, for all of its problems, as the "crown jewel" of Oregon's higher education system.

This case study of OHSU's transformation provides insights into leading and managing change that should interest leaders who want to take their institutions on the bold and risky path to independence. It shows how Kohler's team won the support of Mark Hatfield, Oregon's senior US senator; governors Neil Goldschmidt, Barbara Roberts, and John Kitzhaber; rural and urban, Republican and Democratic legislators; faculty, staff, unions, students; and the State Board of Higher Education and university system chancellors Thomas Bartlett and Joe Cox. Kohler's team also engaged, and in many cases enlisted, many other powerful people in their five-year campaign to transform OHSU, such as state Senate President Gordon Smith and state Senator Eugene Timms (Republican from Burns), cochair of the legislature's Joint Ways and Means Committee; business leaders Fred Buckman, president and CEO of PacifiCorp; John Gray, chair of GrayCo Inc.; Jerry Meyer, chair and CEO of Tektronix; Mark Dodson, a Portland attorney and president of Northwest Natural Gas; and Mike Thorne, former legislator and executive director of the Port of Portland.

Legislators are accustomed to seeing state agency leaders come to them with requests for money. But Kohler didn't do that, says Thorne, the former Senate leader who eventually served on OHSU's board. Instead, the OHSU president came to them with a solution. Once leaders saw where Kohler was headed, Thorne says, "the reasons became obvious."

Given the political paralysis that has gripped so much of government in recent decades, the OHSU story offers a refreshing reminder, says Thorne, that "if people get focused and are willing to commit themselves, you can solve things."[39]

The bill to transform OHSU into a public corporation won all but three votes in the Senate and unanimous support in the House.

NEW HORIZONS

Today, OHSU towers over Portland in a dense complex of medical, classroom, and research buildings on Marquam Hill, commonly called Pill Hill. Old buildings like the sprawling, sand-colored brick medical school mix with new curved, gleaming glass-and-steel towers over 116 acres full of researchers and clinics. From its high perch, the academic health center has a view north over downtown Portland and beyond to the Columbia River and Mount St. Helens. The view opens east to the Willamette River winding into the city and the distant snow-capped Mount Hood and Cascade Mountain Range.

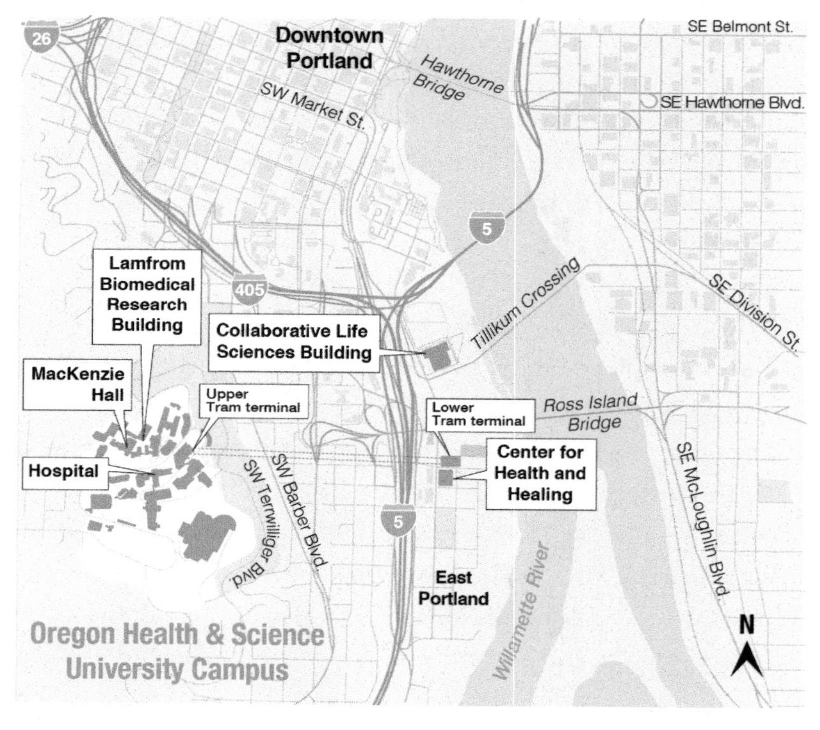

Graphic by Mark Graves.

Despite its lofty location, the medical complex had for nearly a century looked inward and settled for provincial goals, leaving it relatively obscure and unnoticed among the nation's research universities and academic health centers. After becoming an independent public corporation in 1995, however, it raised its sights and profile, expanded dramatically, and became a player on the national stage. Today it looks outward with a national vision more aligned with its commanding view.

Over the last two decades, OHSU's research and operating budgets and its philanthropy dollars grew fourfold, and it doubled the number of people it employs, patients it serves, and degrees it awards. The medical center upgraded its old buildings, overhauled the medical school curriculum, and nearly doubled its square feet of building space, from 3.8 million to 7.1 million. It expanded beyond Pill Hill to the Willamette River waterfront below and added buildings on its 300-acre West Campus near Hillsboro, a city 20 miles west of Portland. There OHSU operates its Oregon National Primate Research Center, Vaccine and Gene Therapy Institute, Neurological Sciences Institute, Institute for Environmental Health and the Department of Biomedical Engineering's Center for Spoken Language Understanding. The university also runs rural health clinics and education and research centers across the state. The once sleepy campus on Pill Hill now pulses around the clock with its thousands of researchers, faculty, and medical students engaged in its primary missions—research, teaching, and health care.

In becoming a public corporation, OHSU was unleashed. It broke from its past and state authority to pursue its independent vision, a break that dramatically changed its culture and trajectory—a break that transformed it.

Notes

1 Marcus Grompe, interview, April 16, 2014.

2 Steve Stadum, interview, Dec. 11, 2014, Peter O. Kohler Pavilion, Oregon Health & Science University (hereafter OHSU).

3 Joseph Robertson, MD (president, OHSU), interview, Aug. 20, 2015, his office in Baird Hall, OHSU.

4 Joseph Robertson, MD, "OHSU as a Public Corporation: Launching a period of growth and programmatic excellence," report printed by OHSU, 2011, p. 1.

5 Eric Orwoll, MD, interview, April 4, 2014, Hatfield Research Center, OHSU.

6 Steven Wartman, MD, interview by telephone with author, March 23, 2015.

7 Roger J. Bulger, MD and Marian Osterweis, "The Organization and Governance of Academic Health Centers: Fundamental Issues in a New Environment," paper published by the Association of Academic Health Centers, Aug. 2003, pp. 6, 7.

8 Steven Wartman, MD, ed., *The Transformation of Academic Health Centers: Meeting the Challenges of Healthcare's Changing Landscape* (San Diego: Academic Press, an imprint of Elsevier, 2015), p. xix.

9 *Academic Health Centers: Creating the Knowledge Economy*, "Facts at a Glance," Association of Academic Health Centers, http://www.aahcdc.org/Portals/0/pdf/FG_AHC_Creating_the_Knowlege_Economy_04-09.pdf.

10 Wartman, interview.

11 Wartman, *Transformation of Academic Health Centers*, p. 3.

12 Charles Kim and Rob York (senior vice presidents for Kaufman Hall), "Strategic Choices for Academic Health Centers," report presented to Kaufman, Hall & Associates, Inc., Oct. 13, 2014, p. 3.

13 "Facts at a Glance," Association of Academic Health Centers, http://www.aahcdc.org/Default.aspx?TabID=177.

14 Wartman, interview.

15 Colleen Flaherty, "Berkeley Announces Major Strategic Planning Process to Address Long-Term Budget Issues," *Inside Higher Ed*, Feb. 11, 2016, https://www.insidehighered.com/news/2016/02/11/berkeley-announces-major-strategic-planning-process-address-long-term-budget-issues.

16 "The 'New Normal,'" *The Chronicle of Higher Education*, Feb. 19, 2016, p. A4.

17 Andy Thomason, "Chicago State Declares Financial Exigency as Budget Standoff Continues," *The Chronicle of Higher Education*, Feb. 4, 2016, http://chronicle.com/blogs/ticker/chicago-state-declares-financial-exigency-as-budget-standoff-continues/108386.

18 David W. Chen, "Dreams Stall as CUNY, New York City's Engine of Mobility, Sputters," *The New York Times*, May 28, 2016, http://www.nytimes.com/2016/05/29/nyregion/dreams-stall-as-cuny-citys-engine-of-mobility-sputters.html?_r=0.

19 Eric Kelderman, "Grim Budget Means More Pain for Louisiana Colleges," *The Chronicle of Higher Education*, March 11, 2016, p. A10.

20 Sarah Brown, "On Her First Day at UNC, Spellings Prepared to Face Critics," *The Chronicle of Higher Education*, March 11, 2016, p. A8.

21 "Kansas' Public Colleges to Lose $17 Million in State Funds," *The Chronicle of Higher*

Education, March 11, 2016, p. A23.

22 Ibid.

23 State Higher Education Executive Officers Association, *State Higher Education Finance: FY 2015*, April 12, 2015, pp. 8, 31–32, http://www.sheeo.org/sites/default/files/project-files/SHEF%20FY%202014-20150410.pdf.

24 Thomas G. Mortenson, "State Funding: A Race to the Bottom," *The Presidency*, Winter 2012.

25 "Trends in College Pricing," *The College Board*, Oct. 2015, http://trends.collegeboard.org/college-pricing/figures-tables/tuition-and-fees-and-room-and-board-over-time-1975-76-2015-16-selected-years.

26 James W. Runcie, Chief Operating Officer, "Letter from the Chief Operating Officer of Federal Student Aid," *Federal Student Aid Annual Report FY 2014, U.S. Department of Education*, Nov. 14, 2014, introduction. The report is available online: https://www2.ed.gov/about/reports/annual/2014report/fsa-report.pdf.

27 Wim Wiewel (president of Portland State University, Oregon's largest university), interview, Sept. 23, 2015.

28 James C. Garland, *Saving Alma Mater: A Rescue Plan for America's Public Universities* (Chicago: The University of Chicago Press, 2009), introduction. Books that raise some of the same concerns as Garland include: Goldie Blumenstyk, *American Higher Education in Crisis? What Everyone Needs to Know* (New York: Oxford University Press, 2015); Richard Arum and Josipa Roksa, *Academically Adrift: Limited Learning on College Campuses* (Chicago: University of Chicago Press, 2011); Richard Vedder, *Going Broke by Degree: Why College Costs So Much* (Washington, DC: American Press Enterprise Institute Press, 2004); Frank Newmand, Lara Couturier and Jamie Scurry, *The Future of Higher Education: Rhetoric, Reality and the Risks of the Market* (New York: Jossey-Bass/Wiley, 2004).

29 US Department of Education, *Digest of Education Statistics 2014*, Table 315.10, https://nces.ed.gov/programs/digest/d14/tables/dt14_315.10.asp.

30 "Non-Tenure-Track Faculty FAQs," *The Delphi Project on the Changing Faculty and Student Success*, a project of the Earl and Pauline Pullias Center for Higher Education at the University of Southern California, http://www.thechangingfaculty.org/ .

31 Emily Mahoney, "Dream Deferred: ASU Facilities Wither Without Maintenance Funding," *The State Press*, Sept. 2, 2014, http://www.statepress.com/article/2014/09/dream-deferred-university-facilities-wither-without-maintenance-funding/.

32 "Sightlines Study Finds $8.4 billion in Deferred Maintenance at Schools of Agriculture in U.S.," *Sightlines*, Oct. 15, 2015, http://www.sightlines.com/sightlines-study-finds-8-4-billion-in-deferred-maintenance-at-schools-of-agriculture-in-u-s/.

33 Chen, "Dreams Stall".

34 Karin Fischer and Jack Stripling, "An Era of Neglect: How Public Colleges were Crowded Out, Beaten Up, and Failed to Fight Back," *The Chronicle of Higher Education*, special report, March 3, 2014, with interactive online graphic showing state revenue declines among public universities.

35 Wartman, *Transformation of Academic Health Centers,* p. 5.
36 "OHSU Hospital," Oregon Hospital Guide, p. 10, http://www.orhospitalquality.org/hospitals/ohsu-hospital/.
37 John Woodward, interview, Oct. 8, 2014.
38 Garland, *Saving Alma Mater,* chapter 14.
39 Michael Thorne, interview, July 16, 2014, River's Edge Hotel, Portland.

Chapter One

Setting the Stage

In the fall of 1983, an Oregon Health Sciences University[1] recruiter invited Jim Walker, chief financial officer for the University of New Mexico Hospital, to apply for the same position at the academic health center's hospital. Dr. Donald Kassebaum, vice president for OHSU's hospital services and director of the University Hospital, was having trouble finding someone for the job. No one wanted to take charge of finances for a hospital that was repeatedly slipping into the red, desperately in need of upgrades and led by a poorly organized team of administrators. What's more, the job was on the frontlines of an ongoing conflict between Kassebaum and the university's president, Dr. Leonard Laster—hardly an appealing place to be.

Walker—a good-humored man with wavy light hair, a mustache, and a ready smile—was only thirty-five, one of the youngest medical center CFOs in the nation, and he liked handling finances for the University of New Mexico Hospital. Though used for teaching by the university, the hospital actually was owned by the county, had its own board of directors, and enjoyed complete autonomy from the university. "I was happy as a lark," Walker recalled. He talked to the OHSU recruiter for about fifteen minutes.

"I really wouldn't be interested," he said.

The recruiter called again the next day.

"I'm happy here," Walker said. "I love Albuquerque."

But the recruiter kept calling. Walker had long wanted to visit the Pacific Northwest and here was a chance for a free trip.

"I'd love to come," he said. "But I'm not interested in the job. I could come only if the director understands I'm not interested in the job."

Within an hour, the recruiter called again and said the hospital would pay for his visit, knowing he was not interested in the job. He told his boss, the hospital's chief executive officer, that he was going to make the trip to get his first glimpse of the Pacific Northwest.

"That place is a mess," his boss warned him, of OHSU. "That is not a place you want to go."

Walker visited the medical center and met with Kassebaum and Dave Witter, chief operational officer for the hospital. He immediately saw why OHSU was having trouble getting a finance officer. In addition to bad relations with the university, the hospital was in a difficult financial bind because of an awkward governance structure that forced it to run everything except patient billing by the State Board of Higher Education.

But Kassebaum and Witter described to Walker efforts under way at OHSU to expand its research capacity. Walker knew the only way a public university could grow in size and excellence was to attract physicians at the top in their specialties. High-performing physicians liked being close to research and were drawn to major research universities where they could keep abreast of the newest ideas. They in turn attracted paying patients. OHSU's commitment to more research piqued Walker's interest. He returned to campus for a second visit and met the people who would report to him.

"I was impressed with them," he said. "That night, my wife and I talked about it. She said, 'This is up to you. Portland would be good for us and the kids.'"

The next morning he went to work, still undecided, still mulling it over.

"I thought the University of New Mexico didn't have the potential to really improve a great deal," he concluded. "But Oregon just might."

He called OHSU and accepted the job. Before reporting to work in February of 1984, Walker and his wife took a two-week trip to Florida to visit Walker's parents. Timothy Goldfarb, an administrator who had joined the hospital a few weeks earlier, repeatedly tried to call Walker on his trip and even left messages with his parents. But Walker told himself he was on vacation and Goldfarb could just wait until he got to OHSU.

On his first day of work, Walker met in the morning with Kassebaum, who emphasized that Walker reported only to him and was to take no guidance from President Laster. That afternoon, he met with Laster who told him he was surprised to see Walker.

"I didn't even know they were hiring a chief financial officer over there," the president said.

Laster made it clear to Walker that he was to report only to him and was not to take his directions from Kassebaum. Then Walker went to see Goldfarb and asked why the hospital administrator was trying to contact him on his Florida vacation.

"I was going to tell you not to come," Goldfarb said. "This place is so dysfunctional. I didn't want someone else making that mistake."

Walker's head was spinning.

"By the end of the first day," he said, "I realized I had made a big mistake in taking this job."[2]

On that first day, Walker had stumbled upon two factors at OHSU that would become important in its transformation to an independent public corporation, a change in which he would play a major role. First, he got a vivid glimpse of the institution's many problems—ranging from internal power struggles and bureaucratic obstacles to financial fragility—that would help President Kohler later make his case for the need to change. Second, he met President Laster, who, despite strained relations with many members of the faculty and administration, had a vision for taking OHSU to a level of excellence. Laster's changes created friction with staff, but they improved the university and put it on a more ambitious trajectory. That set the stage for Kohler, whose vision for the institution fell right in line with his predecessor's.

Laster's administration also brought in people like Walker. While Lesley Hallick, the molecular biologist, was already at OHSU when Laster arrived, Lois Davis, the journalist and lobbyist, and Tim Goldfarb, the hospital administrator, arrived during Laster's tenure. Janet Billups was hired a month after Laster left in November of 1987. Though Kohler didn't hire any of them, he spotted talents in Walker, Hallick, Davis, Goldfarb, and Billups and pulled them together into a powerful leadership team.

Walker soon learned that the acrimony between the president and the hospital director was only one of a growing number of challenges threatening the financial health and future of the institution. Problems had been brewing for years, and many of them were shared by medical institutions across the country. The costs of medical schools and other health professional education had been climbing for decades. With state funding in sharp decline, that problem was coming to a head at OHSU.

Many, if not all, states had found it difficult to sustain a tax base to pay for public and higher education, and an era of free medical school tuition for students in affluent states such as California and Texas was already waning in the 1960s. Even as state support shrank, health professional education needed to expand. The populous Baby Boomers were starting to put stress on the health system. During the 1960s and 1970s, health leaders warned of a looming doctor shortage for the country, so the federal government offered states financial incentives to enlarge their medical schools.[3] The inducements helped launch, but not sustain, the expansion.

Also during this period, medical, nursing, dental, and pharmacy schools—often with the inclusion of a teaching hospital—were being consolidated into academic medical complexes across the country. These new entities, academic health centers, were being created as Medicare and Medicaid became major sources of health care support for the elderly and poor and potentially larger money streams for these institutions. In addition, Medicare provided teaching hospitals extra money to help pay for their physician residency programs.[4] Academic medical centers expanded their clinical activities to serve not only an increase in patients but also to raise more revenue as state support for faculty pay declined. More centers bought city and county public hospitals, often already partially staffed by their faculties, to train their students. But that also meant the responsibility of providing care for poor and indigent patients shifted to these state-owned institutions.

Research became an important enterprise for academic health centers and expanded dramatically during this era, too. The annual budget of the National Institutes of Health (NIH) exploded following World War II. In 1947, it had an annual budget of less than $5 million. When Dr. James A. Shannon became director in 1955, the budget had swelled to $65 million, but Shannon had an even bigger vision for the agency. He believed only government could finance research at the higher levels it needed to reach. He emphasized fundamental research over applied and developmental work as he established new institutes, including the institutes of Child Health and Human Development, which would employ Kohler; of Environmental Health Sciences; and of General Medical Sciences. By the time Shannon left in 1968, the NIH budget had grown to $1.3 billion and its staff had doubled to 13,300 people.[5]

Vannevar Bush, who had been head of the US Office of Scientific Research and Development and chair of the National Defense Research Committee during World War II, also used his influence after the war to press the government into financing more research. He initiated the Manhattan Project during the war, and in a report to President Truman in 1945, he called for an expansion of government funding for science and the creation of a national research foundation. His proposal was enacted in 1950 by Congress as the National Science Foundation.[6]

Rather than create separate research institutes, as was done in France and Germany, the United States turned to academic health centers for its primary medical research sites. The creation of the National Science Foundation, the blossoming of the NIH, and increases in research funding resulted in major expansions of academic health centers, particularly in the basic sciences. With expansion came growing pains. Academic health centers relied on the three-legged stool of teaching, patient care, and research. Research grants, however, came with overhead costs and could not be sustained without additional support. Academic health centers also were expected to provide indigent care. By the 1980s, they were seeing their state support sink as their costs for serving the indigent and supplementing research rose. They collected tuition, but with relatively few students, that accounted for no more than 2 percent to 3 percent of a medical center's budget. So academic health centers increasingly depended on their hospitals and clinics for the revenue they needed to sustain their expanding responsibilities.

THE FIRST PRESIDENT

All of these economic forces were hitting Oregon in 1974 when the State Board of Higher Education approved consolidation of the University of Oregon's medical, dental, and nursing schools along with the medical school's hospital and clinical services into an independent state academic health center. While the new health center operated independently of the University of Oregon, it was initially called the University of Oregon Health Sciences Center. The center would have its own president and remain part of the Oregon State System of Higher Education. The board hired Dr. Lewis William "Bill" Bluemle Jr., president of State University of New York's Upstate Medical Center in Syracuse, to be the Oregon medical center's first president. Bluemle was a tall, distinguished, and innovative nephrologist with a charming demeanor and sharp mind. He used an electric motor from his phonograph to develop a blood pump for the first clinically applicable artificial kidney program at the University of Pennsylvania.

Three weeks after he arrived in Oregon, he was hit with a crisis: the Joint Commission on Accreditation of Hospitals withdrew University Hospital's accreditation for failing to address shortcomings identified three or four years earlier. Part of the problem, Bluemle learned, was in the hospital leadership. The accrediting board felt slighted during its visit to the hospital.

"Some of our people just didn't show up for meetings when the team came on its site visit," Bluemle said years later.[7]

Kassebaum, who was hired by Bluemle to lead the hospital, said the accreditation commission concluded the hospital was badly managed. The commission said, "It's unsafe," he recalled. "It doesn't meet environmental safety standards. The doctors have no discipline. There's no medical staff organization. They don't complete their medical records. You've got 3,500 incomplete medical records."[8]

Without accreditation, the hospital could not qualify for reimbursement from Medicare and Medicaid, which means "we would go out of business," Bluemle said. He scrambled to launch some initiatives and promised improvements that won back temporary accreditation. The crisis revealed a lack of energy and commitment on campus, he said.

> Now, I noticed the first several weekends that I was in my new job that our parking lot was kind of empty from Friday noon on for the rest of the weekend. I had never seen that at the institutions I'd worked at back East. I'm talking about faculty parking lots. And of course the patient parking lots as well because the faculty were taking care of the patients. And that bothered me. That didn't have anything directly to do with accreditation, but it had to do with commitment, and I thought that was a sign that they were a little too laid back, and maybe life was too easy, and maybe they needed a little stimulation to perk up.[9]

Mary Ann Lockwood, who handled public relations for Bluemle, said in a 1998 interview that the new president was bright and "very, very nice," but he had an aloof Eastern manner and distaste for small talk that made him "a bit of a fish out of water" in Oregon.

"He was not good at dealing with Oregon's legislators, and they felt he was patronizing," Lockwood said.[10]

Bluemle hired a pathologist named Dr. Robert Stone as dean of the medical school. Stone, former dean of the University of New Mexico

School of Medicine, had recently served two years as director of the NIH under President Richard Nixon. He was fired, according to author Richard Rettig, for failing to give strong direction to NIH and for promoting medical research instead of the office of the US Secretary of Health, Education, and Welfare.[11] Lockwood said hiring Stone was "a disastrous mistake." Stone had a long, cheeky face, wavy brown hair, and penetrating eyes. He was effective and tough. But he developed a reputation for also being mechanical and impersonal and at odds with many of the school's leaders, including Bluemle. Hallick however, said she liked Stone and his support for expanding the university's research capacity.

Dr. Richard Jones, then the young chairman of the biochemistry department, recalled the first time he met Stone.

"The first thing he did when I sat down across from him was take out his watch and put it on the table in front of him," said Jones. "I kind of had this feeling, 'Boy, I'm working against the clock.'"[12] Lockwood said Stone didn't really like Oregon and thought it was "small potatoes."[13]

Bluemle also found Oregon too parochial, Kassebaum said, and left after less than three years to become president of the private Thomas Jefferson University in Philadelphia, Pennsylvania.

"He didn't like the legislature," Kassebaum recalled. "He didn't like the mindset. He thought that the faculty was weak and the chairs were weak, and he was right. They were inbred. In those days, they just kept appointing from within."[14]

After Bluemle left, Jones, the biochemistry department chair, was appointed interim president for the fourteen months it took the state higher education board to find a permanent one. In 1978, shortly after getting that promotion, Jones fired Stone.

As interim president, Jones decided to move forward with Bluemle's unfinished business rather than launch new initiatives. One incomplete task was building a new Shriners Hospital for Children on campus. Many of the physicians serving as chiefs of staff at the old Shriners Hospital in East Portland worked out of a clinic near Legacy Emanuel Medical Center in North Portland. Those physicians were urging the Shriners to build near Emanuel. City leaders, including then Portland Mayor Neil Goldschmidt also wanted the Shriners hospital near Emanuel, arguing it would create too many traffic and parking headaches on Pill Hill.

The university, of course, saw the hospital as a great asset for its medical school students and clinical services. And the Shriners wanted to put it near the university and researchers. Jones worked out a ninety-nine-year lease agreement with the service organization to build the hospital on the north lower slope of Pill Hill, near Gaines and SW Sam Jackson Park roads. But the city would not issue building permits. The Shriners finally told the city they would build a new hospital in Los Angeles if they were not allowed to build on the hill. Within weeks, the Shriners had their permits.[15]

LASTER ARRIVES

Leonard Laster, a handsome, confident gastroenterologist from the East Coast, became OHSU's second president in 1978. He was a brilliant physician and researcher, born and raised in New York City and admitted to Harvard College in 1944 at age fourteen. He graduated from medical school in 1950 at twenty-one. As a young doctor, he joined the Public Health Service and became a researcher at the NIH when the agency was in its infancy. He stayed twenty-three years during NIH's golden age, as it ushered in the modern era of medicine and later produced nine Nobel laureates.

That period, he said, "was an extraordinarily exciting time" when the institutes of health demonstrated "the benefits to people that come from juxtaposing research, basic research and clinical care. It was a demonstration of how medical care for its own sake, not for profit, the way it is today, could produce some of the most caring and expert care imaginable. It was Camelot."[16] His experience at NIH instilled strong values in him for research and excellence, and a commitment to quality, to exceptional care over marketplace competitiveness, that would shape his leadership in Oregon.

After leaving the NIH, Laster spent several years working for the science adviser to President Richard Nixon, where he was shocked by what he heard from political appointees in budget meetings. At one meeting, they discussed cutting a medical program in half. Laster argued against the idea. An economist turned and looked him in the eye.

"Len," he said. "You must realize that the only cost-effective outcome is death."

"You must be joking," said Laster.

"No, if you think about it, that's the case."

That, Laster said, was when he realized a stark gulf in values separated the world of health care and economic politics.[17]

He moved on to become dean of the medical school at State University of New York Downstate Medical Center, where he soon became frustrated by low state funding and an inability to attract top researchers. He knew he would face the same challenges when he was recruited to the University of Oregon Health Sciences Center in 1978, but at least there he would be president and in a position to do something about it. He didn't know much about Oregon, but he had a fond memory of Portland and the medical university campus, which he once visited to take his board exams in gastroenterology.

"I think it was the one sunny day that Oregon had in the last 50 years," he said in a playful dig on Oregon's abundant overcast skies and rain, "but I remember standing on the steps of Baird Hall, looking out over the city, river, and mountains and thinking, 'How do people get so lucky to work here?'"

Laster's nine-year term at the helm of the university was marked by both conflict and significant growth, especially in research. He was engulfed in controversy even before he arrived thanks to his predecessor. The university provided Bluemle and his wife a house, called the Miller House, near the medical school and perched on Old Orchard Road in Portland Heights, atop the Southwest Hills overlooking downtown Portland. Harold Miller—a prominent Portland owner of a men's clothing store and contributor to the

Medical Research Foundation—donated the house. But the Bluemles didn't want to live in it. They instead rented an attractive gray clapboard home with multiple rooms and bathrooms nearby on Portland Heights owned by the Malarkeys, another prominent Portland family. Some members of the public were offended, seeing the move as ungrateful and wasteful. After the Bluemles left, university leaders decided to sell the Miller house and use the money to buy the Malarkey home, and they promised Laster and his wife that they could live there. But the university had to get approval from the legislature to make the deal. Legislators turned down the request, even though the university already had the money, because many felt college presidents were getting too many perks, said Jones, interim president at the time. The university president's salary, $108,360 a year plus $7,600 for expenses, was the highest in the state, including the salaries of the governor and university system chancellor.[18]

The Lasters had sold their house and were vacationing on Cape Cod, their furniture and goods packed in trucks heading west, when they learned there was no house for them in Portland.

"We scrambled and we scrambled and we scrambled to find someplace because they were ready to come," said Lockwood, the public relations director.

Finally, Lockwood found another house to rent in Portland Heights. Still, some residents criticized the university for being extravagant in selling the generous gift of the Miller House and attempting to buy the Malarkey House.[19] It was a cold reception for the Lasters—literally. Shortly after they arrived, a storm knocked out their power and heat and one of their three children came down with the flu. Still more criticism came when the university bought beds for the Lasters' children and replaced a broken washing machine in their rental with one purchased by the physical plant on campus. There were charges of waste and excess. "The media spin was that patients were being deprived of clean laundry so that the president would not be inconvenienced," according to notes in the university archives.[20] The Lasters later moved into another home on

Montgomery Drive in Portland Heights, which was eventually donated to the university and became Kohler's residence during his tenure.

Laster faced other immediate challenges when he arrived on Pill Hill. In his view, Oregon's only academic health center suffered from a bad self-image. The university offered its best jobs in medicine and surgery to promising doctors elsewhere in the country and were turned down, forcing them to select from within. Bluemle's decision to leave after three years was like being dumped by a parent, Laster said. James McGill, a sixth-generation Oregonian hired by Laster in 1980 as chief administrative and financial officer, said Laster saw the Oregon academic health center as "in the backwater nationally."[21] One veteran staffer took Laster aside and told him, "You know, nobody comes here." When he arrived at the university, it faced "an uncertain future at best and a plodding one at worst," and had become mired in mediocrity, Laster later wrote. "A dispirited institution had lost self confidence and had settled into the central region of the bell-shaped curve."[22]

Laster also found the private sector in Oregon, including the private hospitals, had no respect for government institutions. The enmity between the university and the local hospitals "was palpable," he said. Once, Laster asked the CEO of a large Oregon company for help rejuvenating the health university and was immediately rebuffed.

"You're a state institution," the executive said. "I wouldn't go near state government with a 10 foot pole. You get dirty just thinking about it."

Laster wrote down that prospect as "doubtful."[23]

He also soon discovered that OHSU didn't find much more respect within state government and was "not the favored child" in the state higher education system.

"It was partly because we didn't have a varsity football team," he said, "partly because there was an attitude that really never went away that we were training fat cats, high-income high rollers, and these were not the dirt-under-the-fingernails farmers that are the real people of Oregon."[24]

Similarly, the legislature thought the medical center was too expensive and always asking for too much. During his tenure, Laster said, bills surfaced repeatedly to close OHSU's hospital or the entire academic health center, though none passed. [25] In addition, Laster found himself viewed unfavorably as an outsider simply because he came from the East Coast. During encounters with the Oregon university community, he said, he got a message between the lines that said: "You're an outsider; you don't understand the ethos of this medical school, and you're trying to impose something on it because you're bringing in an outsider's view." [26]

HATFIELD GETS INVOLVED

Early in his term, Laster inherited another conflict carried forward from the interim Jones administration. The medical center was in a battle with Portland leaders, again including Mayor Goldschmidt and Legacy Emanuel Medical Center, over where to build a new Veterans Affairs Hospital to replace the one on Pill Hill. US Senator Mark Hatfield (Republican from Oregon), the state's senior senator, was helping the project with federal money. The university had developed a symbiotic relationship with the VA Hospital and wanted to see it stay on the hill. But the leadership in Portland wanted the VA Hospital, as with the Shriners hospital, to be near Emanuel in North Portland as part of an urban renewal project. Laster, with Hatfield's help, persisted, and the new VA Hospital went up on the hill.

Hatfield began cultivating a working relationship with Laster after the senator had an epiphany upon learning Oregon legislators were thinking about closing the medical school.[27] Hatfield had drifted away from OHSU after a long history with the institution. As a representative in the Oregon Legislature, he helped find state funds to allow the dental school for the University of Oregon in 1956 to move out of its forty-year-old building in Northeast Portland into a $2.2 million ten-floor building on Pill Hill. As a state senator on the Senate Health Committee in 1955, Hatfield carried the bill to the Senate floor that would create a teaching hospital for what was then the University of Oregon Medical School. The bill for the proposed hospital, which would later become University Hospital where Walker worked, drew stiff opposition from the Oregon Medical Association. The association's representatives charged it was a step toward socialized medicine and would create competition with existing hospitals.

Dr. David W. Baird, dean of the medical school, described by many as politically savvy, advised Hatfield as they battled to pass the hospital bill. "David Baird became my tutor basically on how to handle these charges," Hatfield recalled.[28] Baird, who took command as dean in 1943, had led a major expansion of the University of Oregon Medical School. Under his leadership, the school constructed a home for a basic science department and administrative offices in 1949, a building that today bears his name. In 1952, the school built a four-story east wing to Emma Jones Hall, the former nursing dormitory that today serves as home to the OHSU Department of Family Medicine. The medical school's full-time faculty also grew dramatically under Baird's leadership.

Hatfield and Baird became friends, which helped foster Hatfield's affection for the medical school. Later, while governor, Hatfield ended up in University Hospital with what he called "fatigue attacks." Baird came to see him there. Another time during one of his campaigns, Hatfield was hit with vertigo while staying at the Sheraton Hotel near Lloyd Center in east Portland. His wife, Antoinette, called Baird, who came to the hotel to attend on Hatfield.[29]

With renewed interest in OHSU after seeing state legislators try to put it out of business, Hatfield started working with Laster and steering federal funds to projects on Pill Hill.[30] And nobody was in a better position to control the flow of US money than Hatfield, chair of the Senate Appropriations Committee.

"Hatfield's infusion of capital during the 1980s kept OHSU from falling into such a deep hole it would have been impossible to ever recover," Walker said.[31]

THE SOUNDING BOARD

Laster drew fire yet again in 1981 when the institution changed its name from the University of Oregon Health Sciences Center to Oregon Health Sciences University. He tackled the issue in his characteristic style, said McGill, by working the problem intensely through conversations with many people before reaching a conclusion.[32] The change was necessary. The medical center had broken from the University of Oregon as an independent institution in 1974, and it needed to establish its own identity. But it seemed no matter what he did, Laster offended someone. From time to time, he would call on Lesley Hallick, then a molecular biology professor, as a sounding board. She was young, tall, with deep-set inquiring eyes and a disarming smile.

"He would call me in and just chat when he was having a fight with someone," said Hallick. "I was a nobody, you know. I wasn't a chair of a department. I was really safe. And people liked me. . . . But he agonized. I felt badly for him. He would take on one chair as a friend, and he would burn through him. Then he would take on another chair as a friend. But he always had more enemies than he had friends at any given time."[33]

Hallick arrived at OHSU in 1977 after a brief career steeped in academics and molecular biology research. She grew up in Orange, California, the daughter of a World War II fighter pilot, and earned her bachelor's in biochemistry at Pomona College in Claremont, becoming the first person in her family to earn a college degree. She applied for graduate school and was accepted by Harvard University, the Massachusetts Institute of Technology, Rockefeller University in New York City, and the University of Wisconsin. She chose the University of Wisconsin because her boyfriend and future husband was going there.

"As a result [of that decision], I have an absolutely wonderful daughter and two terrific grandchildren, so I don't regret it for a minute," Hallick said years later.[34]

After earning her doctorate in molecular biology, she took a postdoctoral fellowship at the University of California at Berkeley, where she worked with Harry Rubin in virology and John Hurst in chemistry, studying the structures of virus DNA and RNA. She was also able to work on a collaborative project in the laboratory of J. Michael Bishop and Harold Varmus, two inspiring researchers at the University of California at San Francisco who went on to win the 1989 Nobel Prize in physiology. Varmus eventually left UCSF to head the NIH. Hallick taught and launched research that would lead her later to explore virology, simian AIDS retroviruses, and DNA tumor viruses during her twelve years as a faculty member in microbiology at OHSU. By the time she arrived at Berkeley, she was married with a daughter. She and her husband divorced shortly after their move to the Bay Area.

Laster often called on Hallick to head committees and campus initiatives because she had an appealing mix of energy, sagacity, and charm that gave her extraordinary interpersonal and diplomatic skills. As a single mother, professor, and researcher at OHSU, she still managed to earn credentials for preparing income tax returns and tax consulting, work she did nights and weekends. She kept her license for thirty years. She liked numbers, and she liked being around people, especially after spending so many hours isolated in a lab.[35]

Hallick seemed to have limitless energy for handling multiple jobs at once. At Laster's request, she explained molecular biology to a civic group on Pill Hill called the Marquam Hill Society. When the higher education system was slammed with a class action suit, charging discrimination in salary against women, Hallick was singled out as an example. While she was earning $18,000 a year, her male counterpart in biochemistry was earning $21,000. But Hallick did not become a plaintiff, because she didn't feel like she was being discriminated against. She could see that no one, including her boss, knew what other departments were paying their faculty. Still, because she had become viewed by Laster as a reasonable person, he asked her to chair an affirmative action committee to address issues of equity and discrimination at OHSU.

"Mr. President, I don't understand what this committee could do that would be helpful," she said. "It is just going to make everyone mad. It is going to make you mad."[36]

But Laster insisted. So after her sabbatical in the San Francisco Bay area in 1983–84, Hallick took on that mission and recruited an affirmative action officer, established a more open search process to fill professional openings, and created a system that allowed administrators to compare salaries.

POLITICAL PROBLEMS

Hallick got along well with Laster and just about everybody else. But she soon recognized that for all of his brilliance, Laster seemed to have a blind spot when it came to politics and diplomacy with his faculty, legislators, and even the State Board of Higher Education that hired him. He begrudgingly attended board meetings, after being reprimanded for simply skipping them, and behaved as though he had no interest in the board business.[37]

Laster also rubbed faculty leaders the wrong way, probably in part because he pushed them so hard. Dr. Joseph Bloom, chairman of the OHSU Department of Psychiatry under Laster and later dean of the medical school, called Laster a bull in a china shop. "He went a certain distance and kind of wore out his welcome," said Bloom.[38]

Laster could be a compassionate man, but he alienated the faculty, "barked at everybody," and refused to answer his mail—ever, Lockwood said. Dr. John Benson, the university faculty's first full-time gastroenterologist and later dean of the medical school, knew Laster when both worked in Boston. Laster worked well with the community and foundation, he said, but he was not well respected by the faculty.[39]

Dr. Frederick Fraunfelder, who arrived about the same time as Laster to chair the Department of Ophthalmology, found the president so difficult that he agreed to lead a campaign to oust him. He said he collected signatures from twenty-four of the twenty-five department chairs asking the State Board of Higher Education to replace Laster. Dr. George Porter, chair of the Department of Medicine, flew to Washington, DC, and asked Senator Hatfield to support the chairs' call for dumping Laster, Fraunfelder said. But Hatfield shared Laster's vision for OHSU and wanted to see it realized.

"He said, 'No, you are not going to get rid of this man,'" recalled Fraunfelder.[40]

Even so, Fraunfelder thinks his petition reached the state board, though he did not present it himself. Not surprisingly, four years into his presidency, Laster received a less than glowing job evaluation from then Chancellor Roy Lieuallen. He had been accused by faculty and other administrators, the performance review said, of being too abrasive, aloof and intimidating. The chancellor said, "we agree that he must be responsive to them [his critics] and modify his administrative behavior."[41]

The State Board of Higher Education decided to ease friction by assigning James McGill a new title of vice president, with responsibilities to deal with the faculty and internal management. He essentially took over chief executive officer functions, and let Laster concentrate on external responsibilities such as raising funds and working with legislators and the Oregon congressional delegation.[42]

"We turned Leonard loose at what he was good at; fund-raising is his strong suit," said James Peterson, president of the state board.[43]

With the change, deans and clinical chairs could go to McGill instead of Laster to negotiate salaries, purchases, or new initiatives. When Hallick was ready to propose her affirmative action committee's action plan, she went to McGill rather than Laster. The president accepted the state board's intervention. "I'm very demanding," he said in a story in *The Oregonian*, the Portland-based statewide newspaper. "I'm not going to settle for second best."[44]

McGill said he warned Laster the new division of leadership responsibilities may work for a while, but it could not persist. "You don't, over a long period of time, have the CEO of an institution divorced or two arms' length from some of the key day-to-day operation of an institution," he said. The arrangement worked pretty well, he said, for about four years before his relationship with Laster "began to fray."[45]

The president continued to stir conflict both in and outside the academic health center. A year after the board warned Laster to "modify his administrative behavior," Walker arrived to find him still immersed in conflict with Kassebaum. Years later, Kassebaum said he had initially supported Laster, shared his vision for OHSU, even backed his being selected as president, and got along with him well for about three years before their personalities began to clash.[46]

THE MAN WHO LOVES HOSPITALS

Laster's personnel conflicts were apparent to Timothy Goldfarb when he found his way to OHSU through Kassebaum in early 1984. At that time in the summer of 1983, Goldfarb, a young man with dark eyebrows and mustache, and his wife, Laura, were both looking for work in the health field. They had been around one another since they met as adolescents at a church camp in the mountains of Arizona, and they wanted to keep it that way. But after they completed college and married, she found work as a midwife in Phoenix while he landed a job as senior associate administrator of the new hospital at the University of Arizona's medical center in Tucson. Neither could find work in the other's city. They eventually grew tired of being separated and decided one weekend in the summer of 1983 to quit their jobs and find a place where they could both work. OHSU offered such a place. Goldfarb knew OHSU was having internal organizational and financial problems when Kassebaum offered to make him associate director of the University Hospital. But it was a job that would keep him close to Laura, who could work as a midwife at a federally subsidized health clinic in Woodburn, a small city thirty miles south of Portland.

Though he expected problems, Goldfarb was shocked by the dysfunction and disrepair at OHSU, especially in contrast to the new, smooth-functioning hospital he left behind in Arizona. As would be the case with Walker a few weeks later, Kassebaum emphasized he was Goldfarb's supervisor while Laster told the new hire to report only to him. Then Goldfarb was shown to his tiny office on the ninth floor of the hospital. His desk filled the room, so much so that to get to his chair, Goldfarb had to step over the desk.

"They just didn't understand how bad things were or how good things might be," he said.[47]

He was barred from talking to other hospital or university administrators without Laster or Kassebaum in the room. The two executives each worried that administrators might conspire in factions to get rid of them, Goldfarb said. And there were factions. Fraunfelder, the Department of Ophthalmology chair; Porter, the Department of Medicine chair; and other faculty claimed the cafeteria in the old county hospital as a meeting place, Goldfarb said.

"They would go to that cafeteria and kibitz about ways to get rid of Laster," he said. "I kept trying to close the cafeteria to save money . . . They resisted mightily. I never did close the cafeteria."[48]

He and Walker met clandestinely off campus to discuss ways to improve the hospital. "It was exciting; it was kind of dangerous," Goldfarb said.[49]

Despite the university's problems, Goldfarb said, he loved being in the hospital because he grew up in a hospital. Shortly after Goldfarb was born in Jerome, Arizona, in 1949, his father came down with polio, was unable to move his arms and legs and was put into an iron lung to help him breathe. His father spent sixteen years in the iron lung, mostly in hospitals in Cottonwood, which is near Jerome, and in Prescott and Phoenix, before he died of pneumonia, and those hospitals are where Goldfarb spent much of his youth. Since earning his master's in health services administration in 1978, Goldfarb has lived much of his adult life in hospitals too.

When the thirty-four-year-old administrator arrived at OHSU, he set his sights on making its hospital a good place to spend his days.[50]

AN IMPULSIVE HIRE

Lois Davis also joined OHSU during Laster's tenure, though she had no plans to do so when she visited him in October of 1986. She had worked since 1979—first as a press secretary and then four years as chief of staff—for US Representative Ron Wyden, a Democrat from Oregon. She and her husband, Jim, were ready to leave Washington, DC, with their daughter and return to Oregon, where Jim grew up and where both had family. So Davis headed out to Portland to explore employment possibilities. Her first stop was to meet Laster for an informational interview.

She talked with him for about twenty minutes. Then he said, "I have some people I want you to talk to." About 15 minutes later, Davis found herself facing a half-circle of five OHSU administrators, including Dave Witter, then serving as interim chief executive officer for the hospital.

"So tell me why you want this job?" asked Witter.

"What job?" replied Davis. "I didn't know I was interviewing for a job."

The interviewers burst into laughter.

"That's so Len Laster," said Witter.

Laster was looking for a lobbyist for the upcoming 1987 legislative session who could also direct special projects and be a liaison to the faculty and chancellor's office. Davis told the interview committee she could handle government relations but knew nothing about working with faculty, particularly at a medical school. After the interview, she went to Wyden's office in downtown Portland. Minutes later, Laster called her and offered her the job. OHSU had been only her first stop on a networking tour, she told him, and she was not sure this was even the kind of job she wanted. Laster said he would give her twenty-four hours.

When he called the next day, Davis said she needed more time. Laster gave her a week. During that week, Davis flew back to DC and learned Laster had been urging Wyden to encourage her to take the job. She agreed to give the job a six-month trial. Laster left eight months later; Davis stayed for twenty-three years.[51]

The young woman with short brown hair and wide smile was a graduate of the University of Oregon journalism school, had worked as a reporter for the *Springfield News* in Oregon and attended law school for a time before joining Wyden's office. Like Walker, she soon discovered OHSU had rocky relations with the legislature and with the chancellor's office and state higher education system. "We are always a thorn in their side," one university official told her.[52] While most of the state system was focused on its academic mission, OHSU also had to address its research and health care missions.

"None of the Oregon State System of Higher Education personnel were particularly familiar with academic medical centers," Davis wrote, years later. "They did not understand what it took for OHSU to run its clinical enterprise. And they had seven other universities that inevitably resented the 'special' treatment that OHSU sought."[53]

The state system made some concessions to OHSU, but not enough to allow the university to perform at its best. Davis also saw the shaky relationship between the two play out in the legislature. She didn't get much guidance for her new lobbying job. She said she was essentially told, "Here's a map of Oregon. Salem is 50 miles south. Go get us some money."

But she did get one very specific assignment. "I was told to watch the chancellor's staff like a hawk." Witter told her that given the option of more money for the state university system or for University Hospital, the chancellor's office would sell OHSU down the river every time. And Davis saw that play out during her first years on the job. She recalled:

> When the system's budget was under consideration, I could almost guarantee legislative staff members would come to me to tell me

> that the chancellor's office was dealing away the hospital's money in the back rooms. I'm sure these situations were not the result of ill will: It is not hard to understand why the chancellor's staff would prefer to get funds that could be applied generally across all of the Oregon State System of Higher Education institutions. But the net result was to leave the hospital financially vulnerable—a reality that did not win any friends on Pill Hill for the higher education system. [54]

It also did not take Davis long to learn what legislators thought of Laster. The president asked her one day to set up a meeting for him with a state senator, and Davis assumed that would be routine. She conveyed Laster's wish to the senator's office and stopped by the next day to find out when they could meet. A staff member said the senator refused to meet with Laster.

"He said to tell you he will be happy to meet with you anytime," she told Davis, "but he will not meet with Laster."[55]

LASTER'S VISION

At least part of the reason people found Laster difficult to work with was that he set such high standards for the university and for himself. McGill said Laster was "driven." He worked almost every waking hour, even over weekends, and put extreme pressure on himself. And he expected the same of his employees, which put him at odds with "some who were willing to settle for less than first rate, for top quality," McGill said.[56]

In his speeches to the public and to the university, Laster railed against mediocrity and repeatedly emphasized the importance of excellence and quality.

"I know that excellence is becoming trite," he said in a speech to the Rotary Club of Portland, "but I believe the basic problem in this country today, in our businesses, in our governments and in our every societal activity is a falling away from standards of excellence."[57]

In another speech to the City Club of Portland, he hardly talked about OHSU at all, choosing instead to focus on the concept of excellence and how it should be valued in great minds as highly as it is in great sports and entertainment figures.

"Too often, in our national life, we have settled for second best, for mediocrity, and have taught that lesson to our children," he said. "Above almost all other human endeavors, the goal of medicine and the other healing arts must be excellence and dare not be mediocrity."[58]

He again chose to dwell on the importance of seeking "not on how near we could come to average, but rather on how near we could come to the best" in a 1986 speech. "Quality is, indeed, breeding quality," he said. "Achievement is breeding even greater achievement; and excitement is breeding more excitement."[59]

Laster's push for excellence "served the institution well," McGill said.[60] He did manage to forge good relations with some key people and pushed forward with a vision for a more vibrant institution, a vision rooted in those golden years at NIH. He wanted to build some measure of the future of medicine at his institution.

"I thought, 'let's build something that is really of genuine excellence here that will excite the people within; draw more excellence from the outside, as the NIH did,'" he said. "'Let's start a Renaissance and get us known around the country as a center of excellence.'"[61]

He turned to molecular medicine, an emerging discipline, as a place to focus and decided the way to move into that field was to build a research institute. New architecture could also boost the university's self-image, said Laster, who thought the campus had been "uglied up by that big, massive medical school building [Mackenzie Hall]." But to build a research institute, Laster needed money, and he wasn't getting any from the legislature.

Even the Medical Research Foundation was at odds with the medical school. The nonprofit foundation was created by Edwin E. Osgood, one of the university's early researchers, and a group of other physicians and businessmen to raise money to stimulate and support medical research, not just at OHSU but around the state. It would, for example, give young researchers money to build a track record so they could compete for NIH funding. It also served as a fiscal agent to administer grants coming to the faculty.

In the early 1960s, Dr. Don Pickering, a pediatric endocrinologist and researcher, and Dr. Edward S. West, chair of the biochemistry department, received millions of dollars from the NIH to establish the nation's first federally-supported primate center on donated land in Hillsboro, west of Portland. The center would be owned and operated by the Medical Research Foundation largely independent of the medical school save that the school's dean, David Baird, was appointed its principal investigator. Pickering became director of the primate center and wanted to be principal investigator, too. He also spent NIH money on a mainframe computer, which the NIH had not authorized. His actions irritated Baird, who eventually accepted Pickering's resignation, though Pickering continued to work for the foundation. The foundation's board refused to let the Secretary of State's office audit the nonprofit, creating other consequences, recalled Richard Jones, the interim OHSU president and longtime member of the foundation's board.[62]

"The Legislature decided, 'Well, in that case, we can't have the Medical Research Foundation as the fiscal agent for grants coming from the federal government and supporting research at the medical school, because that is a state school,'" recalled Jones.[63]

So the medical school set up a research support office to be fiscal agent for its grants and donations, and the primate center operated independently, through grants administered by the Medical Research Foundation.

"It was civil hatred between [the research board] and the medical school," Laster said. The president turned to other sources for money.[64]

THE VOLLUM INSTITUTE

While serving on the board of directors for an Oregon company called Tektronix, Laster met Jim Castles, a lawyer for Tektronix founder Howard Vollum and a member of the MJ Murdock Charitable Trust in Oregon. Tektronix made oscilloscopes and other electronic measuring equipment. Laster told Castles he was trying to raise money to build a research institute. Castles talked to the Murdock Trust, which then kicked in $500,000 for the institute. Castles also introduced Laster to Vollum, who had a dim view of the medical school and hospital because a pediatrician close to his family had a falling out with its former dean. Even so, Laster and Vollum became friends, and Vollum soon stepped up with a contribution.

"Jean [Vollum's wife] and I are going to start out by giving you $5 million to start an institute," said Howard Vollum as he handed Laster an actual check for $5 million.

"Not many people have that happen to them," the president said.

Later, Vollum upped his contribution to $30 million with only one request to Laster: "Bring seven-foot jumpers to the campus."[65]

Hatfield then found Laster another $25 million in federal support. But the senator said he didn't want Laster to construct just another building; he wanted him to create a new architecture, a new physicality, for the campus. Laster hired architect Pietro Belluschi, former dean of architecture at Massachusetts Institute of Technology. Belluschi came to Portland. One day, as he and Laster walked across the OHSU campus, the president recalled, he pointed to the medical school building and said, "I wish you would have been there when they built this monstrosity."

Belluschi responded, "Before you go further, one of my good friends designed that building. It is actually a school of architecture called Brutalism," a style popular among universities in the 1960s and 1970s, which expressed strength, functionality, and interior people-flows.

"Well," replied Laster, "We have one of the classic examples of Brutalism in the world."[66]

Belluschi and Laster actually must have been talking about the medical school's eight-story Basic Science Building, now known as the Richard T. Jones Hall for Basic Medical Sciences, which opened in 1971, a short ways west of the main medical school building, Mackenzie Hall. The Basic Sciences Building—designed by Campbell Yost Partners, an architectural firm known for its exposed concrete styles—has Brutalism features, including its angular, heavy cement exterior and windows framed and divided by thick bands of steel. Mackenzie Hall was built long before the era of Brutalism, but Laster also didn't care for its design—a squat, three-story, flat-roofed, sandy-brick rectangle, flanked on each side by a square wing with a shallow pitched roof.

As construction got underway on the new research institute, Laster again encountered a groundswell of opposition. Critics on campus called the project a waste of money.[67] He was facing "a faculty revolt," Laster said. "That was a very, very difficult time—and a shock, because I thought I was doing something that would get people starry-eyed."[68]

The faculty had been starved of state funds during the economic recession in the early 1980s and felt the Vollum philanthropy should repair some of that, said Benson, the former medical school dean.[69] Some faculty members also objected to establishing the Vollum Institute outside the medical school as a freestanding research operation, said Bloom, acting chair of the Psychiatry Department during the debate.[70]

Opponents to the Vollum project sent delegations to Washington, DC, to urge Hatfield to redirect the money to other projects. Kassebaum describes a day when all of the vice presidents and deans lined up in Laster's office to meet with Hatfield.

> Hatfield said, "You're giving Laster too much trouble, and you're letting your faculties quibble with him, and so forth, and you either straighten up or get out of here, or I will give all my money to the University of Washington." So he blackmailed us.[71]

After that meeting, Kassebaum said, deans and vice presidents began leaving OHSU, including him. Some faculty members and administrators, however, supported Laster's efforts to build the research institute that would bear Vollum's name. Dr. Howard Lewis, former chair of medicine and in his eighties at the time, visited Laster in his office.

"Len, one, I'm sorry you didn't come while I was still chairman," Laster recalled him saying. "Two, what you're doing is critical for this place. And three, you're going to run into the worst opposition imaginable. People don't take change comfortably here. Don't let them run you down or run you out."[72]

Other faculty members said the project gave them hope at a time when they were considering leaving, Laster said. The president told Hatfield the senator didn't need this conflict and could walk out. He also offered to give the money back to Vollum. But Hatfield and Vollum stuck by Laster.

"Finish this," said Hatfield, "because we have to plan the next one."[73]

Laster observed that the conflict over building Vollum reflected how the OHSU community resisted change and settled for operating with less.

> People had learned to adapt to an unhappy situation. They never really got enough of a budget. Their physical resources hadn't been replenished in I don't know how many years. Their existence was hand-to-mouth, juggling, grants, and it was tough to make it in that environment. But those that had made it had an equilibrium going, and here was an outsider coming in and upsetting things, and that's scary.[74]

Faculty and administrators also worried, Laster said, that if he succeeded in bringing in someone good to run the research institute, that person would be "the favored child," and they would be forgotten as "also-rans." And Laster did succeed. He heard about Edward Herbert, a top-notch molecular biologist at the University of Oregon who had already accepted a position to work for Harvard University in one of its molecular biology research centers at Massachusetts General Hospital. Laster went to see him and made an offer.

"Ed, here is a blank canvas, a new building, an endowment of $30 million, and the freedom to do anything that your creativity will allow," Laster told him.

Herbert turned down Harvard and came to OHSU in 1983 as founding director of the Vollum Institute. And that, said Laster, was the beginning of the turnaround. While Laster gave the university a dream, he said, "Hatfield and Vollum gave it life, and Ed Herbert gave it a soul." Herbert, Laster said, "was a seven-foot jumper."[75]

Herbert was outgoing, helpful to clinicians and basic scientists, and an effective recruiter. He persuaded Dr. Earl Zimmerman, a clinical neurologist and laboratory scientist, to leave Columbia University Medical School to become chairman of Neurology at the OHSU medical school. OHSU also lured Dr. Donald Trunkey from San Francisco to chair its surgery department. Trunkey wanted to be near other neuroscientists as he conducted research on trauma and head injuries.[76]

Success led to more success, momentum began to grow, and the money began to flow. Hatfield was bringing in federal money for new construction on Laster's drawing board: a nursing school building, a library, and a bridge connecting the University Hospital complex to the VA Hospital. Construction of the eight-story building for the Vollum Institute for Advanced Biomedical Research was completed in 1987, just before Laster left to become president of the University of Massachusetts. Herbert died tragically of pancreatic cancer early that year before the institute he had helped create could move into its new building. About two-thirds of the narrow, pink granite building—wedged between the Medical Research Building and Richard T. Jones Hall for Basic Medical Sciences—bows gracefully like a bay window, offering a softer, rounder design in contrast to the angular Brutalism of its neighbor. With its private support and endowment, the institute operates independently on the campus, though it is intrinsically connected with OHSU faculty and researchers. Richard Goodman, a biochemist and molecular biologist and Kohler's first important recruitment, served as its director from 1990 to 2016 and lured many nationally prominent scientists. Among them are Eric Gouaux, who developed new ways to characterize the structure and function of nerve synapses and decode the signals nerve cells use to communicate, and Gail Mandel, who showed how glia and neurons cause Rett Syndrome, an autism-spectrum disorder that strikes young girls. The institute's researchers remain dedicated to the study of the molecular basis of nervous system and brain function, studies that may someday cure brain-related diseases such as multiple sclerosis, autism, drug addiction, and stroke.

A LAWYER ARRIVES

Janet Billups arrived at OHSU about the time the Vollum building was completed. She took a job with the Oregon Attorney General's Office in December of 1987 as the department's lawyer for the health center and for nearby Portland State University. She would be a critical player in giving OHSU a legal path for its transformation into a public corporation.

Billups was a fourth-generation native Oregonian with ancestors who came to the state on the Oregon Trail. She attended a small Seventh-day Adventist college in Walla Walla, Washington, and completed law school at Lewis & Clark Law School in Portland.[77] She passed the Oregon bar exam in 1980, worked as a law clerk and later as a trial lawyer for Multnomah County, which includes Portland, under one of the state's legendary trial lawyers, John Leahy.[78]

That experience would prove valuable for Billups when she took up the challenge of drafting Senate Bill 2, the legislative and legal framework for OHSU's conversion to a public corporation. She had been working for the county eight years when Leahy retired. She decided that was a good time to move on and joined the state Department of Justice as an assistant attorney general. She again was forced into a quick study as she learned the legal terrain of the academic world at Portland State University and of the unique mix of academe and clinical medicine at OHSU. As a practical matter, she spent most of her time at OHSU. The medical center "was very inviting" and "provided the space for me," said Billups, who remains a lawyer for OHSU.[79]

MONEY PROBLEMS

During those years, OHSU had plenty of other problems beyond its struggles between its president and his faculty and administrators. It lacked modern facilities and a critical mass of outstanding doctors who could serve both as faculty and health care providers to draw paying patients and make the hospital profitable. An academic health center needs a profitable hospital to expand. Despite the investment in research driven by Vollum and Hatfield, OHSU's research capacity was small compared to other academic health centers across the country, and that made it harder for it to attract top physicians.

Jim Walker found the university's plants and equipment "abysmal," putting it at a severe disadvantage in the capital-intensive health care industry. Outpatient clinics and services were all in buildings constructed between the 1920s and early 1950s. Many of the hospital wings were putting four patients to a room at a time when the industry standard had become private one-bed rooms or semi-private two-bed rooms. The campus had a great view from its hilltop location, but finding a place to park was exasperating. Walker concluded the clinical faculty had some areas of strengths, but it was nowhere as strong as faculties of top-tier academic health centers across the country.[80]

Private and not-for-profit hospitals run by the Sisters of Providence and Legacy Health System in the Portland area had state-of-the-art facilities and equipment, drawing more paying customers and leaving University Hospital as the primary indigent hospital for the metro area and state. A third of its revenue in 1984 came from uninsured and low-income Medicaid patients, which was three times the proportion of the other metro hospitals and twice the state average.

University Hospital also had limited access to capital, explained Walker. First, it had little or no disposable income to service debt for improving its facilities. Secondly, it had to make its request for capital funding to the legislature as part of the package of construction requests filed by the entire eight-campus university system. The Oregon State System of Higher Education set priorities on capital projects and was not apt to put the University Hospital high on that list.

The chancellor's office, which oversaw the state university system, viewed the hospital as a liability, given its history of financial crises over the years. To grant the hospital more debt would take away from the system's other seven institutions, and the chancellor's office was not confident the hospital would be able to pay its obligations. During the early and middle 1980s, the University Hospital, the primary economic engine of the academic health center, was failing and in constant financial stress. The hospital lost $3.2 million between 1980 and 1984. Patient days, a primary indicator of inpatient volumes, had fallen 17 percent from 1983 to 1986. The hospital occupancy rate was generally in the 71-to-77 percent range during the 1980s and dipped as low as 66 percent in 1985.[81] Rather than an economic engine, the hospital was becoming a financial drain. Administrators were scattered across the OHSU campus, making it difficult for them to communicate, and the hospital administrative culture did not encourage communication. What's more, hospital leaders were not engaged in any strategic planning on how to dig out of this financial hole.[82]

University Hospital, like all state agencies, also had to contend with a cumbersome biennial budgeting process because the legislature met only every two years. So as part of OHSU's two-year budget request, the hospital had to try to predict how many and what type of patients would show up at its doors two years into the future. It frequently missed the mark and had to appeal to the Legislative Emergency Board for more money. Legislators grew weary of the university's constant plea of penury and regularly called university clinical leaders to task for their inability to manage their budget properly.[83]

Mike Thorne, then a state senator from Pendleton and chair of the Ways and Means Committee and member of the emergency board, recalled that the University Hospital seemed to be overwhelmed with indigent care, and Laster offered no solution other than requests for more state money.

"I don't think he had an interest in changing that model," Thorne said. "Pill Hill was a big drain. You would go up there, and it was depressing. It was kind of old and antiquated in so many ways, and it didn't have much of a reputation. It was sort of a place where you sent all of the indigents for hospital care. It was always out of money."[84]

What's more, competing nonprofit metro hospitals such as Legacy Emanuel Medical Center and Providence St. Vincent Medical Center resented state aid to the university's hospital and lobbied against it. Legislators became so irritated with University Hospital in 1985 that they were again talking about closing it. A group of Democratic and Republican representatives sponsored House Bill 2596, which called for creating a "task force to study closing Oregon Health Science University Hospital and to provide indigent care and clinical experience through other hospitals."[85] The bill, which ultimately did not pass, could have taken down the entire academic health center, Billups said.[86]

The strained relationship between the hospital and the university administration came to a head in early 1986, and Laster and Kassebaum agreed on a mutual parting.[87] Dave Witter replaced Kassebaum as interim CEO of the hospital. McGill had been meeting regularly with the hospital administrators to improve relations, and they pulled together, finally, as a real team to plan ways to improve the hospital's performance. Hospital operations slowly improved. Administrators successfully replaced and improved the billing and patient registration systems, enabling the hospital to cut the billing staff by sixty positions while improving bill collections. Goldfarb played a key role in retaining good clinical faculty while recruiting more. Patient volumes started rising after years of decline, and the hospital started operating in the black by the late 1980s. It wasn't earning enough cash to strengthen the School of Medicine or to improve facilities—but it was making money.[88]

McGill resigned in early 1987 to become vice president in charge of finance and other administrative functions at the University of Missouri four-campus system, where he stayed a decade before doing similar work for twelve more years at Johns Hopkins University in Baltimore.

After his departure, Laster asked Walker to join his office as interim vice president of finance and administration. Walker declined, saying he had little academic experience and was more comfortable with the hospital. The next day, Laster called Walker and told him he didn't get to choose. Walker would be joining the Laster team. But not for long, as Laster was about to move on.[89]

A CAMPUS PLAN

By the time he left OHSU in 1987 to take his new job at the University of Massachusetts Medical Center, Laster had developed a long-term building plan for the campus and gotten several other projects underway. He and Hatfield, for example, worked on his dream to build a new library with modern computer technology. Hatfield would get federal money for the library, but construction of what would be called the Biomedical Information Communication Center bogged down in haggling over nearby land that residents were trying to sell at exorbitant prices. Kohler would later decide to build the library near the hospital on land OHSU already owned, allowing construction to proceed. The "library of the 21st Century," which allows distance learning and teleconferencing between rural doctors and

OHSU specialists, opened in 1991 and remains one of the most sophisticated electronic medical libraries in the world. Laster also had laid out plans for a School of Nursing building, but it was Carol Lindeman, dean of the nursing school, who led the effort to turn that idea into a completed building in 1992 with Hatfield's help in securing federal support. The Center for Research on Occupational and Environmental Toxicology, one of the first facilities in the world to combine molecular and cell biology to study adverse effects of chemicals on the human body, also had its roots in the Laster era. So did the 660-foot-long Veterans Affairs Medical Center bridge, a project that Laster put on the drawing board and that Dr. John Kendall, former dean of the medical school, ushered through to construction. Both the toxicology center and bridge were completed in 1992.

Laster, however, was against moving the state's Office of Rural Health to OHSU. Davis recalls the day when Laster revealed his opposition to Senator Eugene Timms, a Republican from the eastern Oregon town of Burns, who would become a major supporter of OHSU's conversion to a public corporation. The large lawmaker got to his feet and extended a big hand as Davis and Laster entered his Salem office, Davis recalled.

"Hi Doc," he boomed. "Hi Lois. Have a seat."

The smaller, nattily-dressed Laster took his chair, and said bluntly, "Lois says I'm crazy not to take you up on your offer to move rural health to OHSU."

Timms reared back, looking startled. Davis was surprised, too. She had made an impassioned case to her new boss for moving the state's Office of Rural Health to OHSU. It would give the university a better toehold statewide and draw more interest from rural legislators such as Timms, broadening OHSU's base of political support. Timms glanced at Davis briefly and then turned back to Laster and leaned forward in his chair.

"You are crazy," he said.[90]

On August 15, 1987, Laster announced he was moving on and gave local reporters a tour through the new Vollum building. He told them dollars and square feet are not what matters.

"It's the people," he said. "Little by little, you get activities going on here so when a young person wants to work in a field, the adviser says, 'Hey, you'd better go to Portland because that's where some of the best work is being done.'"

An account in *The Oregonian* describes Laster taking reporters through a research lab where "a few scientists clad in jeans worked in bright, white light" while rock music blared. They walked to a rounded, fourth-floor window that had a commanding view of Portland. Laster leaned on the bar extending across the window and took a long look, as if for the last time. "There's nothing like it," he said.[91]

Laster had dragged OHSU out of its slumber, pushed it deeper into neural and molecular biology research, pressed it to reach for excellence, and set the stage for its next president. As he said a year earlier in one of his speeches:

"We have set our sights not on the dry dust below us, but rather on the brilliant stars above us."[92]

Notes

1 The university's name was changed to Oregon Health & Science University in 2001.

2 James Walker, interview, June 16, 2014.

3 US Department of Health and Human Services, *The Physician Workforce: Projections and Research into Current Issues Affecting Supply and Demand*, p. 2, http://bhpr.hrsa.gov/healthworkforce/reports/physwfissues.pdf ; see also Public Broadcasting System, *Health Care Crisis Timeline*, https://www.pbs.org/healthcare-crisis/history.htm.

4 Paul B. Rothman, Edward D. Miller, Landon S. King and Ellen F. Gibson, "The Changing Ivory Tower: Balancing Mission and Business," in *The Transformation of Academic Health Centers: Meeting the Challenges of Healthcare's Changing Landscape*, edited by Steven Wartman (San Diego: Elsevier, 2015), pp. 4–5.

5 Thomas J. Kennedy Jr., "James Augustine Shannon, 1904–1994", in *Biographical Memoirs*, vol. 75 (Washington, DC: National Academy Press, 1998), pp. 15–16.

6 Jerome B. Wiesner, "Vannevar Bush, 1890–1974", in *Biographical Memoirs*, vol. 50,

(Washington, DC: National Academy of Sciences, 1979), pp. 98–101.

7 Lewis William Bluemle Jr., interview by Joan S. Ash, May 22, 1998, interview no. 32 5/22, 1998, transcript, OHSU Oral History Project, p. 16.

8 Donald G. Kassebaum, MD, interview by Joan S. Ash, Nov. 7, 1997, the Association of American Medical Colleges, Washington, DC, interview no. 6 11/7, 1997, transcript, OHSU Oral History Project p. 6.

9 Bluemle, interview, p. 17.

10 Mary Ann Lockwood, interview by Joan S. Ash, Feb. 25, 1998, campus of OHSU, interview no. 21 2/25, 1998, transcript, OHSU Oral History Project, pp. 14–15.

11 Richard A. Rettig, *Cancer Crusade: The Story of the National Cancer Act of 1971* (Lincoln, NE: iUniverse, 1977), p. 309.

12 Richard Jones, MD, interview by Joan S. Ash, and Linda Weimer, Jan. 26, 1998, interview no. 16 12/22. 1997, transcript, OHSU Oral History Project, p. 35. Transcript includes interviews on Dec. 22, 1997, Jan. 26, 1998, March 2, 1998, and March 16, 1998.

13 Lockwood, interview, pp. 14–15.

14 Kassebaum, interview, p. 9.

15 Jones, interview, pp. 43–45. Jones said after the city continued to deny permits for the hospitals, the Shriners brought in their Imperial Potentate, a tall, wealthy man from Texas, to meet with Goldschmidt and his staff. They gathered in the mayor's office, and the Shriners explained that their hospital in Portland was one of the first Shriners hospitals ever built, their flagship, and they wanted to replace it and had the money to do so. Why, they asked, couldn't they get responses from the building office?

"Well, there is this problem," began Goldschmidt.

Just then, said Jones, the guy from Texas interrupted and weighed in.

"Well, we understand there are probably some problems," said the Texan, "but I just want you to understand that if we don't get permission within the next couple weeks, we're going to build this hospital down in Los Angeles. They're all ready, and we have permission to go ahead, and I don't know that we'll ever replace the one in Portland."

"You could hear a pin drop," Jones said. The mayor looked over to Angus Duncan, who worked in the city building department.

"Now, what's the problem over here, Mr. Duncan?" Goldschmidt said. "How come this isn't getting taken care of?"

Within weeks, the Shriners had their building permits.

16 Leonard Laster, interview by Joan S. Ash, March 5, 1999, interview no. 64 3/5 1999, transcript, OHSU Oral History Project, p. 4.

17 Ibid., p. 7.

18 Richard Jones, MD, interview by Joan S. Ash and Linda Weimer, March 2, 1998, transcript, OHSU Oral History Project, pp. 56–58.

19 Lockwood, interview, pp. 27–29.

20 "President's Residence, or, House that wasn't Quite a Home", *Historical Notes* (blog), Feb. 13, 2007, *OHSU Historical Collections & Archives*, http://ohsu-hca.blogspot.com.au/2007/02/presidents-residence-or-house-that.html.

21 James T. McGill (former chief administrative and financial officer at OHSU), interview by Joan Ash, March 2, 1999, interview no. 62, 3/2 1999, transcript, OHSU Oral History Project, p. 6.

22 Leonard Laster, MD (president of OHSU), "Attracting Excellent—An Economic Prescription," Peter Kohler collection, OHSU Archives, Oct. 23, 1986. It is unclear where Laster delivered this speech.

23 Laster, interview, pp. 12–14.

24 Ibid.

25 Ibid., p. 13. For example, House Bill 2596, introduced in the 1985 Legislature, called for creating a task force "to study closing of OHSU Hospital and to provide indigent care and clinical experience through other hospitals."

26 Laster, interview, p. 40.

27 Mark O. Hatfield, interview by Joan S. Ash, Oct. 22, 1998, interview no. 51 10/22, 1998, transcript, OHSU Oral History Project, p. 13. Hatfield said, "The state Legislature was debating a resolution to close medical education, health education, for budgetary reasons. In other words, the whole Hill was going to be shut down by this resolution. And it really shocked me. It was like a cold shower; I came to. I'd been in a coma, so to speak, in my loss of connection and knowledge of what was going on on the Hill."

28 Ibid., pp. 8–9.

29 Ibid., p. 10. Hatfield described Baird's curious remedy as follows: "He [Baird] gave me a few eye tests and a few other things. Then he told me to take off my shirt and lie on my stomach. So he got up and straddled me and started giving me a massage, and I said, 'Dean Baird, are you practicing chiropractic or osteopathy?' He says, 'Neither. If you ever tell anybody what I'm doing, I'll tell that you lied.'"

30 Hatfield continued to serve OHSU even after he left the US Senate in 1997. He was a member of the OHSU Board of Directors from Feb. 25, 2000 to May 23, 2008. The chair of the board is called the Mark O. Hatfield Chair in honor of the senator's contributions to the university.

31 James Walker, "OHSU Transition to Public Corporation," an unpublished account in his private possession of his role in OHSU's conversion to a public corporation, p. 3.

32 McGill, interview, p. 6.

33 Lesley Hallick, interview, May 27, 2014, Pacific University, Forest Grove.

34 Ibid., p. 21.

35 Ibid.

36 Ibid.

37 Ibid. Hallick said she was told Laster "would sit there and type, and this was in the days when laptops were pretty noisy and clunky, very obviously not paying atten-

tion and not thinking it was worth his time to be there," Hallick said. "He was just perceived as arrogant."

38 Joseph Bloom, MD, interview, March 11, 2014, Caffe Umbria, Portland's Pearl District.

39 John Benson, MD, interview, March 24, 2014, OHSU's library, Biomedical Information Communications Center. Benson said about Laster, "It was personality. He had a high ego strength. He projected himself a good deal more than the university. He did attract people with money in town and got the foundation started, was successful in beginning to build out a bit of the endowment. But he was not a popular educator, researcher."

40 Frederick Fraunfelder, MD, interview, July 14, 2014, Casey Eye Institute, OHSU.

41 Berney Lerten, "Despite Criticism, Laster to Remain OHSU President," *The [Bend] Bulletin,* March 26, 1982, p. A4.

42 McGill, interview, pp. 9, 10. In 1999, McGill recalled that Laster called him into his office one day to meet with him and Bud Davis, then chancellor or the Oregon university system. "Look, we want to reorganize things a little bit differently in terms of senior administration," Davis told him. McGill would be the inside person, Davis said, allowing Laster to devote more time outside to work with legislators and with the political structure in Washington, DC.

43 Nancy McCarthy, "Laster's Tenure Pushes OHSU Toward Heights," *The Oregonian,* Aug. 16, 1987, p. B06.

44 Ibid. Laster said, "One of the things I demand is that you put the institution above your own self-interest. Two, I want the best you have in you. I'm not going to settle for second best. Three, I want good will and good feeling, because if we don't exude it, how are we going to impart it to the students? For a student to train in a hateful institution is to produce a hateful nurse or a hateful physician or a hateful dentist."

45 McGill, interview, p. 11.

46 Kassebaum, interview, p. 14. Kassenbaum called "the awful Leonard Laster" the "most evil person I ever knew in life." He said, that after a few years, Laster "began to treat people rudely and offensively, and we would refer to being 'Lasterized.' And he developed a personality that was a narcissistic personality. He felt very self-righteous." In her May 27, 2014 interview, Lesley Hallick said Kassenbaum and Laster grew to "hate each other." Years later, she observed another telling example of how Laster seemed to be tone-deaf to political and public relations. She visited Laster shortly after he had become chancellor of the University of Massachusetts Medical Center in Worcester, Massachussets, to learn more about how the center produced spin-off biotech businesses.

"I went into his office, and he has a gigantic picture of Sen. Mark Hatfield on the wall," she said. "I'm thinking, 'I bet this isn't well received in Massachusetts. That should be [Sen. Ted] Kennedy.' You know, why would you do that?"

47 Timothy M. Goldfarb, interview, Oct. 2, 2014.

48 Ibid.

49 Ibid.
50 Ibid.
51 Lois Davis, interview, June 16, 2014, Portland State University.
52 Lois Davis, from her unpublished account of her role in OHSU's transformation to a public corporation, Oct. 12, 2013, p. 2.
53 Ibid.
54 Ibid.
55 Ibid., p. 3.
56 McGill, interview, p. 12.
57 Leonard Laster, MD, speech to the Rotary Club of Portland, Feb. 18, 1983.
58 Leonard Laster, MD, address to the City Club of Portland, June 2, 1983.
59 Laster, "Attracting Excellence—An Economic Prescription," OHSU Archives, Oct. 23, 1986.
60 McGill, interview, p. 12.
61 Laster, interview, p. 13.
62 Richard Jones, MD, interview by Joan S. Ash and Linda Weimer, March 2, 1998, OHSU Oral History Project, pp. 48–51.
63 Ibid., p. 50.
64 Laster, interview, p. 14.
65 Ibid., pp. 16–22.
66 Ibid., p. 21.
67 Ibid., pp. 22, 23. Some faculty said, recalled Laster, "We're not a research center; we're a clinical place. You're going to build this thing, and nobody good comes here, so you're not going to get anyone good to head it. Give us the money. We know what to do with it."
68 Ibid., p. 23.
69 John A. Benson Jr., MD, email to author on June 19, 2014.
70 Joseph Bloom, MD, email to author on June 19, 2014. Laster's "reasoning was that he didn't want the new institute to be lost . . . in the larger medical school," said Bloom. "The older and powerful chairs felt this as a slight on the president's part and an indirect view of how the president viewed the school."
71 Kassebaum, interview, pp. 14–15.
72 Laster, interview, p. 23.
73 Ibid.
74 Ibid., p. 24.
75 Ibid, pp. 24–25.
76 Laster, "Attracting Excellence—An Economic Prescription," OHSU Archives, Oct. 23, 1986.
77 Janet Billups, interview, April 2, 2014, her office at OHSU.
78 Janet Billups, "The Design of the Public Corporation—the Lawyer's Perspective," an unpublished account in her private possession of her role in OHSU's conversion to a public corporation, 2013, p. 3. Billups writes that under the direction of Leahy, "I

was terrified into learning firsthand everything possible about government in Oregon and the laws and constitutional provisions that govern them. My primary career assignment was trial work, but John also introduced me to home rule powers, low-bid contract law, condemnation, immunity from federal antitrust laws, debt financing through bond sales, legislative drafting and analysis, roads and bridges, police and jails and anything else that government undertakes in this state."

79 Billups, interview.

80 James Walker, "OHSU Transition to Public Corporation," an unpublished account in his possession of his role in OHSU's conversion to a public corporation, pp. 2-3.

81 "Table of Selected Statistical Indicators of Patient Activity for Years Ended June 30," chart, Peter Kohler collection, OHSU Archives.

82 Ibid., pp. 2–4.

83 Davis, Oct. 1, 2013, p. 2.

84 Michael Thorne, interview, July 16, 2014, River's Edge Hotel, Portland.

85 H.R. Bill 2596, 63rd Legis. Assemb., Reg. Sess. (Oregon 1985), sponsored by Democratic Representatives Rick Bauman of Portland, Tom Hanlon of Cannon Beach, and Mike McCracken of Albany along with Republican Representative Eldon Johnson of Medford.

86 Billups, interview, April 2, 2014. Billups explained, "If the hospital fails, in this side of the country, you are out of business," she said. "Back East, it is different. Harvard doesn't have a hospital, but it has a medical school. The structure back there is everyone is trained at local hospitals. That is not how it evolved out here. Without a hospital, we don't have training grounds for our medical students and nurses."

87 Kassebaum, interview, p. 15. Kassebaum recalled, "I had been a hospital director for ten years, and I was drifting farther and farther away from the educational center of my academic career. So Laster and I made a deal. I said, 'I'm going to look for a deanship, because we're just squared off . . . and it's very unhealthy and very dysfunctional for the institution.' . . . I found a deanship at Oklahoma, which was good for me."

88 James Walker, interview, Sept. 29, 2014; Goldfarb, interview.

89 Walker, unpublished account, p. 4.

90 Davis, unpublished account, p. 1.

91 McCarthy, "Laster's Tenure Pushes OHSU Toward Heights," p. B06.

92 Laster, "Attracting Excellence—An Economic Prescription," Peter Kohler collection, OHSU Archives, Oct. 23, 1986.

Chapter Two

A Transformation Plan

Oregon Health Sciences University, like the nation's other 124 academic health centers, had become an extraordinarily complex organization by the time Peter Kohler arrived in 1988. It operated on a $254 million annual budget, and employed more than 5,800 workers engaged in multiple missions of conducting research, treating patients, and training doctors, dentists, nurses, and other health workers—about 2,000 trainees in all.[1] It operated two hospitals and was affiliated with three others. It ran clinics, research labs, and classrooms. It collected revenue from its health services, the state, the National Institutes of Health, donors, and other government research grants. It employed a high concentration of bright, highly-educated workers with big personalities and big ambitions capable of transplanting hearts, repairing brains, and probing the frontiers of molecular biology. It enrolled the brightest students of their generation. It functioned both in the lofty world of academe and on the ground, treating sick and injured people in the competitive health care marketplace.

In all that they do, academic health centers walk a tightrope, writes Gregory R. Wegner, as editor of the Higher Education Roundtable's Policy Perspectives. They must maintain a clear commitment to their academic missions, he says, while remaining vigilant about changes in the health care market that can quickly send them into red ink.

"Quite possibly there is no other example of a billion dollar enterprise that has so many layers, so many overlapping lines of authority as commonly appear in an AHC," he writes.[2]

The challenge of making OHSU's moving parts all work together appealed to Kohler, as did its broader mission of improving public health. And he was well prepared to lead the medical center. He had a solid work history in management, research, and patient care, and he also had an unusual grounding in the liberal arts that set him apart from most physicians and researchers and gave him a unique perspective on the value of a well-rounded education.

Dr. Bert W. O'Malley—a longtime close friend of Kohler and an endocrinologist who worked with him at Duke University, the National Institutes of Health and Baylor College of Medicine in Houston—describes Kohler as widely well-liked, even-keeled, unassuming, ethical, and humorous.

"He has a quiet strength about him," said O'Malley, chair of the Department of Molecular and Cellular Biology at Baylor, "combined with a substantial intellect that leads to good decision-making."[3]

Kohler was born July 18, 1928, in Brooklyn, New York, and grew up with one younger brother. His mother, who had a master's degree in literature from Columbia University, worked as an executive assistant to high-powered bosses, including William S. Paley, the chief executive for the Columbia Broadcasting System. While the family was in New York during the summer of Kohler's birth, they ordinarily lived in southwestern Virginia, where Kohler's father was an English professor at Virginia Tech in Blacksburg. During two summers when he was a young boy, Kohler's family returned to live in New York City, where his father wrote plot lines for soap operas. With nurturing, highly-educated, and stimulating parents, Kohler grew up confident and disciplined.

He went off to Charlottesville to study at the University of Virginia. He followed his parents' examples by majoring in English, even though his father had advised him against it. His father thought his talents were better suited to other endeavors, said Kohler. And the fact was, Kohler said, "I hated to write."[4]

Later in school, he came around to his father's view, leaned toward medicine and loaded up on chemistry and biology classes, even while completing his bachelor's degree in English literature. He was inspired by a grandfather who loved being a physician, and he liked the idea of devoting his life to work that could help people and make a difference.

"I thought I would like family medicine," he said. "I could see myself being a family physician. The idea of being a physician appealed to me."[5]

He joined the Delta Kappa Epsilon fraternity and played varsity center and linebacker for the University of Virginia football team. He lettered, he said, though he watched most of the games from the bench. Years later, Joe Cox, chancellor of the Oregon State System of Higher Education, told Kohler that they both had been on the same playing field at the same time during a game between the University of Maryland and the University of Virginia: Cox was on Maryland's sousaphone line. "Our line was heavier than yours," he joked to Kohler.[6]

After graduating, Kohler was admitted to the medical school at Duke University in 1959. His younger brother would follow him there to become a rheumatologist. The Duke medical school, founded in 1944, was young enough when Kohler arrived to still have many of the original faculty. One professor, Dr. Eugene Stead, intimidated students with his brilliance but impressed them with his teaching. He took an interest in Kohler. On one occasion, Stead told Kohler he was exploring the effects of anticoagulation on blood flow, and he wondered whether hemophiliacs have less plaque buildup in their arteries. He invited Kohler to assist him in this venture, but was vague on how. So Kohler dug into some books in the library and found a photo of the aorta of a hemophiliac. The aorta was riddled with plaque, a clear answer to Stead's question. About two weeks later, Stead asked whether he had found anything. He showed the photo to the professor. Stead was impressed, and that would pay off later.

During his freshman year, Kohler stayed in a dormitory for medical students across the street from the nursing students' dorm. The two dorms shared a cafeteria, which led to romance between future doctors, nearly all men in those days, and nurses, nearly all women. One evening, Kohler and another medical student went on a double blind date with two nurses. Kohler became more interested in his friend's date than his own. Her name was Judy Baker, the daughter of a Pennsylvania physician, and after they met, Kohler dated her for nearly 100 consecutive nights. On the day after Christmas that year, in Kohler's freshman year and less than four months after their first blind date, he and Baker married in Judy's hometown of Athens, Pennsylvania. After a "very small wedding," they drove twelve hours back to Duke the next day.[7]

They were both in school for the next eighteen months. During that time Judy developed Graves' disease, which produces an overactive thyroid gland and causes the immune system to attack glands in the neck. The dean of the Duke medical school successfully operated on Judy at the end of her senior year, fixing the problem.

The Kohlers worried Judy might have trouble conceiving because of the surgery and disease, but by December, 1962, she was expecting their first child. Kohler finished school early, and he and Judy moved to Sayre, a town near Athens in northeastern Pennsylvania, where Kohler worked as a pre-intern in the Guthrie Clinic and Robert Packer Hospital. Judy's father, Dr. Dan Baker, an orthopedic surgeon, also worked there, though not directly with his son-in-law. The Kohlers' first child, Brooke, arrived on January 9, 1963, as one of the first babies born in the hospital's new obstetrical suite.

Later that year, the Kohlers moved back to Durham for his internship at Duke. There, Kohler met O'Malley, with whom he still communicates regularly by email or phone. The Kohlers' second child, Stephen, was born the following spring, on March 10, 1964. After his internship, Kohler took a one-year endocrinology fellowship with the thyroid specialist at Duke, and then faced military duty. At that time, all American medical school graduates were drafted. Kohler was picked for the Air Force, and dreaded the possibility he could be sent to the remote Thule Air Base on Greenland. But there was one way around that kind of assignment: he could compete with other medical students for one of the few available slots at the National Institutes of Health in Bethesda, Maryland. "The NIH at that time had its choice of the best and brightest medical school graduates in the US," Kohler said.[8]

He called on Professor Stead, who had a stellar national reputation, to write him a recommendation. Stead also was famous for understating everything, so Kohler didn't expect high praise. But he did say to the professor, "If you just won't say anything bad about me, I will take my chances." Stead must have honored his request: Kohler was selected as a clinical associate.

"We were part of a very collegial group of extremely bright people, many of whom went on to become leaders in academic medicine," he said. Among those colleagues was his friend, O'Malley.[9]

Kohler was already gaining insights from the schools he attended and worked in that would help guide his leadership at OHSU. While at the University of Virginia, the English department invited William Faulkner to be an artist in residence. Kohler noticed that just bringing the literary giant on campus for a spell seemed to raise the national profile and ambitions of the whole school. He would remember that in his efforts to build OHSU's national reputation by luring top researchers. And while at Duke and later at NIH, he noticed the medical school went aggressively after NIH research grants and quickly built up its research capacity. That enabled it to attract top researchers, who in turn won more grants, raising the medical center's reputation more, creating an upward cycle of quality and reputation.

"Watching what they did there has always made me feel we can do some similar things here," he would say later as president of OHSU.[10]

Oregon's academic health center on Pill Hill had shown little interest in NIH grants when Kohler was working for the institutes, and it didn't register on the national radar screen. Dr. John W. Kendall, an endocrinologist who joined the Oregon medical school in 1960 and served as dean from 1983 through 1992, won NIH grants as a researcher. But he could see that Oregon was largely missing out on the rapid expansion of the NIH during the 1950s and 1960s. Though the University of Washington medical school opened more than a half century after Oregon's in 1946, it saw explosive growth with the onset of NIH money during that period as did other younger medical centers at San Diego and Stanford University. While those schools grew, the Oregon medical center drifted, Kendall said, because its older, staid faculty was not interested in NIH money.

> I remember sitting at this lunch table—this would have been in the 50s or 60s—and one of the chairs of a basic science department said, "I don't want any of my faculty to have an NIH grant."
>
> I looked at him and said, "Well, why?"
>
> "They come and go," he said. "The state money is solid. So I won't encourage my faculty to get an NIH grant at all."
>
> Well, hell, the money was pouring into Seattle and San Diego and others around the country while we were bumping along, and this fellow was the most respected research-oriented faculty member on campus, and he was the adviser to the dean on research.[11]

Kohler would eventually bring the Duke model to OHSU. Like Laster, whom he knew at the NIH, Kohler was struck by what the NIH produced when it invested in top researchers and turned them loose to dig into pure science. Like Laster, he would envision bringing NIH-like efforts to produce pockets of excellence at OHSU that would, in turn, lift up the aspirations of the entire university, just as Faulkner did for the University of Virginia. He would understand, as Laster did, that if he was going to attract top researchers, he would have to build first-rate research labs and facilities. And to do that, he would have to expand the medical center's hospital facilities and clinical capacity to help support the research.

While Kohler had planned to stay at NIH in Bethesda only for the two years of his military obligation as a clinical associate, he was invited to stay on as part of the senior staff. He did so for six more years and became head of endocrine service for his unit, which focused on child health and cancer. During his years at NIH, he and his wife had two more children. Todd was born on August 4, 1966, followed by Adam on October 3, 1968.

Kohler not only led his unit, he also worked in the laboratory, exploring cell culture and a variety of things that could affect cells—particularly pituitary cells. He isolated a strain of cancer cells that continue to be replicated and used by scientists all over the world, producing an annual royalty for Kohler of about $1,000 that continues to this day. While running his NIH lab, Kohler also completed his training by working as a resident at Georgetown University.

O'Malley took a job at the private Baylor College of Medicine in Houston, and Kohler soon followed in 1973 to head the endocrinology division. Despite his increasing share of management duties, Kohler received a prestigious Howard Hughes Medical Institute Investigator award to support his research. He developed a reputation for his skill in juggling research, teaching, and management. Baylor also gave Kohler insights to the powers that a private medical center, free of state regulations and bureaucracy, has in competing for research money and patients.

Four years later Kohler left Baylor and O'Malley to move deeper into management as chair of medicine at the University of Arkansas for Medical Sciences in Little Rock. During his nine years in Arkansas, Kohler continued to research and teach, but he also studied how large complex organizations work and bring out the best in their professional staffs. He served his final year as interim dean of the medical school. He finally set research aside when he took a job as Dean of Medical School at the University of Texas medical center in San Antonio. After more than twenty years in research and the classroom, he was ready to move fully into administration.

"I thought I could be more helpful as an administrator than as a scientist," he said. "I thought my science was pretty good, but I couldn't put it in the category of great."[12]

He liked the idea of trying to solve problems for an entire organization, of getting everybody moving in the same direction. He put in 60-to-70-hour work weeks in San Antonio, but still found time to read, fish, go deer hunting—usually taking one of his sons with him—and exercise.[13]

By this time, Kohler had a good appreciation for how tough academic health centers are to manage. In addition to their complexity and mixed missions, they are filled with a rare concentration of extraordinarily bright and accomplished faculty, scientists, and students.

"The more talented they are, the more like prima donnas they can be," Kohler said. "The most ungovernable organizations in the country are our academic health centers."[14]

OHSU CALLS

Kohler had been at San Antonio about two years when Dr. Lynn Loriaux dropped by for a visit. Loriaux had worked with him at NIH, took Kohler's job as head of clinical services when he left and was still there. A week after visiting Kohler, Loriaux visited OHSU to give some talks. At the time, the Oregon State Board of Higher Education had organized a search committee to find a president to replace Laster. A member of the search committee asked Loriaux if he knew of any good candidates. Loriaux suggested Kohler, whom he suspected was restless at San Antonio.[15]

By then, Kohler's name already had reached the search committee, recalled Mark Dodson, a Portland lawyer who at the time was chair of both the State Board of Higher Education and the board's search committee. Dodson, who had been on the board about four years, said he took a hands-on interest in finding OHSU's next leader because he had seen searches for seven university presidents and two chancellors, and "I had seen a lot of them go south."[16]

Dodson grew up and completed high school in Beaverton, a suburb west of Portland, was admitted to Harvard University as an undergraduate and then attended a Baptist seminary for a year. But the seminary "didn't take," he said, and Dodson became the first male in three generations in his family to choose not to become a Baptist minister. Instead, he went to work researching street people in Berkeley, California, while he earned a law degree at the University of California, Berkeley. He moved back to Oregon in 1973 to practice law in Portland, where he and his wife raised two children.

Dodson was determined to find the right leader for OHSU. "It was an institution that could go in either direction very dramatically," he said, and either slide into the backwaters or rise as a national leader in the world of academic health care. The board had hired a national search firm that was good at finding candidates for public universities, but Dodson concluded it didn't have a good grasp on what was required in somebody leading an academic health center. So he met with an OHSU campus search committee charged with giving the state board insights and feedback on the candidates, co-chaired by Lesley Hallick, the molecular biologist who advised Laster. Dodson asked the group to give him ten names. He wrote down each nomination on a blackboard.

"Dr. Peter Kohler," said one committee member. Dodson recalls that the nomination came from Dr. J.S. "Dutch" Reinschmidt, who directed OHSU's regional programs. The group gave Dodson ten names, and he made it a goal to walk the OHSU campus with each of them—and he did.

"That is probably the cheapest, best audit of an institution's potential you are ever going to get, to have those ten people walk the campus and tell you where they see this institution ten or 20 years from now," he said. "They had different visions, but they all saw great potential there."[17]

Dodson's "audit" helped him see the academic health center was not wholly formed, with an undeveloped research arm, no real brand, and some impressive individuals but not yet a coherent, impressive research, clinical, and faculty team. "They needed leadership," he said.

He asked Kohler to apply for the president's job, but Kohler hesitated. He was wary of taking another position so soon for fear he'd get a reputation for frequently jumping jobs. Dr. William Conner—member of the faculty search committee, professor of medicine and head of endocrinology, metabolism, and clinical nutrition at OHSU—called Kohler and also urged him to apply. That pushed Kohler over the edge.

He quickly rose to the top of the list of eighty-four candidates, and of the ten Dodson had collected on his blackboard, and flew to Portland for interviews as one of two finalists. A third anonymous finalist had dropped out. The other was Dr. William N. Kelley, a friend of Kohler's who also had worked at NIH, as a biomedical researcher specializing in biochemical genetics. At the time he applied for the OHSU presidency, Kelley was chair of the internal medicine department at the University of Michigan School of Medicine.

Hallick was chosen to escort Kohler around campus for interviews with a variety of board members and administrators. The easy-going physician with silver hair and fair, freckled skin, impressed her.

> I liked him because he was so honest and so apparently straightforward. I trotted him around, and took him from group A to group B. I had lots of chances to talk with him.
>
> "Why do you want to do this?" I asked him.
>
> "Well, I watched the person doing that at my place," he said, "and I can do that job."
>
> What he was implying was that he could do it better.[18]

Both Walker and Goldfarb at this time were shopping for jobs, but Dodson, who admired the pair both for their work and good humor, told them to back off. "I said, 'You guys aren't going anywhere until we get a new CEO.'" Walker, who held the vice president of finance post that Laster had insisted he take, also met with Kohler during his campus visit. "He was a gentleman," Walker said. "That is how he comes across—a gentleman from Virginia. . . . He also came across as very competent." Walker said he would later learn that the gentleman from Virginia also "can be tough as nails behind the façade."[19]

When Dodson again met with the faculty search group to review their finalists, someone said "Kohler may be a little soft." Then another member, whom Dodson thinks was Reinschmidt, countered: Kohler played as linebacker for the University of Virginia football team. "He is not too soft," he said.

Dodson had settled on Kohler as his first choice and was already worried "we were going to lose him," he recalled. One evening on Kohler's first visit to Portland, Dodson arranged for him to meet with Senator Mike Thorne, the conservative Democrat and rancher from Pendleton who chaired the legislature's Joint Ways and Means Committee—the state's purse strings. Thorne and his wife were having dinner at Portland's upscale Benson Hotel. Dodson knew Kohler was staying there and would soon be back from dinner elsewhere, so Dodson pulled Thorne into the lobby to wait with him to ambush Kohler.

Kohler arrived and the leaders met. Dodson expected Kohler would be impressed by Thorne's legislative power and interest in rural health, and he believed Thorne would find Kohler refreshing. And he was right. Kohler talked about his interest in establishing rural Area Health Education Centers in Oregon as he already had done in Texas. Thorne, who had already been leading discussions about creating the rural health centers in Oregon, loved the plan. "I said, 'You know, I can commit to you now: I'll do everything I can to get that funded,'" he recalled. "He [Kohler] was such a breath of fresh air."[20]

Kohler made two trips to OHSU, but was uneasy with the finalist interview process. He had concluded the state board search committee preferred Kelley.[21] So Kohler withdrew his candidacy. The board, though divided, did first offer the job to Kelley, but he demanded too much in pay and benefits and declined to negotiate. Hallick was relieved. Both candidates "had great visions," she said, "but [Kelley] would have left a lot of blood on the floor. It was just his style. He would just slash and burn, which he did go on to do, absolutely. That was an accurate read."[22]

Dodson turned to Senator Mark Hatfield, whom he knew well, for advice. Hatfield sent him to talk to Dr. Samuel Thier, president of the national Institute of Medicine in Washington, DC, who knew the top candidates. Dodson said he talked to Thier on at least four occasions at Hatfield's suggestion.[23]

Dodson concluded Kelley was "too ambitious, too aggressive." He urged the board to go after Kohler. He told the board that Kohler was perfect because "he would take us one step ahead, one step ahead, and one step ahead, and 10 years later we would turn around and look at how far we'd come," he said. "If we had brought in somebody who didn't have Pete's organizational skills or his demeanor, we could bankrupt the institution." Kohler understood that bringing in too much research too quickly could drown the university in the overhead costs needed to support it. "He gets this; he gets us," Dodson said. [24]

Convinced Kohler was the right man for the job, Dodson set out to persuade him to reconsider. "I never underestimate the value of the dramatic gesture," he said. He arranged for himself and George Richardson, a state board member and lobbyist for Northwest Natural Gas Co., to fly to San Antonio, Texas, to implore Kohler to reconsider.[25]

"If I had to get down on bended knee, I was willing to do that," Dodson said.[26]

But it didn't take that much drama to convince Kohler to take the job.

"It was a move up," he said. "It was a major responsibility. . . . I thought it was a geographically advantaged organization (being in Oregon with its vast wilderness, mountains and ocean.) It is a place you can recruit to. I was sure if things were organized constructively, it would really blossom."[27]

The state board on Monday, April 4, voted to hire Kohler as OHSU's new president. He was given a state salary of $112,680 per year plus an expense allowance of $7,980 and the use of a state-owned house. The OHSU Foundation kicked in another $40,000 to supplement his salary. Still, Kohler would be making less than the $187,750 he was earning at San Antonio.[28]

A special edition of the OHSU newsletter *Campusgram* devoted its cover to the story. The account described Kohler, then 49, as a nationally-known endocrinologist and noted he and Judy had four children, Brooke Kohler-Culp, 25; Stephen, 24; Todd, 21; and Adam, 19. OHSU's Dr. John Benson, who was at the time president of the American Board of Internal Medicine, which included Kohler, declared in the article, "Peter Kohler has rapidly emerged as a leader in American medical education and will serve the citizens and health sciences in Oregon ably and forcefully. A respected clinical investigator and standard-bearer in endocrinology, a congenial former chairman of a large department of internal medicine and now dean of a quality medical school, Dr. Kohler is well prepared to head the university."[29]

In an *Oregonian* article, Kohler's professional colleagues from his work at San Antonio, the NIH and elsewhere, only had praise for the new president: "he's a calm, reasonable man," "an excellent listener," "a true gentleman," "a prince of a person," "a person everyone likes to work with," "exhibits incredible judgment as a physician," "tall, handsome and always smiling," "wry and dry sense of humor," "able to laugh at human folly," "a real down-to-earth guy," "wonderful family man," and "very calm individual, very fair, studious, a real person."[30]

Kohler had researched OHSU before applying for president and knew some of the problems he would be facing. The university had, he recalled, "a very high quality, small faculty and very outdated and poor laboratory space" though the Vollum Institute had just been completed. He knew about building deficiencies, the tussles Laster had had with faculty and the hospital, the hospital's financial challenges, and the friction between OHSU and the legislature and the State Board of Higher Education.

New university presidents typically say they want to spend their first year getting the lay of the land, learning from staff, state leaders, and the public, before setting an agenda. But even before he was hired, Kohler seemed to know exactly what he wanted to do. On March 17, 1988, he outlined his ambitious agenda for the academic medical center in a presentation to the State Board of Higher Education. He said he would not take the job without the board's support of his goals.[31] He said he would seek to:

- Streamline the administrative organization for the university, delegating major responsibilities to vice presidents and the executive council. The administration would rely on consensus building with faculty and constituent groups.
- Upgrade University Hospital to become a premier tertiary care facility.
- Develop Area Health Education Centers (AHECs) to improve health care services in Oregon's less populated regions.
- Upgrade Doernbecher Children's Hospital as a separate facility serving the entire state.
- Expand and coordinate research programs at the Vollum Institute for Advanced Biomedical Research and the Center for Research on Occupational and Environmental Toxicology and develop new research centers.
- Establish a major focus on genetic and gene therapy research.
- Strengthen instruction and make AHECs part of the teaching program.
- Seek state level funding for 30 percent of budget.
- Develop new revenue from federal and private sources.
- Improve and expand facilities, including parking.
- Improve minority faculty, staff, and student recruitment.
- Make OHSU one of the top 20 academic health centers in the nation in terms of NIH research awards.

Dodson welcomed Kohler's agenda. "That is exactly what I wanted to hear," he said."[32]

The State Board of Higher Education voted to support Kohler's agenda, which in many ways carried on President Laster's vision to expand research and facilities and to create focused areas of excellence such as gene therapy research. However, Kohler departed from Laster in fundamental ways, with his emphasis on consensus building with faculty and staff, with expanding OHSU operations into rural areas, and with a statewide mission for Doernbecher Children's Hospital. Unlike Laster, who wanted to keep OHSU's focus on the Hill, Kohler wanted to create a statewide campus. Kohler had concluded that to become better, OHSU would have to get bigger in every way.

"I wanted OHSU to be among the top academic health centers in the country," he said. "It was not going to happen staying small."[33]

COMPLACENCY AND DIVISION

Kohler took command of an academic health center in July of 1988 that was still compromised by mediocre ambition, internal division, and poor relations with the state higher education system and legislature. It had only begun to raise its sights. It lacked the organization that a smooth-running university with so many missions requires.

"When I left, it was still not a coherent organization," said Laster. "One guy got $5 million, I think, from [a foundation] and set up a laboratory without any of us ever knowing it. . . . In those days it was pretty loose and free-wheeling."[34]

Dr. Donald Trunkey, the trauma and general surgeon hired by Laster as chair of the Department of Surgery, arrived in 1986, just two years before Kohler, to find the University Hospital was diverting half of its surgery cases to other hospitals. The hospital was short on operating rooms, surgeons, and computerized tomography (CT) scan capacity, he recalled.

"Nobody was doing general surgery," he said. "It was just a bunch of fiefdoms, just out of control. Three of the fiefdoms—plastic, cardiac, and neurosurgery—were on probation from the Residency Review Committee. . . . I mean, there just was no commitment."[35]

At the time Kohler arrived, the medical school was 101 years old, and the entire academic medical center operated on $254 million a year. It was drawing about $40 million in federal research funds. The university employed more than 3,500 full-time workers, including 800 professors, and more than 1,600 part-time workers, 470 of them faculty members. That made it Portland's third-largest and Oregon's seventh-largest employer. OHSU enrolled 2,066 students, 359 of whom were studying to be doctors, 250 to be dentists, 578 to be nurses, and the rest in other health degrees and fellowship programs. It was among fifty-two of the nation's 125 academic health centers that operated independently of a larger university.

The academic health center had a mediocre national reputation, but it also had its bright spots. For example, one of its earliest researchers, Dr. Edwin E. Osgood—who joined the medical school as student and teacher in 1918—advanced understanding of bone marrow, abnormal blood cell production, and leukemia, research areas in which OHSU continues to excel. In 1958, Dr. Albert Starr launched an open-heart surgery program at the then University of Oregon Medical School and shortly after worked with Lowell Edwards, an electrical engineer, to produce the world's first successful heart valve replacement.[36] By the time Kohler arrived at OHSU, its surgeons had conducted nearly 100 heart transplants.[37] Dr. Kenneth Carl Swan, an ophthalmologist who became the first full-time paid head of a department at the university in 1944, built the Department of Ophthalmology into one of the nation's best. Swan opened the nation's first children's eye clinic, invented the first synthetic tears, developed the Ames Recording Ophthalmoscope, and his department designed the first microscope for ocular surgery. When Kohler arrived, the Vollum Institute had just completed its new building and was in its second year and already gaining national attention for its molecular research of the brain and nervous system.

These successes were not the norm, however. OHSU's research capacity was limited and unexceptional. And its clinical services were struggling with old buildings, insufficient equipment and space, and a large proportion of indigent patients. Most of the buildings had not been updated in decades. The medical center had postponed maintenance for years, racking up more than $350 million in deferred maintenance that needed to be addressed.

"There is a phenomenon I've seen many times," Kohler said. "When you live with something substandard long enough, you get to thinking it is normal. It takes someone with fresh eyes to say, 'This is not normal; it needs to be much better.'"[38]

While the labor and delivery unit offered one of the starkest examples of substandard facilities, the whole campus "was in bad shape overall," Kohler said. On an upper floor of Baird Hall, he said, one of the university's first research areas, the Osgood Laboratory (named for and used by Osgood himself), was dark with old benches and racks. It "looked like it needed to be preserved under glass as a way science was done in the last century," Kohler said. Osgood's lab reminded him of Edgar Allan Poe's room preserved at the University of Virginia, he added.[39]

The hospital roof leaked, and on one occasion, sewage leaked into the Baird Hall conference room. Even the window air conditioner in Kohler's Baird Hall office didn't work. With OHSU so low on the list of the state board and legislature's building priorities, Kohler soon learned that getting help fixing the campus would not come easy. Shortly after he arrived, he traveled to Eugene to meet Representative Carl Hosticka, a Democrat, in his office at the University of Oregon, where he was a professor. Kohler wanted to talk to Hosticka about OHSU's deferred maintenance needs.

"There were two giant holes in the wall of Hosticka's office," Kohler said. "You could see the slats under the drywall. I think I was talking to the wrong person."[40]

When Kohler was hired, the medical center was getting about 23 percent of its budget from the state. Board members had assured him they would do all that they could to push that up to 30 percent. That would help, but Kohler would have to find other ways to start sprucing up his worn campus. He also had much more to learn. Janet Billups, in her first year as the attorney general's representative for OHSU, began meeting regularly with him. In one of their first meetings in his office, he asked about how contracts were written and approved.

"He thought he needed to read and approve every contract at OHSU," she said.[41]

An administrator at one of the health centers Kohler had worked for had become embroiled in a controversy over mismanagement of contracts, and Kohler was determined not to have that happen to him. As a practical matter, Billups told him, he needed to delegate that authority to others, such as a contract officer, or read more than 800 contracts himself. His concern about the contracts reflected his desire to gain a commanding understanding of the institution, Billups said.

"He was clearly really very thorough in understanding this place, understanding how it runs, understanding its business," she said.[42]

After Kohler arrived, acting president Dave Witter took Walker's job as vice president of finance and administration, though he would soon leave, and Walker returned to the job he was originally hired for—chief finance officer of University Hospital. Tim Goldfarb remained permanent CEO of the hospital and clinics. Davis was still handling government relations. Kohler met regularly with Walker, Goldfarb, Davis, and Billups, but Hallick was still grinding away in the classroom and research laboratory.

By the end of 1988, Kohler and his young leadership team, all in their thirties and early forties, had defined their agenda for the 1989 Legislature, which would convene in January. They would seek a better biennial budget, administration of the Office of Rural Health, and a state network of five Area Health Education Centers (AHECs). Kohler began traveling with Davis to Salem to meet legislators individually, including Senator Eugene Timms, the Republican from Burns who would become his key supporter in his quest to make the university a public corporation. Kohler also testified before committees on matters of concern to the medical center, and reached out to Senator Hatfield to nourish the senator's good relationship with the university. He knew that even if the state did increase its support for OHSU, he would need Hatfield's help in getting federal money to turn OHSU into a research powerhouse. State capital did not flow easily to OHSU. Each university in the state higher education system took its turn getting state bond authority for construction. But health care clinical and research buildings cost far more than standard classroom buildings so OHSU's projects often fell to the bottom of the list or were downsized.

Kohler's team set out to educate legislators on the unique demands on a university that, unlike the other seven campuses, included a major health care operation. Legislators had little affection for the higher education system and even less for OHSU, Davis wrote.

> Legislators understood the value of public higher education, but they did not understand how its budget worked or why it cost so much to operate. The budget-setting Ways and Means Committee was used to looking at traditional state agency budgets, which were pretty straightforward. Higher education's budgets were more complicated, featuring everything from state funds to tuition and fees, federal financial aid and federal and private research dollars. Some of the funds were unrestricted, but others were restricted to particular uses. Personnel categories looked nothing like those at state agencies. To frustrated Ways and Means committee members, it looked like higher education's representatives were trying to hide the ball; surely they could present the budget in a fashion more consistent with other state agencies if they chose to.[43]

As Mike Thorne, the Pendleton Democrat who chaired the committee, said: it seemed like Pill Hill was just a big drain.[44]

Kohler's team decided to take a different tack and change the narrative—at least as it related to OHSU. The team would not depend solely on the chancellor's office to carry its message to Salem. It would establish its own working relationship with legislators and their staffs and would explain to them how the academic health care world worked. It also would improve the accuracy and clarity of the financial information it provided, and it would provide as much information as legislators needed when they needed it. If OHSU took on a program or task, it would do exactly what it promised. Finally, it would keep legislators in the loop. There would be no surprises.[45]

OHSU'S RURAL EXPANSION

Kohler also began laying the groundwork for expanding the university's reach beyond Portland into Oregon's vast rural regions. He believed Oregon's sole academic health center needed to serve the entire state. That meant understanding the needs of rural residents by working with them and their health providers. Having grown up in rural Virginia, Kohler also had an affinity and affection for people and their needs across Oregon's countryside. So he strongly supported moving the state's Office of Rural Health to OHSU. When Davis told him that Senator Timms wanted to make that move, Kohler readily agreed. "When can I meet the senator?" he asked.[46]

Kohler appointed Dr. J.S. "Dutch" Reinschmidt to lead OHSU in its expansion to the state's rural reaches. Reinschmidt had joined the University of Oregon Medical School in 1970 as director of its Regional Medical Program and later of its continuing education program. Choosing him to lead OHSU's rural efforts was a "key decision," Hallick said.

> Dutch was beloved. He was a surgeon . . . so he had credentials from both rural and medical arenas. He had run our Continuing Medical Education office, and that meant he stumped the state all the time, little tiny communities, to see what kind of education the doctors wanted and needed. He never stepped on toes. . . . And so he immediately had credibility across the state, especially rural parts of the state. . . . Dutch was a great choice. But he wasn't the kind of choice you'd expect a brand new president necessarily to make. You know, you usually bring in your own person to launch a major new program.[47]

Reinschmidt, who, like Kohler, majored in English along with chemistry as an undergraduate and had a fondness for Shakespeare, grew up in Florida and marched with the US Army across Europe during World War II before entering college.[48] After completing medical school at Vanderbilt University in Nashville, Tennessee, he spent several years in family practice in a small agricultural community called Tekoa in Washington State, near the Idaho border. There he developed an appreciation for the challenge rural physicians faced in keeping up with modern medical developments.

He worked briefly in Pullman, Washington, and then Eugene, Oregon, before he was hired by University of Oregon Medical School to be director of the federally-funded Regional Medical Program, which disseminated the latest knowledge about heart disease, cancer, stroke, and other diseases to rural doctors. The medical school was providing short "circuit rider" courses in rural areas, but Reinschmidt soon concluded "we really needed to broaden ourselves and, as the university developed, to recognize that we had a fundamental responsibility to the entire state."[49]

With help from the Oregon Medical Association, he expanded the program, enlisting university faculty in organizing weekend and week-long courses all over the state. The rural courses evolved into annual education conferences in Bend, Ashland, and at Salishan Lodge on the central coast that would draw hundreds of rural physicians, not only from Oregon, but also other states—all supported by tuition charged to the participating physicians.

When Kohler arrived, Reinschmidt had already been pushing OHSU to look at the federal AHECs, and Laster had pushed back. The AHEC program was developed by Congress in 1971 to recruit and train a health professions workforce committed to underserved populations, mostly in rural America. With a blend of state and federal support, the program helps bring the resources of academic medical centers like OHSU to serve local community health needs. AHECs expose and recruit high school students in underserved areas into the health professions, provide education to rural physicians and future health professionals, and develop strategies to respond to rural health care needs. OHSU medical students are rotated through AHECs, where they are mentored by local physicians and help relieve the health care shortage.[50]

As acting president before Kohler arrived, Dave Witter had been approached by Senator Thorne, the conservative Democrat and wheat farmer from Pendleton, to see what more OHSU could do to support rural physicians, because they were losing them. Rural doctors were leaving because they worked in old facilities, lacked modern equipment, handled heavy patient loads, and had a high proportion of indigent and uninsured patients. A lack of doctors was part of the reason some rural hospitals were closing or struggling financially.[51] Three physicians from Wallowa County had asked Thorne for his help, so he organized a conference in the spring of 1988, just before Kohler arrived, on rural health needs. The conference in Joseph, a small town in Northeast Oregon, drew Reinschmidt, the deans of the medical and nursing schools, nurses, rural physicians, hospital directors, members of the Academy of Family Physicians, and the Oregon Medical Association: more than sixty people in all. The group settled on a plan that included establishing five AHECs across the state.[52]

Kohler embraced the plan. He had helped establish AHECs in the Rio Grande Valley south of San Antonio. One, near Brownsville, has evolved into an academic medical institute. Thorne and those at the Joseph conference wanted to see AHECs in Oregon.

Some rural practitioners and hospital administrators worried that the real goal of the AHEC program might be to provide OHSU with a base from which to set up competitive clinical operations in their areas. Some rural leaders also were wary of OHSU and questioned whether it could credibly and objectively manage the operations of the Office of Rural Health. Since OHSU had relationships with rural doctors and hospitals that referred patients to it, wasn't there a possibility it would favor those over others who were not so connected?

But other rural physicians and legislators, especially Thorne and Timms, defended the rural health education plan. Practitioners in the eastern Oregon district that Timms represented complained the Office of Rural Health was poorly managed by the State Department of Human Resources, and Timms wanted it out of that agency. OHSU assured legislators it would establish firewalls to ensure the office remained at arm's length from its clinical business so that it was not favoring one rural area over another for revenue purposes.[53]

Kohler joined Reinschmidt in travels from town to town across the state to assure legislators, local leaders, health care providers, and the public that OHSU was only looking for ways to help improve local health care. They spoke to Kiwanis and Rotary clubs, chambers of commerce and local newspapers, pressing his message: "I want to know how OHSU can help you." They told rural communities about OHSU's desire to manage and support the Office of Rural Health and launch an AHEC program. People liked Kohler's friendly, unpretentious style, and they listened.

One of Kohler's first trips was in early fall of 1989 to Pendleton, home of Senator Thorne. From the time he met the senator at the Benson Hotel, Kohler had been cultivating a good relationship with Thorne. Kohler flew into Pendleton, a small city on the banks of the Columbia River in north central Oregon, in a twin-engine state plane to speak to the local Rotary Club. He was greeted at the airport by the Main Street Cowboys, a goodwill civic group that welcomes visitors and promotes Pendleton and its famous rodeo and festival, the annual weeklong Pendleton Round-up, which had just ended in late September. The group dressed Kohler in chaps and a cowboy hat and put him in the back of a Round-up float that was playing "Yellow Rose of Texas."[54]

He rode on the float to the Rotary Club meeting, where he talked about OHSU's desire to bring health services and education to rural Oregon in much the same way the Oregon State University Extension Service provided classes and services to rural farmers.

"It was a good way to break the ice," Kohler said of the visit. "Rural Oregonians have tended to be suspicious of people in Portland."[55]

Kohler had other adventures during the winter and early spring of

1989, in visits every two or three weeks throughout Oregon's eastern and southern hinterlands and coast where he got a firsthand view of the state's enormous landscape. Most of the time he talked about OHSU's hopes of expanding services to rural Oregon, but he also made trips to support fundraisers for local hospitals, which were struggling to stay out of debt.

Weather threatened and complicated several trips. On one dark winter night, he was flying to a hospital benefit in Enterprise in northeast Oregon, and it was snowing as his small plane approached the airport. He found it a little unsettling that the airport had no building or tower. The pilot would fly over and flick his lights three times, a signal to whoever was on the ground to turn on the runway lights. The system worked, and Kohler made the visit.

He was going to make a trip by plane to Lakeview, a small town in southeast Oregon, but the state pilot concluded the weather was too dangerous for a trip over the rugged Cascade Range that divided east and west Oregon. But then Kohler got word from a physicians group in Lakeview that Dr. Robert Bomengen—physician, OHSU graduate, and pilot—would fly him over. Kohler made it to the meeting, but the flight back with a commercial pilot had an edge.

"We could hear ice forming on the wing," Kohler said.

Rural residents appreciated his efforts to meet with them, and his travels paid off.[56] The legislature in the spring of 1989 supported moving the rural health office to OHSU and setting aside a state match for federal money to create AHECs in Oregon. OHSU now had the framework to build the 98,000-square-mile statewide campus Kohler envisioned. OHSU's goodwill also had established a supportive statewide political foundation that would become critical in Kohler's quest to make OHSU a public corporation. But Kohler didn't embrace expansion into rural Oregon for political reasons, Dodson said, but because "it was something he had a passion for."[57] The AHEC program continues to operate today in a national network of 235 centers, including the five in Oregon, connected with 120 medical schools in nearly every state.

FINANCIAL CHALLENGES

During the spring of 1989, Kohler got a taste of the financial challenges he was up against in keeping OHSU afloat. The hospital was bleeding out. It was $1 million or more in the red. As so many times in the past, OHSU would have to appeal to the state for a bailout. Kohler, Walker, and Goldfarb went to Salem to meet with then-Governor Neil Goldschmidt, the former Portland mayor, who was in the third year of his first and only term. They met in the governor's conference room, with Walker and Goldfarb at one end of the table, the governor at the other, and Kohler in between. Goldschmidt told the administrators he would help, but he did not want to see them coming for money again. He would not hold the new president responsible for the hospital's financial predicament, he said. He stood, walked behind Kohler, put his hands on Kohler's shoulders and looked over at Walker and Goldfarb.

"This is my guy," he said. "If there are problems, you two guys are gone. The heads that roll will be Tim Goldfarb's and Jim Walker's."[58]

Near the end of 1989, Kohler needed to find someone to replace Dr. Robert Koler, researcher and former chair of the genetics department, who had been serving as vice president for academic affairs since Laster left and was now about to retire. During the university's national search for a candidate, Kohler urged Lesley Hallick to apply. Though she was one of the first people he had met at OHSU as she ushered him about campus for his job interviews, he had seen little of her in his first year. She returned to the classroom and laboratory as a tenured associate professor in molecular microbiology and immunology. But she must have made an impression on the president. In addition, Koler, the outgoing vice president, had worked with Hallick on several issues and committees and praised her strong academic credentials to Kohler. Hallick was shocked when she was actually offered the job, however, because Koler had told her not to get her hopes up.

"You know, I don't think this is a shoo-in for you," he told her.

"I assume I'm a shoo-out," she replied. "I'm not going anywhere . . . I'm fine with that. I have a job. I love my job. That's just fine."[59]

But Hallick had her reasons for wanting to be vice president for academic affairs, a post later renamed provost in keeping with most other academic health centers.

> I didn't really believe the university was a university yet, and it needed to become one. . . . We were sort of fiefdoms, and we needed to integrate and become a grown-up university. We had no infrastructure and none was ever funded. . . . There were just a lot of things about the way [OHSU] worked that weren't very effective in terms of everything from the registrar's office, to student life support or research. It seemed like there were things that could get fixed. I viewed it as a short-term thing. I didn't want to do administration. It sounded really boring. I just figured I would maybe clean some things up and make it better for the university and then go back to my lab and teaching.[60]

With Hallick on board, Kohler had his core inner circle in place. And it wasn't long before he, Hallick, Walker, Davis, Goldfarb, and Billups were talking about the need for more independence for OHSU. While the legislature gave OHSU the rural expansion authority it was after, it didn't give it any more money. It allocated $58 million in state support to OHSU for 1989–90, roughly the same as the previous year. But OHSU's operations, with increased clinical and research revenue, had grown by about $37 million. So state revenue would cover only about 22 percent of the OHSU budget, less than the 30 percent board members told Kohler he could count on. That reality, the hospital's recent financial crisis, and the pressing need to fix buildings and expand OHSU's research capacity all pushed Kohler's team to start talking about the need for another governance model that would give the institution more control over its fate.

Another force fueling that discussion was the rapid spread of managed health care, which penetrated Portland deeper than most parts of the country. In the traditional fee-for-service approach to health care, insurance companies pay doctors according to their services such as stitching a cut, replacing a hip, or knocking down an infection. Under managed care plans, health insurance companies reduce costs by organizing networks of physicians, specialists, and hospitals equipped to give patients whatever care they need for a fixed monthly lump payment on a capitation or per patient basis. These capitation plans, which became popular again under the federal Affordable Care Act signed into law in 2010, try to build incentives for doctors to provide more preventive care and no more services or tests than necessary.

Medicaid, the state- and federally-funded health insurance program for people on low incomes, also uses a managed care approach in many states, including Oregon. The state provides monthly payments to insurance companies that organize managed care networks. Kohler knew OHSU was serving a disproportionately large share of Medicaid patients, as well as low-income non-Medicaid patients who paid nothing. The managed care trend would force the health center to make radical changes in its business model if it were to compete for primary care patients. It would have to become part of private managed care groups, including some that managed Medicaid. The hospital and outpatient clinics would have to work more efficiently together as a system to keep costs down. Most of the health care money under managed care would flow through the primary care clinics and practitioners, Hallick said.[61]

Walker and Goldfarb told Kohler something had to give. OHSU's businesses, its hospital and clinics, couldn't operate in business-like ways in a state bureaucracy under the pressure of managed care. They couldn't survive. They needed to be free of state regulations so they could buy, build, and provide services at a quick, competitive pace. They needed to be independent.

A REBELLIOUS STREAK

The interest of Kohler and his team in more independence for OHSU tapped into a rebellious streak in the medical school that runs back to its origins. The private Willamette University in Salem, founded in 1842 as the first university in the Western United States, opened Oregon's first formal medical education program in 1867. Eleven years later it moved to Portland, which had more and better medical clinics to serve the city's 19,000 residents. Initially, the medical program, called the Willamette Medical Department, operated in a few rooms above a livery stable on SW Park Avenue and Jefferson Street, near where the Portland Art Museum now sprawls. In 1886, the program moved into a Victorian building at NW Fourteenth Avenue and Couch Street in the core of the city. The building featured a 150-seat auditorium, a twenty-table dissecting room, and a refrigerator large enough to store thirty cadavers.[62]

But along with moving, the school reorganized the faculty and appointed a new chair of obstetrics, changes that upset four physicians teaching at the school—Simeon E. Josephi, Kenneth A.J. Mackenzie, H.C. Wilson, and George M. Welles. The four rebelled. They joined four other Portland physicians and won a charter in June 1887 under the Board of Regents of the University of Oregon to open a new state medical school in Portland.[63] Classes opened that fall in two rooms of a former two-story grocery store at NW Twenty-Third Avenue and Marshall Street, the site where Legacy Good Samaritan Medical Center continues to operate today. Students used a block and tackle to pull up cadavers through a trapdoor to the top floor for research and instruction.[64] The school, with eight faculty, offered a two-year course of study, and its first class, a group of seven students who had completed their first year at Willamette, graduated in 1888. The new medical school was not very selective in whom it accepted for admission. Students had to demonstrate a knowledge of arithmetic, geography, and "common English," with a grasp of writing, spelling, and grammar. The school's gross income for 1888 was $2,329.

The following year, the school moved its building one block to Lovejoy Street and replaced it in 1893 with a well-equipped medical college building. The medical school established by four rebellious physicians as part of the University of Oregon would evolve into Oregon Health & Science University.[65]

Josephi—distinctive with his wire glasses, white hair, and long white goatee—was elected dean of the new medical school. The other three dissenters served on its faculty. By 1909, the school had arranged for its students to learn in Multnomah County Hospital at First Avenue and SW Hooker Street, about four blocks from OHSU's South Waterfront campus today. Eight years after the dissenters started the UO Medical School, the Willamette Medical Department moved back to Salem. By 1912, the UO Medical School had established itself as a solid academic program with a full-time laboratory staff, support from the state legislature, and a public mission to serve the indigent through its affiliations with a teaching hospital and an outpatient clinic called the People's Institute and Free Dispensary in downtown Portland. Mackenzie replaced Josephi as dean, and in 1913, the Willamette Medical Department merged with the UO Medical School as the state's sole medical education program.[66]

Mackenzie, who had curly dark hair and a bushy mustache, was among the first of a long line of leaders longing to see the medical school expand and excel. He wanted to see it moved to a quiet, pastoral setting more conducive to learning and reflection, away from the noise and grit of the city. He moonlighted as chief surgeon of the Oregon–Washington Railway and Navigation Company and persuaded the company in 1914 to donate twenty acres of land on Marquam Hill, inaccessible to its trains, for a new medical school campus. An old wagon road was the only way to get to the hilltop, about 1.5 miles from downtown Portland. Critics called the new campus "Mackenzie's Folly," charging it was too remote to be practical. But the next year, the legislature appropriated $50,000 for a new medical building on the site, and the three-story Mackenzie Hall was completed in 1919. The medical school opened on the hill with ten full-time faculty serving fifty students, including some women and many returning war veterans. A janitor kept the key to a closet-sized room where it initially stored its medical textbooks.[67]

Rather than become forgotten and isolated, the medical school became a beacon for other health-related enterprises and rapidly expanded over Pill Hill. Four years after it opened, Multnomah County built a new hospital on the hill so that it could contract with the medical school to serve its patients. In 1926, Doernbecher Memorial Hospital for Children rose on the hill, financed primarily by a donation from a charitable trust managed by the heirs of Frank Silas Doernbecher, a prominent Portland businessman who established Portland's leading furniture factory. He had stipulated in his will that the $200,000 be given "to some charity for the benefit of the people of Oregon." The medical school took over operations of Doernbecher, the first full-service children's hospital in the Pacific Northwest, two years after it was built.

In 1931, the school built a clinic building for outpatient services. The University of Oregon opened a nursing school on the hill the next year. In 1938, the medical school added a library and auditorium building, a three-story laboratory wing to Mackenzie Hall and an eighty-bed University State Tuberculosis Hospital, later converted to the Campus Services Building. The private North Pacific Dental College in Portland became part of the University of Oregon in 1945 and moved into a new building on the OHSU campus eleven years later. Baird Hall rose in 1949 as a building for administrative offices and basic sciences departments, including Osgood's research lab. A Child Development and Rehabilitation Center was built on the campus in 1954. Multnomah County decided to get out of the inpatient care business and sold its hospital in 1973 for $1 to the state, which then turned its operations over to the medical school. The school then merged its hospital, the county hospital, and the university's outpatient clinics into University Hospital.

The medical school in 1974 pursued more independence in a move it had been contemplating for years, with support from the State Board of

Higher Education. It broke from the University of Oregon to become an independent institution within the state university system. It merged its dental, nursing, and medical schools into the University of Oregon Health Sciences Center to create the state's only academic medical center, and the state board hired Dr. Lewis William Bluemle Jr. to run it.[68]

Now, sixteen years later, Kohler and his team were looking at another split, this time from the state bureaucracy and higher education system. Any doubts Kohler's team had about the need to make that break vanished when Oregon voters approved Measure 5 in November, 1990.

MEASURE 5

The Oregon Department of Revenue divides the history of property taxation in Oregon between before and after Measure 5. The landmark property tax limitation legislation dramatically shifted the way the state funded public and higher education. Before Measure 5, Oregon had a pure levy-based property tax system. Each taxing district—whether for water, recreation, community colleges, schools, or other services—calculated its own tax levy based on its budget needs. The levy for each taxing district, say, Portland Public Schools, was then divided by the total real market value in the district to arrive at a district tax rate. The tax rate times the real market value equaled the amount of money that Portland schools or any other tax district could collect. Most levies were limited to an annual growth rate of 6 percent, and any increase greater than that required voter approval.

This system created great inequities in public school funding. Taxpayers living in districts like Portland with high property values could raise far more money for their schools with a given tax rate than could property owners in rural areas such as Burns with low property values. The result was Portland school district was so awash in money that it could afford, for example, to provide musical instruments for all interested students, run its own repair shop to fix those instruments, and bring in local performing artists to teach children how to use them. Some rural districts, by contrast, struggled to keep their schools opened for a full school year.

That all changed under Measure 5, which went into effect during the 1991–92 fiscal year. The measure limited tax rates to $5 per $1,000 of real market value for school taxes and to $10 per $1,000 real market value for general government taxes. This applied only to money raised for operating costs. Schools and other government agencies could still ask voters for approval to levy taxes to pay for maintenance and construction bond sales.

With the Measure 5 limits, most school districts could not raise enough money to sustain their budgets. The measure required the state to make up the sizable difference. In doing so, the state equalized spending, meaning rich districts like Portland got less while poor rural districts got more. The State of Oregon assumed the major burden of supporting public schools, which now get half their money from the state, 35 percent from local property taxes, and 15 percent from the federal government. Without a sales tax, the state relies on an income tax for 89 percent of the revenue it uses to support all state services, including prisons, social services, and higher education. Measure 5 forced the state to use a big share of that income tax money to also support public schools, which meant less money was available for the other agencies, including state universities.[69] Governor Barbara Roberts, elected on the same day Measure 5 passed, ordered state agencies, including the universities, to cut their state funding requests by 25 percent.

It was now clear to Kohler and his team that they were going to have to find another source of money if the university was to survive, let alone grow and prosper. The state was giving too little and expecting too much of the medical center, said Hallick.

"So when Measure 5 hit, and it was obvious it was just going to get worse, and very quickly, we were already in the conversations [about independence] and very quickly went to, 'OK, what are the extremes here and what is in between?'" she said. "That's when we started talking to various business leaders."[70]

Neither Kohler nor members of his leadership team recall precisely when or how the term "public corporation" surfaced as they explored ways to deal with declining state revenue. The notion of breaking away or becoming more independent of the state goes back to the academic health center's origins. Bluemle left the Oregon medical center knowing it needed "a new paradigm for financing," he said years later. The new paradigm, he said:

> had to be a change the legislature would support, a radical change, which would make the institution more dependent upon itself to survive. That's the only way you can build the incentive to do—or encourage people to do—the hard work, to generate the resources to make it first class. You can't do it any other way. And I guess that's one reason that [the private Thomas Jefferson University in Philadelphia] appealed to me, because it had to rely on itself to generate its resources. . . . But you had to change, you had to depend more on yourself, you had to give up your old biases. You had to scramble, you had to become competitive, and you had to rely on yourself to win. And that would have taken a lot longer than three years [that he headed OHSU].[71]

Donald Kassebaum also recalled exploring with Bluemle and a member of his staff, John D'Aprix, the public corporation option:

> We were going to do it for the hospital. We went to the Port of Portland. We studied the model of the public authority, and we proposed it to the Oregon State System of Higher Education and to the Oregon Legislature. . . . they simply gave us a lot of freedoms and said, "We really don't want to talk about that now."[72]

Bluemle's successor, Leonard Laster, said he and his staff also talked about taking OHSU more private, but didn't see that as a realistic option. "Things that we talked about as just ridiculous ideas, like making the hospital private, have come to pass," he said. "It couldn't have been done in my time—I really would have been run out of town."[73]

Memories differ, but several people point to Brian Booth, attorney and a founder of the Tonkon Torp LLP law firm in Portland, and member of the OHSU Foundation board, as one of the first to talk about restructuring the academic health center in a way that would give it more independence and control over its fate.

In the months before Kohler joined the university, Booth talked to Billups and interim President David Witter about whether OHSU—or at least its clinical operations—would be better off as a hospital district.[74] Conversations about how a different structure could benefit OHSU and the state continued to percolate after Kohler arrived. A number of universities around the country were divesting—or discussing divesting—themselves of their hospitals, and there were questions about whether this would make sense for OHSU. Most of those early conversations occurred at the Oregon State System of Higher Education level, among close associates of the university, or, in some cases, with legislators or legislative staff who had some knowledge of the health care field. Although none of these discussions led anywhere, they did keep the need for change alive in people's minds—including that of Kohler.

The term "public corporation" appears as a broad, generic label in Oregon statutes and court cases to apply to a wide range of public institutions. Early court decisions, such as McClain v. Regents of the University of Oregon in 1928, refer to state universities such as the University of Oregon as "public corporations." A more descriptive term for what Kohler's team was seeking would be an independent public university.

But Kohler had not been president long before the idea of a public corporation surfaced. Wendy Robinson, assistant Oregon attorney general, wrote an analysis in 1989 that reached Kohler's office. Robinson outlines the qualities and powers of a "public corporation."[75] She notes a public corporation is: created by government in a public process, gets at least some support with public money, has a board of directors, is subject to public records laws, is exempt from public contracting rules, and carries out public functions that would otherwise be performed by the state.

Kohler and his team also considered spinning the hospital off as an independent operation divorced from OHSU, but Kohler had reservations. The hospital would have its own board and director independent of the university and would be in control over how much of its revenue would flow to support the university and its medical school. Kohler wanted to retain that control. His effort to move OHSU to the top echelon of the nation's academic health centers would be limited if he were to lose command of the hospital, a potential major moneymaker if operated well.

But he and his team were willing to take a hard look at every option, whether creating some kind of hospital district, becoming part of the state health department, going completely private, or becoming a public corporation. They quietly began running those ideas by leaders in the medical center and by legislators such as Thorne and Timms, civic leaders, and others who had a stake or interest in OHSU. Kohler talked to Dodson about making OHSU a public corporation when Dodson still chaired the State Board of Higher Education. Dodson still subscribed to the old system—you go to the legislature to get money. He pushed back.

"Look, you've been right about everything up to this point," he told Kohler, "but I really have got to ask you, 'Do you know what you are doing here? Is this really the right thing? Because you know, you are going to cut yourself off from a lot of state funding.'"[76]

Pursuing any of the various options Kohler and his team were considering would take time, and they had more immediate challenges commanding their attention. Measure 5 put a tremendous strain on the state budget, and in such times, higher education usually took hard hits because legislators knew that unlike most state agencies, universities could raise money by charging students tuition. And among higher education institutions, OHSU was likely to suffer even more because it also could earn money through its hospital and clinical services. Early in 1991, Roberts, in her proposed budget to the legislature, appropriated

$665 million to the state's eight universities for 1991–93, $28 million less than they had been getting.[77]

At the same time, OHSU was launching major initiatives. It was establishing AHECs around the state. Its new medical ethics center, created to ensure patients receive compassionate and ethical care, had just opened the previous year. The medical school had received a foundation grant to overhaul its curriculum. And the university complex was in the midst of a building boom, including many projects Laster had planned with Hatfield's support. An article in the *Sunday Oregonian* on August 5, 1991, noted buildings were multiplying on Marquam Hill "like bacteria in a petri dish."

> On the east edge of campus, the concrete frame of the [privately-funded] $23 million Casey Eye Institute is rising on a brow of the hill overlooking Portland. Higher on the hill, beyond the hospital, a towering crane pivots over the reinforcement rods sprouting from the foundation of the new $20.4 million Biomedical Information Communications Center. . . . To the south, the university just broke ground for a $14 million nursing school building.[78]

Hatfield over the previous decade had funneled $91 million into construction at OHSU, including federal money for the already completed $42 million Vollum Institute for Advanced Biomedical Research and a $10 million renovation of the hospital's south wing.[79] And as Laster had envisioned, the new space was enabling the university to attract researchers. The Vollum Institute, under Richard Goodman's leadership, had quickly filled its four floors with eighteen bright young scientists, many of who would reach national prominence, since it opened three years earlier. One of them, Michael Forte, a geneticist from Case Western Reserve University in Cleveland, turned down two other jobs to come to Portland and probe fruit flies and secrets of the brain at the molecular level. A team led by Olivier Civelli had already found a way to reproduce a substance that nerve cells make to communicate with one another. The university also had recruited Dr. Neil Swanson, a skin cancer expert, from the University of Michigan and Dr. Melvin Ball, an expert in brain diseases from the University of Western Ontario.[80]

CREATING THE FREEDOM TO COMPETE

Even as the university expanded its research capacity, Kohler knew that to sustain OHSU's growth in quality and size in the face of declining state support, the university would need to compete more aggressively for paying patients. In late 1991, he assembled a task force of business leaders, legislators, and representatives from OHSU, the university system, governor's office and community to study and recommend a course of action. The committee, which included Brian Booth, the lawyer, studied the pros and cons of four possible paths: stick with the status quo, merge with the Oregon Health Division, become fully private, or transform into a public corporation.[81]

The group considered how each of these courses would affect OHSU's faculty, staff, patients, taxpayers, the state higher education system, state government, and the academic health center's commitment to research, education, and patient care. It did so in the context of four key issues:

- The two-year cycles of budget reductions and uncertainties complicate long-term planning.
- Overall state support had dropped from 42 percent of OHSU's operating budget in 1975–76 to 17.5 percent in 1991–92.
- While OHSU had made some significant expansions with the help of federal grants and private donations such as Vollum's for the Vollum Institute, the academic health center still needed to address deferred maintenance on its existing buildings and to expand its clinical and research capacity. Its attempts to get help in capital investment from the state for

these needs were regularly delayed and often deferred indefinitely.

- The state management system creates delays and inefficiencies that work against the health care needs of an academic health center.[82]

The group quickly rejected maintaining the status quo as unworkable. The health center could not count on increased revenue from the federal or state governments. So to cover increasing costs, let alone grow, it would have to raise more money from its health services. State regulations constrained its ability to compete, raised its administrative costs and prevented it from responding swiftly to capital development needs. And there were political barriers. The state higher education system was focused on academics, not health care. Legislators sometimes criticized the university medical center for competing with private hospitals, though nearly all in the Portland area were nonprofits.[83]

The committee also rejected the idea of merging with the Oregon Health Division. That would essentially amount to replacing one bureaucracy with another. The division was more aligned with other state agencies than with a business enterprise like clinical care. While the division did overlap with OHSU in some areas of health care, the two operations were different enough that merging would probably lead to more, not fewer, problems.[84]

The medical school did not have a large enough private endowment to make full privatization practical. It could spin off the hospital as a private operation, but Kohler didn't want to give up that control or invite the conflict that would naturally arise from splitting the hospital and university. What's more, university and state leaders likely would oppose full privatization, making it politically nonviable.[85]

So transforming to a public corporation quickly emerged as the best choice. It would keep the academic health center whole and give it the freedom and flexibility to trim administrative costs and engage in private business practices while retaining its public mission, access to some state support, and public accountability. While exempt from state agency status, the health center would still be bound by laws that affect all public bodies such as civil rights, affirmative action, anti-discrimination, the Public Records Act, the Open Meetings Law, the Public Employees Rights Law, the Municipal Audit Law, and the Ethics in Government Act. Its assets would still belong to the people of Oregon. It would not be a privately held business, but remain a unit of government. It would have its own governing board, bonding authority, and responsibility for its own budget and spending. But it would still have the protection of state tort liability limits and retain immunity from federal antitrust laws.

The public corporation option seemed in many ways to offer the best of the public and private worlds, but the committee cautioned that there could be drawbacks, too. Plunging so heavily into the marketplace was financially risky, and funding could be fragile. The university likely would feel pressure to raise tuition. Further, making the transformation would require major legislation, and it was unclear whether it would draw sufficient community and political support.[86]

Though this was a radical move for such a large, complex organization, one never tried by any other academic health center, it had precedents both in Oregon and elsewhere in the country.

The Port of Portland, the Oregon State Accident and Insurance Fund Corporation (Oregon's workers' compensation program), and TriMet, a transit authority spread over three counties in the Portland metropolitan area, all had both corporate and public features.[87]

Rutgers University in New Jersey and many Pennsylvania universities—including Pennsylvania State University, Temple University, and the University of Pittsburgh—essentially operate as public corporations. But these all started as private institutions that gained a public corporation status as their state ties and financial support and public missions grew.[88]

The Pennsylvania Legislature, for example, approved the Temple University-Commonwealth Act in 1965, converting the university, created in 1874 as a "corporation," to an "instrumentality of the Commonwealth to serve as a state-related university in the higher education system."[89] The university would have its own board and control over its financial affairs while receiving the benefits of state support and bonding authority. But some of its powers, such as setting tuition, were turned over to the state.

Earlier, in 1929, the New Jersey Legislature replaced Rutgers University's private governing board with a New Jersey State Board of Regents appointed by the governor. By 1955, Rutgers was getting half of its money from the state. In 1956, the New Jersey Superior Court upheld a challenge to a governance overhaul that gave Rutgers two governing boards, a Board of Governors and a Board of Trustees, with duties divided roughly along its public and private missions. The court refers to the university in its decision as a "corporation," and notes it "shall be and continue to be given a high degree of self government and that the government and the conduct of the Corporation and the University shall be free of partisanship."[90]

Kohler's task force recommended OHSU become a public corporation. On April 3, 1992, Kohler sent an eleven-page memo to Thomas A. Bartlett, the new chancellor of the Oregon State System of Higher Education, outlining "suggested actions" for enabling OHSU to operate more effectively, either as a "component" of the state higher education system or, "alternatively, as a public corporation."[91]

Notes

1 OHSU, "Growth & Change at OHSU at a Glance: 1987–88," available through OHSU Strategic Communications.

2 Gregory R. Wegner, *Academic Health Center Governance and the Responsibilities of University Boards and Chief Executives*, Occasional Paper Series, Association of Governing Boards of Universities and Colleges, Oct. 2003, p. 4.

3 Bert W. O'Malley, MD, interview, June 18, 2014.

4 Peter O. Kohler, interview, Dec. 5, 2014, his office at OHSU.

5 Peter O. Kohler, interview, May 17, 2014, Portland, Oregon.

6 Joseph Cox (former chancellor of the Oregon State System of Higher Education), interview, April 9, 2014.

7 Kohler, interview, May 17, 2014.
8 Ibid.
9 Ibid.
10 Peter O. Kohler, MD, interview by Charles Morrissey, April 21, 1998, president's office at OHSU, interview no. 27 4/21, 1998, transcript, OHSU Oral History Project.
11 John W. Kendall, MD, interview by Joan Ash, June 23, 1999, Biomedical Information and Communications Center, OHSU campus, interview no. 75 6/23, 1999, transcript, OHSU Oral History Project.
12 Kohler, interview, May 17, 2014.
13 Jim Hill, "'Calling Dr. Kohler,' To Cure, Prevent OHSU Ills," *The Oregonian*, April 10, 1988, p. C01. Kohler also found time to exercise. "I play a poor game of tennis," he told Jim Hill in this article. "I play racquetball a little better. I've tried golf, but I'm dangerous."
14 Kohler, interview, May 17, 2014.
15 Lynn D. Loriaux, MD, interview, March 24, 2014, his OHSU office.
16 Mark S. Dodson (attorney), Feb. 23, 2016, interview, Multnomah Athletic Club, Portland.
17 Ibid.
18 Lesley Hallick, interview, May 27, 2014, Pacific University, Forest Grove, Oregon.
19 James Walker, interview, June 16, 2014.
20 Michael Thorne, interview, July 16, 2014, River's Edge Hotel, Portland.
21 Peter O. Kohler, interview, April 11, 2014. "I think honestly they would have preferred to have him [Kelley] based on what criteria they were using," Kohler said.
22 Hallick, interview. A year after he rejected OHSU's offer to be president, Kelley was hired as chief executive officer of the University of Pennsylvania Medical Center and Health System and dean of the school of medicine. In February of 2000 he was fired after a flurry of hospital purchases and other expansions left the health system with a $198 million loss, forcing it to eliminate 2,800 jobs to balance its budget.
23 Dodson, interview.
24 Ibid.
25 Ibid.
26 Ibid.
27 Kohler, interview, May 17, 2014.
28 Jim Hill, "OHSU Foundation to Buy Land For Expansion," *The Oregonian*, Sept. 29, 1988, p. D02.
29 "Texas Medical School Dean Chosen New President of OHSU," *Campusgram*, OHSU, April 4, 1988.
30 Jim Hill, "'Calling Dr. Kohler'," p. C01.
31 Jim Hill, "New Chief Has Agenda for OHSU," *The Oregonian*, April 5, 1988, p. D14.
32 Dodson, interview.
33 Kohler, interview, April 11, 2014.
34 Leonard Laster, MD, and Ruth Ann Laster, interview by Joan Ash, March 5, 1999,

Woods Hole, Massachusetts, interview no. 64 3/5, 1999, transcript, OHSU Oral History Project, p. 28.

35 Donald D. Trunkey, MD, interview by Dr. Richard Mullins, June 21, 2005, Oregon Medical Association headquarters in Portland, Oregon, pp. 24–25.

36 Nick Budnick, "Famed Heart Surgeon Rejoins OHSU Faculty," *The Oregonian*, July 25, 2011, local news section.

37 David Austin, "100th Heart-Transplant Patient Leaves OHSU," *The Oregonian*, March 21, 1990, p. D04.

38 Kohler, interview, April 11, 2014.

39 Ibid.

40 Ibid.

41 Janet Billups, interview, April 2, 2014, her office at OHSU.

42 Ibid.

43 Lois Davis, from unpublished account of her role in OHSU's transformation to a public corporation, Oct. 12, 2013, pp. 5–6.

44 Thorne, interview.

45 Davis's unpublished account, p. 6.

46 Ibid., p. 4.

47 Hallick, interview.

48 J.S. "Dutch" Reinschmidt, MD, interview by Joan Ash and Linda Weimer, Sept. 3, 1997, Mackenzie Hall OHSU, interview no. 2 9/3, 1997, transcript, OHSU Oral History Project, p. 1. Reinschmidt got his nickname on the first day of his freshman chemistry class at Vanderbilt University. His professor "kind of wiggled his mustache a bit and said, 'that's the first Dutchman we've had around here in years,'" Reinschmidt recalled. Classmates started calling him "Dutch," and the name stuck.

49 Ibid., p. 10.

50 Information on OHSU's Area Health Education Centers program is available online at: http://www.ohsu.edu/xd/outreach/ahec/.

51 Bill MacKenzie, "Hospitals Battle Own Grim Reaper," *The Oregonian*, Aug. 13, 1989, p. B1. Rural areas continue to struggle with doctor shortages. As Olga Khazan describes in "Why Are There So Few Doctors in Rural America?" (*The Atlantic*, Aug. 28, 2014), 6,000 federal designated areas have a shortage of primary care doctors, and 4,000 have a shortage of dentists. About a fifth of Americans live in rural areas, but only a tenth of doctors practice there. See: http://www.theatlantic.com/health/archive/2014/08/why-wont-doctors-move-to-rural-america/379291/.

52 Thorne, interview.

53 Davis's unpublished account, pp. 7-8.

54 Peter O. Kohler, MD, interview, July 3, 2014.

55 Ibid.

56 Ibid.

57 Dodson, interview.

58 Timothy M. Goldfarb, interview, Oct. 2, 2014; Walker, interview.

59 Hallick, interview.
60 Ibid.
61 Ibid.
62 OHSU, *Reflections on Yesterday*, OHSU School of Medicine History, 2012, p. 9.
63 Ibid.
64 Don Hamilton, "OHSU Sets Centennial Graduation," *The Oregonian*, June 9, 1988, p. B02.
65 OHSU, *Reflections on Yesterday*, pp. 9–11.
66 Ibid., pp. 10–15.
67 Ibid., p. 15; Hamilton, "OHSU Sets Centennial Graduation".
68 OHSU, *Reflections on Yesterday*, pp. 15–26.
69 Oregon Department of Revenue, *A Brief History of Oregon Property Taxation.*
70 Hallick, interview. Hallick noted that while the state was giving less, it still expected a lot of OHSU. "We were still expected to carry the indigent care load, and there was no place else to send them. We were the place of last resort. And we wanted to do it because it was great for a teaching hospital. It was the right thing to do, but it wasn't reimbursed so it felt very unfair."
71 Lewis W. Bluemle Jr., MD, interview by Joan S. Ash, Thomas Jefferson University, Philadelphia, when Bluemle was president there, March 22, 1998, p. 35.
72 Donald G. Kassebaum, MD, interview by Joan S. Ash, Nov. 7, 1997, the Association of American Medical Colleges Washington, DC, interview no. 6 11/7 1997, OHSU Oral History Project, p. 19.
73 Laster, interview, p. 33.
74 Janet Billups, "The Design of the Public Corporation – the Lawyer's Perspective", an unpublished account of her role in transforming OHSU into a public corporation, 2013, p. 1.
75 Wendy Robinson (assistant attorney general), *The Benefits and Pitfalls of Public Agency/Private Joint Ventures*, internal report to OHSU, p. 1. Peter Kohler collection, OHSU Archives.
76 Dodson, interview.
77 Jim Hill, "Education Board Approves Tight Budget," *The Oregonian*, March 2, 1991, p. D01.
78 Bill Graves, "Federal Largess Benefits OHSU," *The Oregonian*, Aug. 5, 1990, p. D01.
79 Senator Mark Hatfield, during his career, led Congress to appropriate more than $300 million dollars to Oregon for health care research and infrastructure development, according to Oregon's Office of the Governor. Governor Theodore R. Kulongoski's Executive Order No. 08-12, May, 2008.
80 Ibid.
81 Billups account, p. 2, and Davis account, pp. 9-10.
82 Barbara Archer, "Transformation in Public Organizations," (doctoral dissertation presented to the faculty of the School of Policy, Planning and Development, University of Southern California, Dec. 2002), Appendix B; *Oregon Health Sciences University*

Update on Report to Reorganization Planning Committee, March 30, 1992.

83 Peter Kohler, MD, Lois Davis, and Elaine R. Rubin, *The Oregon Health Sciences University Becomes a Public Corporation*, report for the Association of Academic Health Centers, (Washington, DC: 1996), pp. 5–6.

84 Ibid.

85 Ibid.

86 Archer, "Transformation in Public Organizations," Appendix B.

87 *OHSU: The Case for Restructuring*, draft report for OHSU administration, March 10, 1994.

88 Ibid.

89 Temple University–Commonwealth Act, P.L. 843, No. 355, § 2510-2, p. 20.

90 Trustees of Rutgers College in New Jersey v. Grover C. Richman, Jr., Attorney General of the State of New Jersey, 125 A.2d 10, p. 22.

91 Peter O. Kohler, memo to Thomas A. Bartlett, chancellor of Oregon State System of Higher Education (OSSHE) on "Suggested Actions by the State of Oregon and OSSHE to Improve the Operating Effectiveness of OHSU and its Hospital and Clinics," April 3, 1992, Peter Kohler collection, OHSU Archives.

Chapter Three

Selling the Plan

George Pernsteiner, associate vice chancellor of the Oregon University System, held up a small jar of water before the Oregon Legislative Emergency Board on January 8, 1993, and gave it a little shake. Flecks of rust fell through the water like flakes in a snow globe, clouding it red. The water, Pernsteiner explained to the board, came from the water pipes of the Multnomah Pavilion, also known as the north hospital, the former Multnomah County Hospital built in 1923. Among other clinical and hospital services, the old building housed on its fourth floor the Oregon Health Sciences University Labor and Delivery Department. Rusty water, Pernsteiner said, was just one symptom of bigger problems OHSU was having with providing medical services in an increasingly competitive and unstable market.

He was appealing on behalf of OHSU to a dozen members of the emergency board, chaired by Senator John Kitzhaber, a Democrat and physician who graduated from OHSU and would soon be elected governor. The room included Jim Walker, the hospital financial chief, and Tim Goldfarb, the hospital director who gave OHSU lobbyist Lois Davis the vial of rusty water for Pernsteiner's presentation. President Peter Kohler was at a medical meeting out of state. The university wanted to use $18 million in gifts, bonds, and cash from hospital earnings for the first phase of a $25 million project and $7 million in bonds for the second phase. The project would make repairs and add five stories to the nine-story C-Wing of the newer University Hospital, also called the south hospital. Two of those floors would be devoted to modern labor and delivery, mother and baby care, and neonatal services.[1]

OHSU had set aside money to launch the expansion project seven years earlier. But it needed state permission to proceed. In 1987, it asked for that authority from the State Board of Higher Education. But the board did not forward its request to the 1987 Legislature, which needed to approve its request to sell state bonds. The board again failed to refer it to the legislature in 1989. After more delays, OHSU finally won approval to sell state bonds to build the new wing, but it still had to get permission from the emergency board for the specific plan and dollar amount for the new labor and delivery wing.

As Kohler and his leadership team set out to make their case for converting OHSU into a public corporation, the worn, outdated maternity ward became Exhibit A. It provided a vivid image of OHSU's state of disrepair and of how the state bureaucracy mired the medical center in regulations and delays that made it nearly impossible for it to upgrade its facilities so it could compete for patients.

The existing outdated birthing wing had only one bathroom and shower and five delivery rooms for the entire fourth floor in the north hospital. It lacked space for family member visits and packed at least two, and as many as four, women per room. It had the capacity to deliver 1,800 babies a year, yet 2,800 babies were arriving, forcing some women to deliver their babies in the hallway when all delivery rooms were full. Even then, the hospital was forced to divert one-third of its pregnant mothers, most of whom were indigent, to other hospitals to deliver their babies.

Laura Goldfarb, wife of the hospital director, gave birth to twin daughters in the old maternity ward on August 4, 1987. The twins were delivered by cesarean section, and the room was suffocating, said Tim Goldfarb.

"I was so nervous, and I was standing on a table and chair to take pictures of the twins being born," he recalled. "I was pouring sweat. It was so hot in her room. There was no air conditioning, no ventilation. It was like being in a battle zone."[2]

Mothers needing ultrasound or other imaging services would have to go outside to the nearby and newer University Hospital, the south hospital, built in 1956. One day, Kohler was showing a woman from the office of Governor Neil Goldschmidt around campus. They happened to be standing outside in an area between the two hospitals when suddenly they heard someone shout "gangway." It was a hospital worker pushing a mother on a gurney up a steep ramp from south hospital to north hospital above. He had to get a running start to make it up the hill.[3]

As lobbyist for the academic health center, Lois Davis felt compelled to deliver her son, Matt, in the university's primitive labor and delivery wing in September of 1988.

"How could I go to Salem and tell everybody what an amazing place this was and why it should be supported if I wasn't even prepared to have my baby there?" she said.[4]

But she also had been the one who got Pernsteiner his rusty water sample.

"We actually had people come and take a tour and see where the pipes were rusting," she said. "Really, as a pregnant woman, I was afraid to drink the water at the university because it was so bad. That was before the days of bottled water so it was difficult."

She asked Goldfarb to promise her she would not have to deliver in the hallway and that she would have a full-fledged anesthesiologist rather than an intern or resident in training. She had delivered her daughter by cesarean years earlier in a teaching hospital in Washington, DC, and the anesthesiologist, a resident, put the epidural into her bloodstream instead of her lower spine, a potentially devastating mistake.

At OHSU, she was admitted into a room with peeling paint, a hole in the wall, and another pregnant mother. The women shared a bathroom down the hall. Davis delivered again by cesarean, and this time the anesthesiologist, a doctor on fellowship, performed well, as did everyone else. She had wonderful care in grim surroundings, Davis said.[5]

A few years later, Susan Stanley, a Portland freelance journalist, spent three weeks in the OHSU Labor and Delivery Department, and wrote a book called *Maternity Ward: Behind the Scenes at a Big City Hospital.* She described it like this:

> Put plainly, the best that can be said is that L&D [Labor and Delivery] looks like some turn-of-the-century charity hospital. "Spare" would be about the kindest description. The five delivery rooms, with the exception of the room called "Special Delivery," are entirely too small, scarcely accommodating the delivery bed and chair or two for the family and friends who so often nowadays are part of the show. Tuck a couple of residents, a nurse or two, a medical student, and perhaps a student nurse into one of those rooms, and it's a mob scene—untidy, confusing, and very possibly unsafe.
>
> All too often, the PAR—the post-anesthesia recovery room—and the prep room down the hall are redefined as delivery rooms. Sometimes, normal vaginal deliveries take place in one of the two operating rooms, simply because the other rooms are filled. (For that matter, in a pinch, the hallway has had to serve, a screen dragged over for a modicum of privacy if there's time.)[6]

After Pernsteiner's dramatic presentation with the vial of rusty water, the emergency board approved OHSU's project with an estimated completion date of July 1994. But there were more delays. The City of Portland in January of 1994 denied OHSU building permits for the project until it paved remote dirt parking lots. In a letter to Commissioner Charlie Hales, Kohler pleaded for a break. To pave the lots, he said, the university would have to raise fees for employees, who had not received a cost of living increase in two years. If the project did not get underway by January 31, he said, the contract bids would expire, and the university would have to spend more money to rebid. The bids did expire before the city finally issued permits, and the Attorney General's Office said OHSU should start over. So the university bid the project again in February of 1994 and selected a contractor, but the Department of Administrative Services and the Department of Justice took issue over the award process OHSU followed, though it had been approved by the university system. The dispute was settled in June. The contract was finally awarded, and the hospital expansion project was completed in the fall of 1995—nine years after it began. The delays had cost OHSU millions of dollars a year in lost business.

Kohler called it a horror story and one of his favorite examples of what would change if OHSU were allowed to become a public corporation.[7] The story made it clear to state leaders why the university could not compete in a rapidly changing health care market as part of a state agency, Pernsteiner said years later. Legislators worried OHSU was going to go broke and take down the whole eight-campus Oregon University System, he said.

"For a lot of financial reasons, state [leaders] worried they could get stuck with the bill," he said.[8]

In retrospect, Goldfarb said, it was probably a bad business practice to so dramatically display in public the bad water coming from the taps of a hospital desperate for more paying patients. But he and the others on Kohler's leadership team were young, bold, and still a little green.

"We were all kids," said Goldfarb, who was thirty-three at the time.[9]

In the summer of 1992, six months before the emergency board meeting, Kohler's team was poised to launch a major push for converting OHSU to a public corporation in the 1993 Legislature. The task force that studied restructuring options had just recommended the university take that path. It was time to take action. Kohler and his leadership team—Goldfarb, Davis, Jim Walker, provost Lesley Hallick, and attorney Janet Billups—were taking stock of what they were up against and trying to define more clearly what becoming a public corporation would mean.

As they did so, the daunting scope of what they were taking on settled in. Some academic health centers facing economic problems during this period had spun off their hospitals as private, nonprofit operations to give them a fighting chance to compete. But no state had turned loose an entire public academic health center—the hospitals, clinics, schools of medicine, nursing, and dentistry, and research enterprises—to operate independently. There was no precedent. For all its problems, OHSU had become a massive enterprise in Oregon as the state's only academic health center and the fifth-largest employer in the Portland metro area with 6,600 workers and rural health services across the state. Among others, Herb Aschkenasy, chair of the State Board of Higher Education, called OHSU the "crown jewel" of Oregon's university system, and Kohler and his team were asking Aschkenasy and the board to give it up. They also had to convince the legislature and the governor to surrender control.

The university's push to separate from the state bureaucracy and university system was seen as an insult by the people who worked in those systems, Walker said. "We were saying we can't get our business done because we have to go through these state agencies."[10]

What's more, they were asking taxpayers to trust them without the oversight of the state board or legislature. And they had to sell the plan internally to OHSU faculty, unions, staff, and students. The faculty would worry about the academic mission being compromised for the bottom line. Students would worry about higher tuition. The unions would worry about job security.

On an optimistic day, Walker said, he put the university's odds of winning approval to become a public corporation at about 50–50. More often, he said, it looked like a long shot, maybe a 20 percent or 30 percent chance. But he and the others all concluded they had little choice but to try.

"I was firmly convinced it was the right thing to do," he said.[11]

Though the team could clearly see it faced an "uphill battle," Davis said, it also could see that giving the university more independence made sense.

"We just didn't acknowledge to ourselves that we wouldn't be successful," she said. "We were going to make this happen."[12]

Hallick said she hadn't been out of the laboratory and classroom for long and was "pretty naïve politically." She recalled:

> I think what drove us all was not so much confidence that we could make it happen, but a belief that if we didn't the institution wouldn't survive. We really thought it was critical that we had to get some operating freedom so that we could be more efficient. . . . We were going to have to compete in the business world with other health systems and provide uncompensated care at the same time that the state with Measure 5 was trying to pull out all of the state money in the hospital and in the education mission for that matter. We just didn't think it was doable. So some of it was just backs-together desperation that we had to do it. . . . We had to figure out a way to make it happen.[13]

DRAFTING A PUBLIC CORPORATION

The leadership group talked for months about how it should sell the public corporation model to the state board, legislators, the OHSU workforce, and others. But then it turned inward, Hallick said, to focus on writing what it thought the public corporation should be. Once they had a good grasp of the change they were proposing, they could more convincingly sell it to others. By the summer of 1992, Janet Billups was deeply immersed in writing what would become Senate Bill 2.

She had been working since Kohler's arrival at OHSU as a representative of the Attorney General's Office. But in March of 1992, Kohler hired her to be OHSU's lawyer and to help him draft legislation to make the university a public corporation, even though the task force had not yet recommended that course. Letting OHSU hire its own attorney was frowned upon by the Department of Justice. In fact, two months earlier, Donald Arnold, administrator for the Department of Justice's General Counsel Division, sent out an interoffice memo saying he wanted to know about any state agencies contemplating reorganization.[14]

He wanted to know about OHSU's proposed reorganization early so he could stop it, Billups said. That created a conflict for her because while she was still working for the Department of Justice, her client and soon-to-be employer was OHSU.

"I was in such an awkward, difficult situation," Billups said, "I knew I had to leave. I wanted to leave and come to OHSU."[15]

Fortunately, the interim attorney general at the time, Charles S. Crookham, a judge, had been like a mentor to Billups and granted her permission to leave the Department of Justice to serve OHSU as in-house counsel. But he told her not to hire any outside attorneys. Typically, an attorney entrusted to design the legal architecture for restructuring a major public institution would have assembled a team of lawyers. But Billups was on her own to write OHSU's public corporation law. She had no staff; no partners. She did, however, turn to Douglas Goe, a bond attorney at the Ater Wynne firm in Portland, to help her craft the law's borrowing authority provisions. One of OHSU's chief objectives in becoming a public corporation was to gain authority over its own debt financing, but Billups lacked expertise in that area. Goe agreed to help her for free. Mark Dodson, who also worked at Ater Wynne, said he too did some work on the bill, including one part that proposed allowing OHSU to keep secret all but the final stage of its searches for new presidents.[16]

But Billups wrote most of the bill herself. She drew on her twelve years of legal experience, crowded her dining room table with a heavily used copy of Oregon's Local Government Law Manual and a two-foot stack of the gray, hardback volumes of the Oregon Revised Statutes and went to work. She combed through the manual and every book of statutes, researching what laws would need to be modified to make OHSU a public corporation. Key appellate cases surfaced as she read, and she found those cases and read those too, and cases that related to them. She reshaped the university in the law as a public body that would meet the academic and business needs identified by Kohler's leadership team. The team wanted to be sure the law would:

- Retain the university's public character as it would remain the property of the people of the State of Oregon.

- Establish governance and leadership focused on the mission and success of OHSU.
- Keep intact the integrated OHSU missions of health care, research, and education.

Billups also scoured federal laws, primarily those relating to health care financing, and looked in Oregon and elsewhere for organizations that might be similar to the public corporation model OHSU was proposing. She concluded the Port of Portland offered the best model. Other universities, such as Rutgers and the University of Pennsylvania, evolved over decades from private to public institutions and did not provide good comparisons. The University of California system has its own authority as a constitutional fourth branch of government, but taking that path would require changing the Oregon constitution. Changing laws to make the university a public corporation accomplished the same thing.

Billups wrote a solid bill that would only see small modifications as it moved through the legislature. The law addressed the overall philosophy of the public corporation, the powers of an OHSU board of directors, how OHSU would coordinate with the Oregon State System of Higher Education, OHSU's powers for debt financing and stock ownership, its obligations to the state Public Employees Retirement System, and its state protection from federal antitrust laws. While long and complex, the bill provided clarity and detail about precisely what OHSU was proposing to become.

The bill gave comprehensive powers to what would be OHSU's board of directors. Billups gave the board every logical power and authority she could find in Oregon statutes for both public and private organizations. She included a provision common in governance statutes that required the law to be liberally construed so that the board's authority would be broadly interpreted. Her bill also drew on what the statutes said about articles of incorporation and on bylaws from other universities, hospitals, and scientific research institutes.

The state's governance role over OHSU would come through the governor's authority to appoint board members. The governor would be able to remove board members, but that authority would be based on "cause," minimizing political interference into the institution's research, education, and health care operations. The State Board of Higher Education included two student members, which had proved valuable, so the OHSU board would also include a student member. No constituencies were promised board seats; each board member would represent OHSU as a whole.

The chief mission of Billups' bill was to free OHSU from state bureaucratic entanglements. So Senate Bill 2 exempted OHSU from any statute that applied only to state agencies or that required the exclusive use of state-mandated centralized services. Under its own board and governance structure, OHSU could enter the market with freedom to buy goods and choose professional and trade services as it saw fit.

After completing a draft of the bill, Billups would meet with Kohler, Walker, Goldfarb, Davis, and Hallick to thrash out each section. They met every week for months. One week, they might focus on the powers of the board. The next, they might review the low-bid contract law. The following meeting might turn to the Public Employee Retirement System. They debated concepts and big questions such as, "Should we retain a few state services or cut the cord entirely?" They had even more discussions during hallway encounters. Through it all, Billups gained deep respect for the group. She said it was the most "cohesive, gifted, creative team of people" she would ever work with.[17] The bill may be her career legacy, Billups said, but she was proudest of how well her colleagues learned its every detail:

> By the time the bill was introduced, the team—none of them lawyers—not only knew what the bill said, they also knew the legal reasoning for why it was said. I once watched while Dr. Kohler explained that the bill had to include condemnation authority in order to help avoid the fatal flaw of violating the special legisla-

> tion prohibition. He then went on to describe that an alternative to condemnation authority would be to grant OHSU taxing power, and, oh, by the way, the special legislation prohibition is one reason why the bill had to make clear that OHSU would be a statewide resource without territorial boundaries. It was a proud moment.[18]

Kohler didn't know so much about the bill, which Billups was still writing, when he and the team prepared to make a push for it in the 1993 legislative session. The conventional wisdom was that it would take three sessions of the legislature, which met every two years, to get a major initiative like the public corporation plan approved. Kohler began speaking publicly about it. He described the public corporation proposal in a speech to the Portland Rotary Club on July 14, 1992, drawing a short story inside *The Oregonian* the next day.[19] But there was little public discussion of the proposal after that. That's partly because just as Kohler and his team were starting to make their first push for the 1993 Legislature, Governor Barbara Roberts asked them to stop.

She opposed turning OHSU loose from the state higher education system, and she didn't want its campaign to become a public corporation overshadowing her drive for tax reform. She didn't want people to think government wasn't working, she recalled.

"We were trying to keep everything as stable as we could keep it," she said, "so people felt good that we were doing a good job so that they could look at tax reform."[20]

She had called the legislature into a one-day special session on July 1, 1992, with hopes lawmakers would support a tax reform package that she wanted to present to voters on the November ballot. Her plan included a 3.5 percent sales tax, which Oregon voters had rejected repeatedly in earlier proposals, along with cuts in personal income and property taxes. The plan would raise $950 million in new taxes to help offset revenue losses under Measure 5. The Oregon House crushed her plan by voting 33–26 against it. But Roberts didn't give up. She planned to craft a new, more modest tax package, which would also include a sales tax, for the 1993 Legislature.

So Kohler and his team retreated.

"We turned inward," said Hallick. "We didn't stop working internally, but we sort of slowed down the external pitching."[21] They talked quietly and informally among the various constituents and leaders they would need in their camp. Kohler, Davis, and others on the leadership team all had individual conversations with legislators and other leaders in hallways and offices.

"We were very straight with people," Davis said. "We said, 'The governor has asked us to back off. We're not pushing to do this right now, but we do think it needs to be looked at because we are not convinced that there will ultimately be any other solution.'"[22]

That's why there are few public records of OHSU's quest for public corporation status during this time, notes Barbara Archer, a professor at Concordia University in Portland who wrote her doctoral dissertation on OHSU's transformation and what she calls its "divorce" from the state and university system. She writes:

> The process chosen for the divorce was very quiet and diffuse. The process allowed OHSU to effectively control and manage the overall process. Instead of bringing groups together and having large discussions, behind-the-scenes quiet diplomacy was the approach used. . . . Much of the process was one-on-one or small group, informal discussions.[23]

While the Kohler team continued to soft-pedal its plan, Roberts took hers to the 1993 Legislature for a long seven-month battle. And she won. The legislature narrowly agreed to put a 5-cent sales tax proposal on the November ballot that would raise $1 billion a year. Like sales tax measures put before Oregon voters eight times before, this one went down in flames by a 3-to-1 margin, leaving the state with a $1.2 billion budget shortfall. That would mean big cuts for all state agencies, including OHSU. And that added urgency to the quest by Kohler's team to give the university freedom to compete for money on its own. As Hallick said, they "had to do it."

OREGON HEALTH PLAN

Another development adding to the team's pressure for change was the 1993 Legislature's eleventh-hour approval of a bill that would provide $66 million, most coming from a 10 cents per pack cigarette tax increase, to launch the Oregon Health Plan. The plan expanded those eligible for Medicaid, a state and federal supported health program for low-income residents, from households earning under 58 percent of the federal poverty level to all under the poverty level. The change added about 120,000 more Oregonians. It also created a state high-risk insurance pool for those whose pre-existing medical conditions shut them out of other insurance plans.[24] In addition, it required most employers to provide medical coverage to full-time workers beginning in 1997. These features would appear later in the Massachusetts health care plan developed by Governor Mitt Romney and the Affordable Care Act steered through Congress by President Barack Obama.

The Oregon Health Plan had emerged in the 1989 Legislature through a series of bills, but only now was being funded. It would be implemented on February 1, 1994. Kitzhaber, first elected to the legislature in 1978, led the design and legislative passage of the health plan as Senate president. The OHSU alumnus, who had worked as an emergency room physician in southern Oregon, wanted to see good health care across the state and became an eloquent spokesman for health care reform.

The most innovative, and controversial, feature of the plan was that it created a priority list of the health services it would cover based on efficacy and cost, with the most effective and least expensive services at the top. State officials, after a series of public hearings and focus groups, prioritized a list of 709 medical conditions.[25]

The cutoff line fell at 587. Medicaid money would cover those conditions up to 587, but not above.[26] The cutoff line would fluctuate from year to year with the state budget. The plan put a priority, as would Obamacare, on preventive care—physicals, prenatal services, mammograms, immunizations. It covered dental care, doctor visits for diagnosis of any condition, and follow-up medical treatment for most conditions, including the costs of hospitalization. It covered surgical care for treatable cancers, repair of deep and open wounds, appendectomies, treatment for burns, and services that could prevent death, restore health, or improve the quality of life. Also covered were prescription drugs, psychological treatment for conditions ranging from depression to schizophrenia, treatment for drug and alcohol abuse, gynecological care (including tubal ligations and abortions), organ transplants and other non-cosmetic surgery, physical and occupational therapy, and hospice care for the terminally ill.[27]

Among services above the 587 cutoff were treatment for infertility, restorative breast surgery, medical treatment for diaper rash, stripping of varicose veins, and health services that may have uncertain or limited value. Newborn care was covered; intensive neonatal treatment for extremely premature babies was not. Drug therapy for HIV infection made the cut; but only comfort and hospice care—not aggressive treatment—were included for those in the last stages of AIDS or cancer.[28] A majority of Oregonians supported the plan, but critics, including some congressional leaders, attacked it as health care "rationing." In a speech to the Association of Canadian Medical Colleges, Kohler noted that health care has been "implicitly rationed for years." Medicaid and private insurance plans ration by specifying what they will pay for, Kohler said, but legislators did not appreciate or understand the implicit rationing.

"[They] often took up the cause of a particularly sympathetic individual needing a glamorous or at least newsworthy procedure such as an organ transplant," he said. "At the same time these same legislators seemed oblivious to the thousands of women who were not receiving prenatal care or other preventative services."[29]

The primary feature of the Oregon Health Plan, the expansion of Medicaid, hit OHSU right between the eyes. Compared to other hospitals, OHSU handled the highest proportion of Oregon's Medicaid patients, earning $40 million in the prior year for those services. But it would be in danger of losing those patients and that revenue stream if it didn't develop more cost-efficient care for a much larger statewide population of Medicaid patients. The health plan spawned a number of new health maintenance organizations (HMOs) that would contract with the state to manage Medicaid patients, including some of those who had been going to OHSU. The new HMOs were reluctant to include OHSU in their networks. They saw the academic health center as more expensive, partly because it provided so much indigent care, Kohler said.[30]

OHSU needed to be included in the Medicaid HMO networks, and to do that, it would have to contract with doctors and hospitals across Oregon—all within a five month deadline established by the legislation signed in August of 1993. Under state rules, it would have to issue a request for proposals (RFPs) to the hundreds of providers, mostly primary care doctors, with whom it would attempt to forge agreements. Putting out RFPs in rural communities would be "nonsense because there would be only one provider," said Hallick.[31] The university would never meet that deadline unless the state gave it an exemption from the onerous contracting rules it had to follow as a state agency. State officials initially refused to exempt it. OHSU administrators put in hundreds of hours to finally get the exemption the medical center needed from Governor Barbara Roberts' office. The academic health center couldn't have asked for a better example of how being part of a state agency hampered its ability to succeed. It cited the example in a four-page treatise it would later use to make its case for converting to a public corporation:

> The contracting issues had nothing to do with the development of a quality health care program. It was exclusively a debate about how state regulations directed at traditional government activities should be applied to a unique public institution, which must operate in a competitive industry. The delay put the University significantly behind schedule, placing at risk the continuity of care of the thousands of Medicaid patients historically treated by OHSU physicians.[32]

The burden of the new health plan, probably more than anything else, helped make OHSU's need for change clear to Governor Roberts. Kohler and some members of his leadership team met with Roberts and told her it would be nearly impossible to participate in the Oregon Health Plan under the state contracting requirements, Hallick said. No one on the team remembers when that meeting was, but it may have been February 10, 1994, when Kohler's calendar shows him meeting at 3:45 p.m. with Roberts and Gary Weeks, then director of the Department of Administrative Services, on the 1995–97 budget. The group met again on February 23. In any case, Roberts came to understand that "they were not only handicapped, in a sense discriminated against, compared to the other medical operations in the area. I remember now listening to that and thinking, 'that is not right. They should not be penalized for their structure when their intentions are good.'"[33] She expressed that realization to Kohler in a rhetorical question:

"You really need this public corporation, don't you?" she said.

She not only gave OHSU the waiver it needed to carry out the Oregon Health Plan, but also agreed to include a note in her 1995–97 budget to the legislature to propose a public corporation bill for the 1995 session. Legislators and state leaders took budget notes seriously. That promise gave the university a green light and a deadline for selling its plan. Walker said it was more like a yellow light. Roberts was allowing OHSU to openly resume its public corporation quest, but she wasn't necessarily endorsing it, he said. In her 1995–97 budget plan, however, Roberts did pledge support for making

OHSU a public corporation, though not for giving more autonomy to the entire university system.[34]

TAKING THE PLAN PUBLIC

With Roberts' blessing, Kohler and his team in early 1994 geared up for their campaign to make OHSU a public corporation. Kohler anticipated some opposition. He explained in an email to the team that Kitzhaber, well into his campaign for governor, was concerned the unions and other health systems might fight the public corporation plan.[35] The team quickly needed to gain union leadership's support, Kohler wrote, and to inform the major Portland health organizations such as Kaiser Permanente and Providence Health & Services about OHSU's quest to become a public corporation.[36]

Other possible competition also was surfacing. As the state wrestled with a budget squeezed by the property tax limits of Measure 5, other higher education leaders were weighing in with plans of their own to privatize public universities. In January, Michael D. Mooney, president of the private Lewis & Clark College in Portland, told *The Oregonian's* editorial board that Oregon should make all of its colleges and universities private and focus on providing financial aid so more students could afford to attend them. The colleges could tap their alumni for donations as private colleges do and raise tuition for those who could pay. "Higher education can help itself," he said.[37]

About a year earlier, Kohler and Myles Brand, president of the University of Oregon, explored whether there was enough private philanthropy in Oregon to support their institutions if they went private. They concluded there was not. But in March of 1993, Brand was again talking to the State Board of Higher Education about making UO more independent. Representative Carolyn Oakley (Republican from Albany), who would chair the Ways and Means subcommittee on education two years later, asked the state board to describe the merits of turning the 16,700-student

Eugene university over to a private board of directors that would run it as a public corporation as OHSU was proposing. The change would be risky, Brand reported, should be considered only as a last resort, and would demand the university remain small, raise tuition, and take fewer Oregon students in favor of higher-paying out-of-state students. Becoming more independent could mean the university would lose students and research and descend into ruin, Brand said. But with sufficient donors and tuition, it could reduce state funding by half and allow the university to raise its quality to "sterling" levels.[38] In the following January of 1994, the University of Oregon produced a report which projected that if UO became a public corporation, then it would see healthy annual increases in revenue despite declines in state support, largely because of tuition increases.[39]

In April of 1994, Thomas A. Bartlett, chancellor of the State System of Higher Education, announced he wanted to make the entire system a public corporation because Measure 5 had produced a $92 million cut in state money for the 1995–97 higher education budget.[40] The state's support of higher education had dropped over four years from 30 percent of the total university system budget to 25 percent. It soon would fall to 20 percent. The system had cut $65 million from its 1993–95 appropriation, which was initially $732 million, and eliminated scores of positions, programs, even departments.[41] Under a public corporation system, Oregon's eight universities could save $20 million in two years, Bartlett predicted. All of the universities could be more businesslike and efficient with "greater authority to manage day-to-day operations," he said. His proposal "would fundamentally change the administrative relationship between the public institutions of higher education and state government."[42]

The chancellor's office, Davis said, "knew we were making headway with Senate Bill 2, and [it] wanted to say, 'No, we can take care of it. Just make us all a public corporation, and it'll take care of everything.' It was clearly an attempt to keep us within the system."[43]

Like Roberts, Kitzhaber, who would succeed her as governor in January of 1995, did not support making the whole university system a public corporation. It made sense for OHSU to gain more autonomy, he said, because the State Board of Higher Education wasn't equipped to oversee OHSU's large clinical and research operations. But the state board did have appropriate expertise and authority to oversee undergraduate education, the primary business of the other universities.

Other legislators also had doubts about giving the other universities more independence. Representative John Minnis (Republican from Wood Village) said he was skeptical, noting it was already "unbelievably difficult" to get the state board to respond to the legislature.[44] But *The Oregonian* editorial board came out the next day in support of the plan. "The [university] system could end up offering the Legislature a continuing education on how all state government could run better," the board said.[45]

CAMPAIGN GEARS UP

In January of 1994, Kohler began meeting with business leaders and created the Public Corporation Advisory Committee, which would be chaired by former Governor Neil Goldschmidt. He also began working on a document that would outline in detail why OHSU should become a public corporation. In the following months, he met repeatedly with legislators in Salem, and he traveled to small towns across the state such as Ashland, Lincoln City, Klamath Falls, Medford, Bend, Sunriver, Eugene, and La Grande to speak to rural health meetings, legislators, newspaper editorial boards, chambers of commerce, and radio interviewers. He talked with Senator Brady Adams (Republican from Grants Pass), Representative Dick Springer (Democrat from Portland), Representative Eugene Timms (Republican from Burns), Senator Lenn Hannon (Republican from Ashland), US Senator Mark Hatfield, Portland Mayor Vera Katz, and Janice Wilson, president of the State Board of Higher Education. Kohler understood the value of meeting people on their home turf and did so regularly, no matter whether the legislature was in session, Davis said.

"He'd go to Burns to meet Gene Timms," she said, "go to Pendleton to see Mike Thorne, because it said, 'We respect you.' It said, 'We actually are statewide. We aren't just statewide during the legislative session when we want your help.'"[46]

Kohler's leadership team also was selling the public corporation. Team members launched an "all-out" public campaign in 1994, said Hallick, and met with "every legislator or potential legislator" to describe why OHSU needed to become a public corporation.[47]

In February, Commissioner Earl Blumenauer, now an Oregon Congressman, proposed a Portland City Council resolution to urge the governor, legislature and State Board of Higher Education to let OHSU spin off as a public corporation on July 1, 1995. He said the resolution could "get the ball rolling" on what he called the "OHSU spin-off."[48]

Kohler's team also started collecting ammunition for its upcoming battle in the legislature. Steven Forrey, who worked for Walker, sent out an email on January 24, 1994, to three dozen OHSU administrators and employees seeking anecdotes about work slowed by the state bureaucracy that would help make the case for converting to a public corporation. The request was part "of the ongoing investigation into the value of functioning as a public corporation," he wrote.

Jim Walker provided an example on March 18 in a memo to Forrey, Davis, and Billups. He noted the Oregon State System of Higher Education conducted an internal audit of $2,827 in credit card purchases by the OHSU business office. The inquiry resulted in a six-page report, which cost more than the $2,827 worth of transactions being audited.

Kohler raised the profile of the OHSU public corporation proposal by making his pitch on May 25, 1994, to more than 1,000 business people, politicians, and community leaders gathered for the Portland Metropolitan Chamber of Commerce's annual membership meeting at the Portland Hilton. He said OHSU was "swimming against twin tides"—a rapidly changing health care environment and budget cuts resulting from Measure 5.

"After almost three years of planning, we have begun to talk about the idea of converting to a public corporation, either as part of an umbrella corporation formed by the State System of Higher Education or independently on our own," he said. "We're not talking about a private corporation, but a public one. . . . We would continue to fulfill our statewide public mission of education, indigent patient care, research and outreach."[49]

But, Kohler added, OHSU also runs a health care business.

> Remember, OHSU receives 60 percent of its revenue from a business enterprise which must operate in a business environment by the same rules as the other players in the marketplace. It receives another 26 percent of its revenues from gifts, grants and contracts, the majority of which come from the federal government or other out-of-state sources. Only 13.8 percent of its budget comes from the state general fund, and that percentage will drop in the next biennium given Measure 5.[50]

In an article about Kohler's speech the next day in *The Oregonian*, reporter Steve Woodward noted that "the idea of spinning off OHSU from state control is a couple of years old, but Kohler took the opportunity to push the idea afresh."[51]

That evening, Kohler gave a tough speech to the OHSU medical staff at a faculty dinner in which he appeared to be preparing them for work in a corporation. He stated bluntly that they either must improve the quality and production of their clinical services or move on. With state money declining, the university had to adjust to the emerging managed care market and compete, he said. "Clinical income," he said "has become the life-blood of OHSU."

As health maintenance organizations expand, he said, OHSU was running a system of care that is "often a non-system" characterized by poor coordination and internal communication. He ticked off other problems:

- Service was often not up to our customers' expectations.

- Accountable faculty care was often lacking—many patients were unable to identify the faculty member responsible for their care.
- Numbers of faculty were out of balance. OHSU needed either more clinical activity or less faculty.

Kohler said researchers were going to have to support themselves with grants; faculty must do the same with clinical income.

"We cannot support those faculty who do not contribute," he said, "and those who do not contribute should expect to leave OHSU. . . . Those who cannot—or will not—support themselves by seeing patients or through grants are in trouble."[52]

DEMANDS OF LEADERSHIP

Kohler set high expectations for himself, too. He devoted a big chunk of his time to selling the public corporation, but he also was swamped by the demands of running a complex medical university. One way he managed to do so much was by sleeping less than most people. He could work late into the evening and still rise every day at about 4:00 a.m. He'd turn to snacks for a morning boost. Carol Reinmiller, his secretary, said he had a sweet tooth and was a "Diet Coke addict." Each morning and afternoon, he'd take a walk from his office down the old corridors of Baird Hall to the cafeteria where he would get a cookie. He often ate lunch at his desk, regularly choosing a tuna fish sandwich with chips and an apple. Though he looked trim, his wife, Judy, was repeatedly telling him he needed to go on a diet. He was also inclined, maybe too inclined, to say yes to everyone who wanted to meet with him, Reinmiller said.

"His days would be just jammed with things he really should not have been bothered with," she said.[53]

He worked on building and writing projects, speeches, letters, meetings with national health and political leaders. He met regularly with his deans, vice presidents, and other staff members about a variety of initiatives unfolding at OHSU, such as construction projects for the Mark Hatfield Research Center and a new Doernbecher Children's Hospital, a merger with the Oregon Regional Primate Research Center, a medical school curriculum overhaul, and a nursing school program expansion through partnerships with other universities across the state.

He also had duties off campus. During the years leading up to the 1995 Legislature, he held leadership posts with numerous professional organizations. He served, for example, as an endocrinology executive committee member with the American Board of Internal Medicine, vice president of the American Clinical and Climatological Association, board of director member for the Association of Academic Health Centers, a council member for the Endocrine Society, and chair of the board of scientific counselors for the National Institute of Child Health and Human Development. He also served on numerous boards of directors, including those for the Alzheimer's Disease Center of Oregon, Health Bridge Northwest, Standard Insurance Company, HealthChoice Inc., the Mayor's Business Roundtable, and the Oregon Health Council, which he chaired 1993 through 1995.

He stayed involved with national health care issues and connected regularly with Hatfield and the Oregon congressional delegation. He, for example, extended his support to the national health plan that First Lady Hillary Clinton was designing. "At a time when the National Health Security Plan will soon be released, your support is very important to me," Clinton wrote him.[54]

And when anything went sideways on campus, Kohler had to deal with it. On January 25, 1994, for example, OHSU surgeons cracked open the chest of Mark DeSylvia, a fifteen-year-old boy from Scappoose, a town twenty miles northwest of Portland, to give him a new heart. The high school freshmen, member of the swimming team, suffered from a form of cardiomyopathy, a genetic condition that killed his mother and aunt. But as DeSylvia lay on the operating table, doctors realized the heart came from a donor with blood type A, and the boy had blood type B. The heart was incompatible. Dr. Adnan Cobanoglu, head of the transplant team, called off the operation. The team sewed up DySylvia's chest and waited for a new heart. None came. Ten days later, the boy died.[55] Kohler announced the university would conduct an "independent outside review" into the blood type mix-up. Procedures were changed. The boy's family filed a lawsuit, and two years later, settled with OHSU for $250,000. Like other academic health centers, OHSU handled the region's most complicated medical procedures, often to address imminent life-threatening conditions. And that meant it also sometimes faced heart-breaking tragedies. It fell to Kohler to lead the university forward through those dark patches.

OHSU'S IMPROVING HEALTH

Through regular meetings in 1993 and 1994, Kohler and members of his leadership team honed their message in preparation for the 1995 legislative session. As they pressed their case internally and externally for making OHSU a public corporation, they portrayed the university as an institution that was gaining health and momentum. But they argued it could not sustain that momentum without more freedom to grow and earn money. Kohler struck a delicate balance between showing OHSU on the path to prosperity and in danger of decline, even collapse, if it could not break free from the weight of state controls to compete in the managed care market. And as noted by former Oregon Senate leader Mike Thorne—by this time head of the Port of Portland, another public corporation—what impressed lawmakers was that Kohler was not begging for money from a strapped state. Instead, he was offering a solution.

Kohler's strategy, like that of Laster before him, was to build new research laboratories and upgrade the hospitals and clinics so the university could attract better researchers and faculty, which would in turn attract paying patients and increased revenue. Walker and Goldfarb embraced that strategy, too.

Even before Kohler arrived, improvements were underway. Walker and Goldfarb had begun coordinating and streamlining the disorganized hospital management system. "The management was awful," recalled Walker. The patient billing system, for example, was overly complex and antiquated. Walker and Goldfarb bought a new computer system around 1986 that reduced the number of workers needed to handle patient accounts from 156 to 55. The new system saved money and allowed the health center to more efficiently bill patients and track bad debt, which could then be sent to collections, Walker said.[56]

As finances improved, Walker and Goldfarb began sinking whatever money they could into attracting faculty and researchers with national reputations. Shortly after Kohler arrived, the university got a big boost with the completion of the Vollum Institute in 1987 and the Physicians Pavilion in 1993.[57] The first brought in some high-powered researchers; the latter provided modern outpatient services. Both made the university more attractive to faculty and patients.

In addition, several other facilities were completed during this period that helped raise OHSU's profile. The privately-supported Casey Eye Institute and the Biomedical Information Communication Center, the electronic library conceived by Laster and Hatfield, opened in 1991. In the following year, the Center for Research on Occupational and Environmental Toxicology building opened and the 660-foot-long suspended, enclosed pedestrian sky bridge, the longest in North America, both physically and symbolically tied University Hospital to the Veterans Affairs Medical Center.

OHSU's forward-thinking revised medical school curriculum was drawing top students and national attention. "Dutch" Reinschmidt and John Kendall, dean of the School of Medicine, had led an overhaul in the early 1990s of the old curriculum, which they had concluded was too packed, lecture heavy, and inflexible. With grants from the Charles E. Culpeper and

Robert Wood Johnson foundations, the faculty dramatically changed the way it taught, putting more emphasis on problem solving, clinical practice, and family medicine. The students also spent time working in rural hospitals as part of their study rotations. Reinschmidt explained:

> One of the major tenets at the time was to reduce lecture time by 50 percent or more and replace that by self-directed learning and group learning activities so that there was direct involvement of the students in the educational process. So they see patients in their first two weeks—very superficially, but they have exposure to clinical situations so that they see the connection between what they're learning in the basic sciences and what's happening to this person's heart and cardiovascular system, as an example.[58]

US News & World Report in March of 1994 ranked the nation's 126 medical universities in two categories: research, which included sixty schools such as Harvard and Stanford universities that received the most NIH research money; and comprehensive, the sixty-six schools like OHSU that were more oriented toward training primary care doctors. As evidence of the impact of its curriculum changes, the magazine ranked OHSU the top comprehensive medical school in the nation, giving it top ratings in reputation and student selectivity.[59]

The university on Pill Hill also was becoming the hub of a statewide campus: the State Office of Rural Health became part of OHSU, and Area Health Education Centers opened across the state. The School of Nursing, operating in a new building, created a statewide integrated nursing education system, an initiative led by Chancellor Bartlett and Carol Lindeman, dean of the nursing school. The OHSU nursing programs were connected with those at Eastern Oregon University in La Grande, Southern Oregon University in Ashland and the Oregon Institute of Technology in Klamath Falls. These rural expansions helped Kohler cement favor with rural legislators.

In the first five years of Kohler's presidency, the university had dramatically increased its complexity, research capacity, staff, and reputation—all of which helped stabilize it financially. OHSU's revenue had climbed 75 percent, from $261 million to $458 million; its research awards had increased 80 percent, from $41 million to $74 million.[60] By 1993, both Walker and Goldfarb had been promoted. Goldfarb had risen to chief executive officer of the hospital. Walker initially turned down Kohler's offer in 1992 to make him vice president of finance for the entire university. But after Kohler told him he would have to hire someone else who would become Walker's boss, Walker took the job.

As university clinical and laboratory space improved, Goldfarb and Walker concentrated on finding good people to fill it. They leveraged their relationship with the Veterans Affairs Hospital to pool money and offer attractive salaries to faculty and researchers whom the university and VA could share. The hospital also started kicking in money so the dean of the School of Medicine could offer salaries attractive enough to attract top faculty. They would, for example, recruit a top orthopedic surgeon, who in turn attracted faulty who wanted to work with him.

"We wanted physicians who were cutting edge," said Walker.[61]

In addition to recruiting Dr. Neil Swanson from the University of Michigan and Dr. Melvin Ball from the University of Western Ontario, OHSU also hired Dr. Lynn Loriaux, a gland expert and longtime friend of Kohler's from the NIH. As more experts joined the university and its reputation grew, more paying patients started seeking out its care. New faculty came with "fresh blood and eyes," Goldfarb said. They brought new ambition, saw new possibilities and raised the university's aspirations.

"It was just an unbelievable, young, aggressive, ambitious smart faculty that even got the old guys to believe," Goldfarb said.[62]

The impact of this "fresh blood" was reflected in the hospital's bottom line. The hospital is the university's economic engine, and for a long period, it was sputtering at 65 percent capacity, meaning a third of its beds were empty. Occasionally, it slipped into the red. By 1989, University Hospital had stabilized and was posting consistent net income with 85 percent occupancy. Through the 90s, it sustained an average 80 percent capacity, enough to allow it to cover all fixed costs and still make money.[63] Between 1991 and 1994, the hospital achieved an average 5.6 percent net income, unheard of in OHSU history.[64] The effects of new buildings, better faculty, and more patients produced an upward spiral toward financial health.

Walker and Goldfarb's interest in seeing the university become a public corporation sharpened when they saw how quickly and smoothly the Physicians Pavilion went up in 1993 with private money. Brim Inc., which managed small hospitals in twenty-two states, served as general partner and developer for the 80,000-square-foot, four-story medical pavilion built on top of an existing parking garage. Brim financed the construction, conducted by Walsh Construction, and then OHSU leased the building from Brim.

The building rose within two years, on time and within budget, even as the project to build a labor and delivery unit on the existing University Hospital had not yet begun after more than six years of waiting for the state's okay. The pavilion project showed Walker and Goldfarb what would be possible for OHSU if it were free of state regulations to build like a private company, said John Woodward, who at the time was a public debt banker with Paine Webber's San Francisco Office.[65]

In late 1993, Walker and Goldfarb invited Woodward to look at OHSU's finances and public corporation model to see if the university could obtain debt financing from Wall Street on its own. Woodward concluded the university was undercapitalized with a significant backlog of deferred maintenance. The relatively short-term debt on its capital projects could be refinanced and stretched out so that it was less of a burden, he said. He agreed that the university would need to break away from the state and borrow on its own faith and credit to get the capital it needed for upgrades and expansion.

But could OHSU raise money on its own? This was a time of great financial turbulence for academic health centers. Walker speculated at the time that as many as 45 of about 125 were in danger of failing financially if they could not adjust to the health care environment that was moving headlong toward managed care. State legislatures had permitted other academic health centers, such as the University of Arizona in Tucson and the University of Colorado in Denver, to spin off their hospitals as private, independent operations because they were seen as financial drains, Woodward said.

"In almost every instance," he said, "the reason it was done was the Legislature was fearful of the liability that it could cost for the state to operate."

But that was not the case with OHSU, he said. The Oregon academic health center wasn't digging out of a hole, but instead "clearly on the rise as far as reputation."[66]

While not easy, Woodward concluded it would be possible for the university to get the terms it needed to make bond financing on Wall Street economically viable. The university was stable financially, growing and valued by state leaders and the populace. Woodward had heard it called the "crown jewel" of the university system more than once. "People were not going to walk away from this," he said. Still, there were risks. OHSU was essentially proposing to launch an unprecedented start-up, and it had no credit history, Woodward said.[67]

The university also was going through an internal debate on how best to position itself. With the rise of managed care and its emphasis on primary care, Goldfarb was pushing for a big shift to primary care. He argued the university should open primary care clinics off the hill where they would be more accessible and people would be more apt to use them, and allow the university to compete in the managed care market. But Walker could see the university was building a significant competitive advantage over other health care providers in the region with its expanding array of specialists and experts. OHSU was no longer only the service of last resort, where you go when you were poor or without insurance. It was becoming the first choice for paying patients looking for the doctors most familiar with the latest research.

"The only advantage you had in an academic health center, especially an academic health center on a hill, was in the tertiary, specialty care," he said. "You have physicians who want to stay on the cutting edge. . . . That is an economic advantage you are going to have . . . and that is the only advantage you have."[68]

OHSU did expand its primary care operations with some clinics in Portland during this period, though not as much as Goldfarb wanted. But it was that competitive advantage that Walker described, the medical center's subsequent dramatic expansion of specialists and a capacity to handle the most complex cases, that allowed it to prosper.

By 1994, as Kohler and his team made its public push for the public corporation, Walker and Goldfarb could show the university was financially solid and capable of securing its own capital in the market. But again, the team had to strike a balance—show that while it was positioned to succeed in the capital market, it could do so only with authority to go to Wall Street and borrow money on its own. That authority would come only if it could be freed from state restrictions to operate as a public corporation. Otherwise it would have to rely on the slow state bonding process that had forced it to wait nine years to replace its outdated maternity ward. It could not compete with other area hospital networks if it didn't have the authority and independence to move faster, to control its purchases and streamline its operations, to expand its research laboratories and clinics. Its recent gains and future prospects would fade like an old photograph.

SHORING UP SUPPORT

By late 1994, Kohler also was winning the support of key leaders at every level of government. After Kitzhaber was elected governor in 1994, state Senator Gordon Smith, a Republican from Pendleton, replaced him as Senate president. Both would support the OHSU public corporation proposal. So did Hatfield, who understood that OHSU was strapped by state regulations and a weak economy and needed more autonomy to breathe and blossom. Kohler happened to be meeting with Smith in his Salem office in late 1994 when Hatfield called Smith to say he wanted to see Senate Bill 2 introduced in the legislature.

But there was another surprise meeting that reminded Kohler and his team not everyone was behind them. On December 6, 1994, Dave Frohnmayer, the former state attorney general who had become University of Oregon president five months earlier, invited Kohler, Walker, and Hallick to his room at the Hilton Hotel during a stay in downtown Portland. He supported Chancellor Bartlett's proposal to make the entire university system a public corporation, which Bartlett's successor, Chancellor Joe Cox, was planning to push in the 1995 Legislature. Frohnmayer thought the University of Oregon had made a mistake by letting the medical school become independent, Davis said.

"He knew the status of the [Oregon University System] would be diminished by losing OHSU," she said.[69]

He also thought Bartlett's plan would prevent OHSU from breaking free on its own. And he could see Kohler's team was gaining momentum.

"Don't do this," he told Kohler and his team.

Hallick said she was shocked to hear him threaten to undermine the effort if OHSU persisted. But Frohnmayer also understood the merits of what OHSU was trying to do. Fifteen years later, shortly after he retired as UO president, he would at the request of Chancellor George Pernsteiner write a report recommending that Oregon convert its largest universities—the UO, Portland State and Oregon State—into public corporations so they would have more freedom to raise money and revitalize the state's stifled higher education system.[70]

By late 1994, Billups had completed several drafts of Senate Bill 2, Davis had prepared attractive documents on the importance of OHSU and the case for making it a public corporation, and the Public Corporation Advisory Committee was wrapping up its work. But there was still one group OHSU had to get on board—the State Board of Higher Education.

During a meeting on November 18, 1994, at what was then called Western Oregon State College in Monmouth, the State Board of Higher Education took up the public corporation proposals of OHSU and of the chancellor's office. Cox told the board that he and Kohler could not come to an agreement on the two bills. He said he agreed OHSU needed more freedom from state rules to compete in the health care market, but he argued against giving OHSU a clean break from the system. He said state money for education needed to continue to flow through the state board, and he was troubled by OHSU having its own governing board. He questioned how the two boards could set priorities and how both would try to influence the legislature.

"Can there be two boards of higher education—one board of higher education that is nonmedical and one board of higher education that is medical?" he asked.

Kohler was at an American College of Physicians meeting in Philadelphia, so Hallick stepped in to make OHSU's case for full autonomy. She argued the university needed the independence to compete as the health care market tilted toward managed care, but noted it would remain a "unit of government totally accountable to the public good." The wisdom with which the university reorganized "will determine whether or not we thrive or go into bankruptcy," she said. "It's as dramatic as that."[71]

The board agreed to try to resolve the issues at its meeting in December. Before that meeting, Cox, Kohler, and Governor-elect Kitzhaber met to find a solution. Kitzhaber agreed to support Kohler's bill, Senate Bill 2. He also agreed to allow the university system to float its proposal, though he did not support it.[72] Cox and Kohler acknowledged OHSU would continue to have a relationship to the state system if it succeeded in becoming a public corporation. OHSU would fully control the hospital and clinical programs, but the university would remain connected to the state system and share joint responsibility with the state board in changing or closing academic programs.[73] The state money for OHSU's instructional programs would flow through the state board as a line item, and the amount would be fixed at the 1995–97 levels through 1997–99, after which state support would be scaled down.[74]

The state board also added it wanted to retain final approval on OHSU education programs and tuition and fees. It then voted unanimously to ask Kitzhaber to introduce both bills in the legislature.[75]

Cox subsequently spoke in favor of the OHSU bill. He said he and the state board "reached the conclusion mutually, that one size was not going to fit all; that the unique nature of Oregon Health Sciences University did require that we go further in the direction of a true public corporation, further than OSSHE [wants] to go with the other seven."

SELLING THE PLAN INTERNALLY

As Kohler's leadership team sold its public corporation proposal across the state, members also carefully explained the plan to everyone at OHSU—students, management, the unions, and faculty. Sometimes Kohler or Hallick or Billups alone would talk to a group of faculty, staff, or students on how the public corporation would benefit them and the university; other times they would make presentations together. They also talked with leaders of the unions—the Oregon Nurses Association and the American Federation of State, County and Municipal Employees (AFSCME) Local 328. Kohler, Walker, Hallick, and Goldfarb had been meeting regularly for years with officials of AFSCME Local 328, the union representing OHSU workers, as a formal labor-management committee. The four union officials included Doug Hurd, president, and Diane Lovell, field staff representative, both of whom would testify in favor of Senate Bill 2. OHSU leaders had developed a good relationship with union members so they were receptive, but cautious, when administrators proposed the public corporation early in 1994. Kohler's team promised that the public corporation would give union members better job security. It also would help to "get their salaries up to market," Hallick told them.[76]

And that argument hit home with the union, which had long struggled to get better salaries from the state, recalled Lovell. The state classified workers by title and paid them accordingly, but many of the AFSCME employees at OHSU had specialized training that was not reflected in their state title. Radiology technicians, for example, might be classified simply as technicians or medical workers and not get the pay they deserved for their expertise. Discussions with AFSCME were cordial and productive, and union officials showed a good grasp of the difficulties an academic health center faced fitting into a state system.

But the union had concerns about how the public corporation model would affect its contracts, bargaining, salaries, and job stability. Would the university try to outsource jobs, break the union, or cut off access to the Public Employees Retirement System? The AFSCME 12-to-15 member executive committee studied the proposal with help from its national office and concluded the move to a public corporation would be good for its workers.

OHSU in Senate Bill 2 assured the union its workers could participate in the Public Employees Retirement System and engage in collective bargaining directly with OHSU rather than the state, which the union preferred. The union also shared OHSU's concern that the university could get dragged into the financial problems that were hitting other academic health centers around the country. And the union trusted Kohler and his team, Lovell said.[77]

Students also were relatively easy to bring on board in favor of the public corporation, Hallick said. OHSU had only about 2,400 students, all working on graduate or medical degrees, and graduate students are typically too busy to become involved in issues such as restructuring the university. "They are just focused on trying to survive their curricula," she said, "and it is a very intense thing so they are sort of oblivious to the whole thing."[78]

Students were represented by a council comprised of elected members from all the schools. As provost, Hallick served as chief supporter and liaison to students and their deans. Students were concerned that becoming a public corporation would drive up tuition, though OHSU already had gained authority to set tuition in 1991. Students also wanted to have two representatives on the university board when OHSU became a public corporation, just as there were two students on the State Board of Higher Education, one of whom at the time was Ronda Trotman Reese, an OHSU dental student. But Kohler and other leaders wanted to keep the board small enough to be able to act swiftly in making critical financial decisions. After hearing many proposals and going through many discussions, students and the leadership team agreed the OHSU board would have one student member. Trotman Reese became an advocate on behalf of students for the public corporation, and she would testify effectively in the legislature in support of the proposal.

The faculty was the most difficult group to get behind the public corporation. Initially, the faculty was in an uproar, Hallick said.

"They were convinced that it would be the death knell of our education mission," she said, "that we would just turn and focus entirely on business, and we wouldn't care about the education mission or the public mission."[79]

Faculty at most universities, including OHSU, are notoriously independent and resistant to change. David Korn, dean of the medical school at Stanford University, once observed his faculty members were anarchists united only by a common parking problem.[80] But faculties also are bright and can appreciate reasoning and a good argument. So Hallick presented a strong, rational case for a public corporation to the faculty council and Faculty Senate leaders. The Faculty Senate appointed a task force to study the impact of the public corporation proposal on the university and faculty. The task force concluded the university's future "was rather bleak" if it did not have more freedom to raise capital and invest in its clinics and hospital, said Dr. Jerris Hedges, who chaired the faculty group. It also believed the Oregon State Board of Higher Education "did not demonstrate a strong understanding of the unique nature of health sciences education," he said.[81] Provided the faculty could preserve its role in university governance and retain its health, retirement, and other benefits, the task force concluded, it would support a move to the public corporation model.

On the eve of OHSU's 1995 legislative battle for Senate Bill 2, Kohler made the case for converting to a public corporation in his annual OHSU Convocation. The October 7, 1994, presentation was titled "OHSU in the 21st Century: Changing the Way We Do Business Without Changing the Business That We Do." He began by describing the threats to the university.

> We are in the midst of a period of dramatic, historical change. State and federal revenues are declining. National health reform has an unclear future. And the health care marketplace is being turned on its head. Fee-for-service is on the decline, being replaced by capitated payment and contractual arrangements. Insurance companies are no longer just payers—they're also providers, and they're partnering with individual health systems to the potential exclusion of others. Health systems are scrambling to lock up primary care networks and to cut off referrals to competitive systems or facilities. It's an environment of take no prisoners and may the best person—or in this case system—win. Faced with this brave new world, the OHSU community has two choices: we can go up or we can go down. What we cannot do is stand still.

The university already was making big changes, he said, with revisions of the curricula for the dental, medical, and nursing schools, expansion of its rural health programs, the Biomedical Information Communication Center's growing electronic communication network, increasing research, and the university's move into the world of managed care through agreements with Multnomah County, ODS Health (now Moda Health), and providers all over the state to form networks and health maintenance organizations. But state support was still falling, Kohler said, and the university needed to be more innovative because its state agency role "has worked against us in our effort to reinvent ourselves." He talked about state delays in getting contracting exemptions for its Medicaid patients and for building a new maternal-child unit. He quoted Roger Bassett, Oregon's community college commissioner: "It is hard to be aggressive with your foot in a bucket."

OHSU needed to become a public corporation, he argued. He described what that would mean, and how it would not change the university's core mission of care, research, and education. He noted the plan Chancellor Bartlett had introduced to free the whole university system from state regulations would not come close to giving OHSU the freedom it needed.

Legislators would support the OHSU plan, Kohler said, because they could see that with declining state revenue and a rapidly changing health care marketplace, the university would fall into a downward spiral, depriving the state of direct services, faculty, and out-of-state revenues.

"We do not want to abandon our mission, we want to enhance it," he said. "The public corporation will also be the only way for us to do business successfully in the future."[82]

Kohler and his team had led the university through more than two years of debate and discussion. They had won the internal support of deans, administrators, faculty, unions, and students, and the external support of the governor, key legislative leaders, the State Board of Higher Education, and top business leaders. One of the final and decisive debates unfolded the day before Kohler delivered his convocation speech, when the Faculty Senate took a vote on the public corporation proposal. The head of the nurse midwifery program spoke. She didn't like the idea of a public corporation, she said, but without it, she didn't think the university could survive to carry out its education mission. The Senate approved the change.

Kohler and his team were ready to introduce Senate Bill 2 and make their case to the legislature.

Notes

1 "State to fund OHSU work on hospital," *The Register-Guard,* Jan. 8, 1993, p. 5B.
2 Timothy Goldfarb (former OHSU hospital director), and Laura Goldfarb (his wife, former OHSU nurse), interview, Oct. 2, 2014.
3 Peter O. Kohler, MD, interview, April 11, 2014.
4 Lois Davis (former OHSU communications director, vice president for communications at Portland State University), interview, June 16, 2014, in her Portland State University office.
5 Ibid.
6 Susan Stanley, *Maternity Ward: Behind the Scenes at a Big City Hospital* (New York: William Morrow and Company, Inc., 1992), p. 20.
7 "Maternity Wing's gestation a case in bureaucratic point," *The Oregonian,* Jan. 23, 1995, p. B01.
8 George Pernsteiner, interview, March 25, 2014.
9 Timothy M. Goldfarb, interview, Oct. 2, 2014.
10 James Walker, interview, Sept. 29, 2014.
11 Ibid.
12 Lois Davis, interview, Oct. 3, 2014, in her office at Portland State University.
13 Lesley Hallick, interview, Oct. 1, 2014.
14 Donald C. Arnold (administrator, General Counsel Division, Department of Justice), interoffice memo, Jan. 2, 1992. Arnold wrote: "I want to be informed of any inquiries from agencies, board or commissions on the subject, and to review any advice concerning reorganization issues *before* it is provided."
15 Janet Billups, interview, April 2, 2014.
16 Mark Dodson, interview, Feb. 23, 2016, Multnomah Athletic Club, Portland, Oregon.
17 Ibid.
18 Ibid.
19 Patrick O'Neill, "Corporation Route Mulled for OHSU," *The Oregonian,* July 15, 1992, p. D03.
20 Barbara Roberts (former Oregon governor), interview, April 29, 2016.
21 Hallick, interview.
22 Davis, interview.
23 Unpublished written statement provided by Barbara Archer during interview at Concordia University in Portland, Oregon, May 7, 2014.
24 Patrick O'Neill, "Variety of Groups Criticize Oregon Health Care Plan," *The Oregonian,* May 13, 1992, p. C01.
25 Ibid.
26 Ibid.
27 Joan Beck, "Oregon Health Plan Faces The Reality of Care Rationing," *The Chicago Tribune,* March 2, 1992, http://articles.chicagotribune.com/1992-03-02/news/

9201200194_1_preventive-care-prenatal-services-basic-care-packages-oregon-list.

28 Ibid.

29 Peter O. Kohler, MD, "The Oregon Health Plan," speech delivered to the Association of Canadian Medical Colleges, April 23, 1994.

30 Peter O. Kohler, MD, interview, Sept. 17, 2014.

31 Hallick, interview.

32 OHSU, "From State to Public Corporation: A Better Way To Do Business, A Smarter Way to Serve Oregonians," p.2, 1994, OHSU legal department.

33 Roberts, interview.

34 Barbara Roberts, "Roadmap for Oregon's Future: 1995–97 Budget Plan," Oct. 19, 1994, p. 19. The report says, "There has been a great deal of discussion about 'privatizing' all of higher education. Because of concern about how that change would affect the goals of higher education, Governor Roberts does not support this change. However, Governor Roberts has endorsed changing the status of the OHSU from a traditional state agency to a public corporation, so that it is better able to meet its mission as an educational institution and health care center."

35 John Kitzhaber (interview, Feb. 12, 2016, Portland), said the unions and other hospitals had concerns that Kohler had to deal with right away. The unions "don't want to be disadvantaged in terms of organizing. . . . Even if you don't agree with the union position, they have a lot of juice in the Legislature so you need to deal with them. You need to get them to the table. I think probably the hospitals were concerned again about market share and competition." He noted that during this time, there was a debate in the Portland area about having three heart transplant centers. That, Kitzhaber said, was the "craziest thing in the world."

36 Peter O. Kohler, MD, email to Janet Billups, Lois Davis, Jim Walker, Tim Goldfarb, Lesley Hallick, and Steve Forreys, Feb. 1, 1994.

37 Bill Graves, "Educator: Privatize Oregon's Universities," *The Oregonian*, Jan. 26, 1994, p. C05.

38 Bill Graves, "UO Chief Lists Costs, Benefits of Going Private," *The Oregonian*, March 13, 1993, p. D04.

39 University of Oregon, "An Analysis of the Alternative of Establishing the University of Oregon as a Public Corporation Independent of the State System of Higher Education," Jan. 1994.

40 Bill Graves, "Oregon Panel Says Incorporate to Educate," *The Oregonian*, April 13, 1994, p. B1.

41 Kit Lively, "Autonomy Comes at a Price for Oregon's Public Colleges," *The Chronicle of Higher Education*, July 14, 1995.

42 Ibid.

43 Davis, interview.

44 Norm Maves Jr., "Higher Education Idea Stirs Surprise," *The Oregonian*, April 14, 1994, p. E07.

45 "Higher Ed, Lower Overhead," *The Oregonian*, April 17, 1994, p. F02.

46 Davis, interview. Davis said, "By [Kohler] going out there, it built relationships with the local community and the local community leaders that those legislators turn to for advice. There was a deliberate building. At first it was the one-on-one conversations, and then as you got closer and closer, then you were talking to the leaders or hospital folks. Simultaneously, it was internal, so you were talking to the labor unions, talking to the faculty and staff. . . . Obviously, if the internal community was not with us, we wouldn't be able to do it any more than we would able to do it if the legislators weren't supporting it."
47 Lesley Hallick, interview, May 27, 2014.
48 Earl Blumenauer, letter to Peter O. Kohler, Feb. 24, 1994.
49 Peter O. Kohler, MD, "A Time for Change," speech to the Portland Chamber of Commerce, May 25, 1994, Peter Kohler collection, OHSU archives.
50 Ibid.
51 Steve Woodward, "OHSU Chief Suggests Public Corporation," *The Oregonian*, May 16, 1994, p. F06.
52 Peter O. Kohler, MD, "A Message from OHSU President Peter Kohler, M.D.," excerpts from Dr. Kohler's speech to the medical staff on May 25, 1994, *UMG News*, June 1994, pp. 1–3.
53 Carol Reinmiller, interview, Oct. 21, 2014, Baird Hall at OHSU.
54 Hillary Rodham Clinton, letter to Peter O. Kohler, Sept. 10, 1993.
55 Spencer Heinz, "Time Runs Out for Scappoose Teen," *The Oregonian*, Feb. 4, 1994, p. A1; Spencer Heinz and Patrick O'Neill, "Blood-type Mistake Halted Heart Transplant," *The Oregonian*, Feb. 10, 1994, p. A1.
56 Jim Walker, interview, June 16, 2004.
57 Ibid. Walker said, "That was the first new outpatient building in probably 40 years or so. This was a whole new step up for OHSU."
58 J.S. "Dutch" Reinschmidt, MD, interview by Joan Ash and Linda Weimer, Sept. 3, 1997, Mackenzie Hall OHSU, interview no. 2 9/3, 1997, transcript, OHSU Oral History Project, p. 21.
59 Oz Hopkins Koglin, "OHSU Gets Top Billing as Comprehensive School," *The Oregonian*, March 12, 1994, p. D02.
60 OHSU, "At a Glance" facts for 1988, 1993, and "Growth and Change at OHSU," 1990–2004, available from OHSU Strategic Communications.
61 Jim Walker, interview, Sept. 29, 2014.
62 Goldfarb, interview.
63 OHSU, Table of Historical Utilization, "Selected Statistical Indicators of Patient Activity for Years Ended June 30," table, Peter Kohler collection, OHSU Archives.
64 Jim Walker, "OHSU Transition to Public Corporation," unpublished written account, 2013.
65 John Woodward, interview, Oct. 8, 2014.
66 Ibid.
67 Ibid.

68 Jim Walker, interview, Sept. 29, 2014.

69 Davis, interview, Oct. 3, 2014.

70 Bill Graves, "Frohnmayer: Make Oregon universities public corporations," *The Oregonian*, Nov. 18, 2009.

71 Oregon State Board of Higher Education Minutes, Nov. 18, 1994, pp. 587–592.

72 John Kitzhaber (in an email to the author on Feb. 20, 2016), explained why he supported allowing OHSU but not the whole university system to become a public corporation: "The case for OHSU was based on the fact that their educational mission was only a small part of the overall enterprise," he wrote. "I have always been a strong supporter of a true system of higher education rather than a group of competing institutions. Moving all those institutions into a public corporation would run counter to that goal and exempt them from many of the tools necessary for a coordinated and cooperative system with a strong mission to provide quality postsecondary education, especially to Oregon high school graduates. The creation of the Higher Education Coordinating Commission [which Kitzhaber created in 2012 to replace the State Board of Higher Education] is a reflection of that view."

73 John Kitzhaber (interview, Feb. 12, 2016, Portland), said Kohler had agreed that OHSU needed to keep its academic connections to the State Board of Higher Education.

74 Oregon State Board of Higher Education Minutes, Dec. 16, 1994, p. 640.

75 Ibid., pp. 641, 642.

76 Lesley Hallick, interview, Oct. 1, 2014.

77 Diane Lovell, interview, Sept. 23, 2014. Lovell said, "We made sure all of our concerns were addressed before we supported the legislation. We did not believe that they (OHSU) would successfully break out of that kind of downward spiral (hitting other academic health centers) as long as it was part of the state and governed by all the state restrictions, including collective bargaining. . . . (Kohler's team) was very forward thinking, which I respected a lot. I had relationships with them previously, so there's a good, trusting relationship between the union and OHSU leadership that really helped."

78 Hallick, interview.

79 Ibid.

80 Peter O. Kohler, MD, email, Aug. 30, 2016, recalled incident in which he was present when Dean Korn made this comment around 1995.

81 Jerris Hedges, MD, email to author on Dec. 13, 2015. Hedges wrote: "Considerable work was done to ensure the conversion of health, retirement and other benefits for employees, but given greater administrative flexibility in the public corporation model, these transitions went smoothly. Although some faculty members belonged to the State of Oregon's higher education faculty union, the direct involvement of faculty members in the transition discussion and the inclusion of executive leaders such as deans and associate deans as faculty members at OHSU avoided a divisive situation whereby isolated faculty members might have focused the work of the task

force upon the status of the individual faculty member rather than on the overall health of the institution and thus the ability of OHSU to benefit the larger faculty needs and meet its mission for Oregon."

82 Peter O. Kohler, MD, "OHSU in the 21st Century: Changing the Way We Do Business With Changing the Business That We Do," a speech delivered at the annual OHSU Convocation, Oct. 7, 1994.

Chapter Four

The Legislative Battle

On January 23, 1995, the eve of the opening of the Oregon biennial legislative session, Oregon Health Sciences University's Public Corporation Advisory Committee released its final report at a news conference in the state capitol in Salem. The committee, led by former Governor Neil Goldschmidt and composed of seven prominent business leaders, recommended OHSU be cut loose from the state system of higher education and the state Department of Administrative Services to become a public corporation—a public agency, not a state agency. The university could not prosper under the existing structure, the panel concluded in its report, but as a public corporation, it could compete, reduce its costs, and grow while continuing to fulfill its public mission both in Portland and in rural areas.[1]

"OHSU has the potential to become one of the top-10 biomedical research universities in the country, a national model for academic health centers, and a powerful catalyst for developing Oregon's biotechnology industry," the committee said. Under the existing structure, OHSU "is not capable of turning that vision into reality."[2]

The committee noted OHSU's annual state appropriation had climbed only slightly from about $52 million to $65 million between 1984 and 1994, yet its total revenues had climbed from $176 million to $463 million. As a result, the institution's share of support from the state had dropped from 30 percent to less than 14 percent during that period.[3] The state could not afford to support OHSU if it failed in the marketplace, the panel's report said. The ability of OHSU to compete was hampered by "unnecessary layers of approval, cumbersome administrative processes and restricted procurement and personnel requirements" and laws preventing it from holding stock or entering partnerships that could enable it to raise money. "OHSU must be free to run its business activities in a more business-like manner," the committee concluded.[4]

The advisory group considered whether OHSU would be better off as a private nonprofit, but concluded that would undermine its public academic and research mission. The panel recommended that OHSU be exempt from the state's public records and open meetings laws for business negotiations and records and for new president searches, and that the president serve as a member of the OHSU governing board—all conditions requested by neither President Kohler nor members of his leadership team.[5]

The firm endorsement from a panel that included a former governor and well-respected top business leaders added to growing momentum in support of OHSU's public corporation proposal. As the legislative session approached, Kohler had amassed an impressive array of backers, ranging from faculty, staff, unions, and students to the governor and the State Board of Higher Education. Governor Kitzhaber said OHSU could serve as a laboratory to test whether the public corporation structure would work. Joseph Cox, in an *Oregonian* article anticipating the release of the advisory committee report, said he was behind OHSU's plan. "I came to be persuaded that [OHSU] had to be sprung even further from the nest than the other [universities]," he said.[6] Another key legislator, Senator Tom Hartung (Republican from Portland), chair of the Senate Education Committee, also expressed his support. "This fits right into our philosophy of making government smaller, more efficient and more productive," he said.[7] Further, the Portland City Council on January 11 unanimously passed a resolution in support of OHSU's quest to operate as an independent, public institution.[8]

Most legislators and state leaders also supported OHSU's public corporation proposal. The medical university showed both a clear need to make the change and the capacity to earn money and survive on its own.

And most leaders could see the urgency of its plan. The skeptics were mostly liberal Democrats. They worried "the further OHSU got away from the state, the less likely it was to continue its mission for the poor and its other very public missions," said Davis.[9] They feared it would focus primarily on the bottom line.

Republicans, who controlled both the House and Senate, were largely enthusiastic about the public corporation plan. Like Hartung, they saw it as the embodiment of what they had been pushing for across all government programs: a more businesslike approach to providing services. And they trusted Kohler. He had built political support by delivering on his promise to bring more health care to rural Oregon, which was dominated by Republican legislators. Since OHSU took over the Office of Rural Health and launched its five Area Health Education Centers (AHECs), rural areas had gained sixty-one physicians, seventy-seven nurse practitioners, and seventeen physician assistants; provided clinical services to fifteen towns; and arranged for twenty-nine family medicine residents to complete at least twenty weeks of clinical rotations in rural AHEC practice sites.[10]

THE PERFECT CHAMPION

OHSU had the perfect champion in one rural Republican—Senator Eugene Timms, who was born and raised in Burns. He graduated from Burns Union High in 1950, earned a bachelor's degree in business at Willamette University and married his lifelong friend, Edna Evans, in 1953. He served a stint in the military before returning to Burns and his family's business, Alpine Creamery. Timms was civically active and served in the state Senate twenty-two years. He proved an ideal advocate for OHSU with his avuncular, friendly style: a legislator well liked by his community and by both Republicans and Democrats. He worried about the chronic shortage of health providers in rural Oregon and saw OHSU as an ally in addressing the problem. He worked with Kohler almost from the day the president arrived to establish AHECs and other medical services in rural Oregon.

Timms probably did more than any other single leader in Oregon to help OHSU gain authority to operate as a public corporation, which he viewed as "an exciting opportunity for this Legislature and the people of Oregon." Kohler needed someone with Timms' clout to usher the university's public corporation bill, Senate Bill 2 (SB 2) through the legislature. Most bills die in committees without even a hearing. As cochair of the Joint Ways and Means Committee, Timms had the power to insure SB 2 got on the Senate Education Committee's agenda. He made the proposal personal by telling the committee "Oregon Health Sciences University is as much a Burns university as it is a Portland University."[11]

As the legislature went into session, Kohler and his team continued to solicit support from other quarters of the state. Early in the year, Portland Mayor Vera Katz sent a letter to Hartung and the Senate Committee on Education, urging it to support OHSU's public corporation proposal. She noted the university was the metro area's largest employer, bringing in more than $150 million a year to Oregon from out-of-state sources. "Members of Portland's City Council are convinced that with the changing realities nationally for health care systems and academic learning centers," she wrote, "becoming a public corporation is a critical move if OHSU is to remain successful and competitive."[12]

A short time later, two weeks after the 1995 legislative session opened in January, Kohler's team staged a second news conference in Salem. Kohler, Governor Kitzhaber, Timms, Goldschmidt, and eight other legislative leaders announced they would be introducing bills to make OHSU a public corporation. Timms would sponsor and introduce SB 2, which was joined by twenty-seven cosponsors. Governor Kitzhaber would introduce a nearly identical bill, House Bill 275, to show his support for the proposal and to provide a separate vehicle for it should anything go wrong in the Senate.

As the news conference began, Kitzhaber rose to go to the podium, leaned over to Kohler and whispered, "By the way, I am going to announce we will keep our budget flat through the 1997–99 biennium."[13]

This came as a surprise to Kohler. He knew OHSU had agreed to accept the 15 percent cut the governor had proposed for the entire higher education system for 1995–97. But he had somehow missed that the state higher education board had agreed to a four-year freeze on state revenue at its December meeting. In the moment, there was nothing he could say, so Kohler just nodded slightly as the governor stepped to the podium.[14]

The two public corporations bills were formally introduced on February 2.

Though Kohler's team had gained wide support, not everyone supported OHSU's quest. David Frohnmayer, president of the University of Oregon, made it clear at the meeting in his hotel that he was against the plan. Attorney General Ted Kulongoski opposed the public corporation structure, and some Democratic legislators argued OHSU would lose its commitment to its public mission if it were no longer a state agency.

So Kohler's leadership team was taking no chances. In addition to the business advisory committee's report and a news conference showcasing the support of the governor and other key legislators, the team led efforts to compose an executive summary of the bill, a section-by-section analysis, a list of questions and answers, a two-page fact sheet, a four-page white paper, a highlights document with a list of key supporters on the back, and a booklet describing OHSU called *One of a Kind in Oregon*. One four-page treatise described how OHSU under a new governance structure would both save money and remain accountable to the public. It argued that a public corporation was "a better way to do business," "a smarter way to serve Oregonians," and would "unleash OHSU to succeed."[15]

"Making OHSU a public corporation would not change its missions, just how it achieves them," it said. "It would unleash enormous potential the university has to compete in the marketplace and to expand its reputation as one of the nation's premier academic medical centers."[16]

Kohler's team met regularly to discuss details of their public corporation plan and strategies for selling it. Kohler's calendar shows scheduled public corporation meetings, usually on Tuesdays, thirteen times during the first half of 1995, but team members said they met far more often with each other and with legislators and other leaders. By this time, Walker and Davis had offices in Kohler's presidential suite in the northwest corner of Baird Hall. Their offices fringed a lobby area where secretaries were clustered in a warren of desks. Billups and Hallick had offices in a suite about ninety feet down the hall. Goldfarb's office was in the hospital, but he often spent time with the rest of the team in Baird Hall. So it was easy for some or all of the team members to strike up informal meetings about issues pressing on the public corporation. Sometimes they met in Kohler's office, other times in the conference room. Often bursts of laughter would roll out from wherever they were meeting.

"We liked each other; we respected each other," said Davis. "We took our work very seriously. We did not take ourselves very seriously. . . . One of the ways we dealt with this high stress situation was that we could laugh about it."[17]

Meetings often lasted an hour, sometimes two, and the topic of the moment would dictate who dominated, Billups said.[18] Once the legislature got underway, the team often was scattered so they would meet in conference calls. Walker said he must have attended 100 to 200 meetings on the public corporation. "It is a blur," he said.[19]

Team members met with legislators and staff to solidify votes from members who had already said they were supportive—and to secure votes from those who were on the fence or in the "no" column. Davis went nearly every day to Salem, putting in sixty-hour weeks while she and her husband, who was also lobbying in Salem, raised two small children and juggled ways to get them to and from daycare. Hallick and Kohler regularly rose at 4:00 a.m. to tackle their multitude of duties. Sometimes Davis was up at 4:00 a.m., too.

Kohler traveled to the capitol about once a week, and Davis and some other lobbyists working for the team made up to 100 trips by the time the session ended in June. Kohler made at least twenty-six trips to Salem during the session and met personally with at least nineteen legislators, including all five members of the Senate Committee on Education, at least nine members on the Joint Committee on Ways and Means education subcommittee, and the cochairs of the full Ways and Means Committee.

He and his team members were prepared to talk about any feature down to the smallest technical detail about the public corporation plan, but they repeatedly blundered in coordinating their carpooling. Those traveling to Salem on any given day had agreed to meet at the Howard Johnson's motel at the I-405 exit off Interstate 5 on the south side of Portland. Somebody invariably would fail to show up for the rendezvous at the appointed time, which would vary slightly from day to day.

"So at least once a week," recalled Billups, "some collection of us sat stressed out in a motel parking lot [in the days before cell phones] wondering about our colleague's whereabouts and whether we would make it to Salem on time."[20]

Walker recalled that on one winter Monday morning, possibly before the session began, he and Kohler were to meet at the motel and drive to Salem to meet with Timms and some other legislators. They woke to four inches of snow, which paralyzed Portland because it is not well-equipped to plow. Hardly anyone was driving, but Walker, who lived in Lake Oswego, a suburban city south of Portland, and Kohler each pulled on high boots and got in their cars. Walker strapped chains on his tires, and Kohler had snow tires. They rendezvoused at the motel and drove to Salem. With only about an inch of snow in Salem, a few legislators, including Timms, had showed at the capitol.

"They were in unbelief, shocked that Pete and I had made it," Walker said. "It made a big impression on them."[21]

FIRST HEARING

Senate Bill 2 made its legislative debut at 8:00 a.m. on February 23 in a public hearing conducted by the Senate Committee on Education. Kohler, Hallick, Walker, and Billups all for the first time formally made their case before legislators for converting OHSU into a public corporation. They had cleared their first hurdle by getting the bill on the agenda. Now they had to persuade the committee to support it and send it to the Ways and Means Committee. That committee would put the bill on the calendar of its education subcommittee. The subcommittee could kill it or refer it to the full committee with a recommendation for passage. If the full committee supported it, the bill would then go to the Senate floor for a vote. If the Senate supported it, the bill would go to the House for a vote that would bring either final passage or defeat.

Timms put his clout behind the bill by introducing it to the five-member Committee on Education. He sat at a small table for people testifying to the lawmakers. The panel members sat behind the hearing room's arcing, blonde-wood desk, which was raised like a judge's bench so that they all looked down at Timms. The senator said OHSU had reached the limit of what it could accomplish as a state agency and was offering a way to make government more efficient by rethinking the way it provided services. Freed from state strictures, OHSU could become one of the top biomedical universities in the nation, he said.[22]

Kohler then took a seat at the table to testify. He described the problem OHSU faced with increased competition in a marketplace shifting to managed care. "Those who cannot be responsive and efficient, and those unwilling to embrace change, will simply not survive," he said.[23]

OHSU was poised not only to survive but also to thrive if it could be freed from the state bureaucracy and gain more flexibility, he said. Oregon's only academic health center had become one of Portland's largest employers, with a staff of nearly 7,000 people. It brought in $150 million a year from out-of-state sources and had tripled its research dollars over the previous eight years, even as its state support had fallen to less than 14 percent of its budget. OHSU was rated as one of the most efficient academic medical centers in the nation, he said.[24]

"We have downsized central administration by almost 50 percent by combining hospital and university administration in a way that is unique in the country," he said. "We are visited almost weekly by other institutions trying to understand our lack of time-consuming turf battles."[25]

He explained that without more state support or more freedom, OHSU could not sustain its services and role as an economic catalyst. The university was "in essence an important business enterprise supporting its education activities." State regulations and procedures were designed for traditional government, not the biomedical research and patient care that dominated the university's work. The public corporation model offered the best solution for keeping the university healthy while allowing it to fulfill its public missions of providing indigent care and education. Kohler described how a public corporation would work and how it would save the university money and allow it to flourish. He concluded:

> OHSU can be one of the country's top biomedical research universities and a model for academic health centers. It can continue to improve health care services in rural Oregon and serve as a catalyst for economic growth statewide. It can achieve all this without additional state support, but not without the tools provided by the public corporation proposal.[26]

Hallick testified next. She identified herself as the provost, an academic title sometimes referred to as vice president for academic affairs. "There are other names used, but I won't mention them here," she joked. She emphasized that the university's academic mission would remain "in the public corporation our first and primary mission." She described the university's schools and programs and noted "we have been under siege for a few years here" because of a decline in state support, which is "the underpinning of many of the educational programs." Despite that decline, the university had not eliminated a single educational program. Instead, she said, the university had cut and consolidated its administration, creating "the leanest administration of any academic health center in the country." Data from two years earlier showed OHSU's administration leanest next to Mississippi. "They have not undergone this last round of cuts nor the next one," she said. "So we are reasonably confident that we are the leanest, and that isn't all good."[27]

Walker took his turn before the Senate committee. He described university finances, the threats of managed health care, and OHSU's difficulty forming a statewide health maintenance organization with Multnomah County because of cumbersome state contract regulations. He said OHSU carried about $110 million in debt, was strong enough to access the private debt market and wanted the option of issuing bonds through the state.[28] He implied a threat loomed over OHSU by describing how academic health centers can slip into a downward spiral when their buildings and equipment age, and they start having difficulty attracting patients and sustaining research.

"The business erodes, the research erodes," he said. "The patient care isn't very good, they don't have the research dollars coming into the state, and they have very little research going on. . . . It all interrelates."[29]

OHSU, on the other hand, was getting financially stronger, Walker said, because Kohler had put money into maintenance and good faculty and adopted a strategic plan that brought all of the university schools and departments together under a consolidated administration and common vision.

"You have to get the business side healthy," he said. "You have to start investing in faculty and be able to make the unit run as a whole . . . If you don't have the quality faculty, patients aren't going to come up to our institution."[30]

He warned declining state revenue threatened OHSU's ability to make those investments. As the Public Corporation Advisory Committee had reported, OHSU could not compensate for less state support and sustain its financial health in an increasingly competitive market without more freedom to reduce its costs, raise its own capital, and expand so that it could attract more high-quality faculty and doctors, who would in turn draw more paying patients.

DEFINING CHANGE

Next Billups, who identified herself as OHSU's Legal Policy Advisor, took a seat at the table and calmly and confidently walked the committee through the ninety-two-section bill, section by section. She made it clear to committee members and the audience that OHSU's proposal was what it claimed to be, nothing more and nothing less. There was no subtext, no secret plan. If people had questions, the OHSU team would answer them. If they had concerns, the team would do its best to address them. Senator Ken Baker (Republican from Clackamas), raised one concern as Billups described section 2 of the bill as "intended to define or at least explain what kind of creature we are creating here."

Baker asked, "Have we anywhere else in Oregon statutes defining what we mean by independent public corporation?"

"No, and that's a bit of a problem," said Billups, "and that's one reason it is difficult to . . ."

"So, wouldn't it be good," said Baker, "if we are going to do this like we did on SB 271 [the chancellor's public corporation proposal for the whole university system] to have a definition to use sort of as a template?"[31]

Baker had a point. Public corporation was not explicitly defined in the bill, and it needed to be. By the next meeting five days later, Billups had a definition:

> A public corporation is an entity that is created by the state to carry out public missions and services. In order to carry out these public missions and services, the public corporation participates

> in activities or provides services that are also provided by private enterprise. A public corporation is granted increased operating flexibility in order to best insure its success while retaining principles of public accountability and fundamental public policy. The Board of Directors of the public corporation is appointed by the governor and confirmed by the senate but is otherwise delegated the authority to set policy and manage the operations of the public corporation.[32]

During the first hearing, Billups took the committee through other features of SB 2, describing the composition of the board and its powers, state statutes that would still apply to the university and those from which it would be exempt, and how OHSU would pay for state services it used. The state personnel system would remain in place until OHSU developed its own, which would preserve collective bargaining rights and employee access to the Public Employees Retirement System.[33]

Senator Cliff Trow, a Democrat, history professor, and administrator at Oregon State University in Corvallis, asked if severing OHSU from the rest of the state university system would disrupt cooperative research among faculty of the state institutions, a concern that came up in Goldschmidt's advisory committee. Kohler went to the table and said OHSU would remain involved with the state university system's academic programs, noting that cooperation among researchers depended more on their initiative and the strength of their research programs than on administrative efforts to foster collaboration.

The committee did not raise many other concerns in the first meeting, but Hartung scheduled the next meeting five days later to start at 7:00 a.m. so the panel would have time to probe the proposal more deeply. One striking feature of these meetings was how much OHSU's image had changed in the eyes of lawmakers. No longer were lawmakers looking at the university as a mismanaged drain on the system. Instead, they spoke about it with respect.

"It is just amazing to me the public perception on what you are doing up there, and doing very well," said Hartung in his committee's second meeting on the bill. "In this process, we do not want to denigrate that or downgrade it. I wish we could have the same public perception on education K-12."[34]

On the other hand, word began reaching Kohler's team during this time that some legislators saw OHSU denigrating state government and its employees with its arguments about being stalled and held back by state bureaucrats. The team scrambled to meet with legislators one-on-one to clarify that they were not criticizing state government, but making the point that 60 percent of their money came from a competitive business enterprise with other health care providers, not other state agencies.

Kohler also looked for chances to sell the public corporation elsewhere. During the first half of 1995, as the legislature pored over SB 2, Kohler managed to give at least nine speeches to various groups. He spoke on "The role of OHSU for the New Health Care Environment" to the Clackamas County Medical Society and on "The Changing Face of Medical Education in the Decade of the 90s" to a medical group in Seattle. He spoke to the Portland City Council, to a Kiwanis group in Portland, to the American Lung Association, and to the Jewish Federation of Portland.

On February 10, he agreed to pinch hit for University of Oregon President Dave Frohnmayer, who had a conflict, as speaker at the weekly meeting of the City Club of Portland, an influential group of civic and business leaders and citizens. The talk was broadcast on Oregon Public Radio. Kohler talked about the importance of higher education on the economy and the workforce challenges of the changing world of health care. As in most of his talks, he took a few minutes at the end of his presentation to mention OHSU's quest to become a public corporation.

"There is a lot of talk about reinventing government," he said. "There aren't many effective examples yet. OHSU will be one of the first; and, we believe, one of the most successful."[35]

Kohler was to speak on April 19 on "What happens to Teaching in Managed Care" to a black tie dinner in Oklahoma City, two days before the Ways and Means Committee would take up its final vote on SB 2. But his speech was canceled after Timothy McVeigh earlier that day bombed the downtown federal building.[36]

UNIVERSITY SYSTEM PLAN

As OHSU pushed for more independence, so did the Oregon State System of Higher Education with Senate Bill 271, also called the Higher Education Administrative Efficiency Act for the 21st Century. The legislation, introduced by Chancellor Thomas Bartlett, and then carried forward by his successor, Joseph Cox, proposed making the entire eight-campus university system a public corporation. It reflected a national unrest in higher education. Public universities, academic health centers, and university systems in other parts of the country also were casting about for more autonomy. Higher education leaders in Florida were proposing to privatize some university operations, and leaders in Virginia were seeking more autonomy for some of their colleges.[37] The University of Wisconsin and the University of Maryland had recently won legislative approval to spin off their hospitals as a "public authority or public corporation" with their own boards and operating flexibility. Governor Christine Todd Whitman was proposing to eliminate the New Jersey Department of Higher Education.[38] Academics were writing about these winds of change in articles such as one by Fred Evans, a professor at Eastern Washington University, titled "The Coming Privatization of Higher Education." State higher education leaders also were reading David Osborne and Ted Gaebler's best-selling book *Reinventing Government: How the Entrepreneurial Spirit is Transforming the Public Sector.*[39]

But unlike SB 2, the state board's plan had been getting a cool reception from politicians, campus leaders, and editorial boards from the day Bartlett floated it. Many were uneasy with the magnitude of the proposal. The term "public corporation" was part of the problem, Cox said. "It confounded our friends and confused our critics," he said.[40]

He and other university system administrators emphasized the plan was not radical and not privatization. They modified the proposed bill in September for the upcoming 1995 legislative session. Their new bill would convert the state system into "a semi-independent state agency." But legislators still worried about giving up too much authority over higher education. Representative Tony Van Vliet, a Republican and former Oregon State University professor who left the legislature in 1994, expressed the view of many state leaders. With their lump-sum state budgets and authority to set tuition, he said, the state's universities had enough independence.

"They want all the perks that go with a public agency, such as access to funds, but the advantages of the private sector," he said. "It doesn't give much accountability either way. They can't be neither fish nor fowl."[41]

While SB 2 stayed on track in the 1995 Legislature, the Higher Education Administrative Efficiency Act for the 21st Century foundered. When Cox heard a rumor that the Efficiency Act already was dead, he invited about a dozen legislative leaders to a breakfast, described by reporter Kit Lively, in *The Chronicle of Higher Education*:

> It was an intentionally frugal affair, with boxes of Danish pastry and juice served in a cramped basement room of the State Capitol. After everyone was settled at a Formica-topped table, Mr. Cox closed the door and asked what was going on. Brady Adams, the Senate Majority Leader and an old friend, said he was sorry, but the bill did not have the support it needed to survive. The chancellor froze.
>
> Suddenly, the Senate's new president, a businessman named Gordon Smith, said he wasn't quite ready to call the coroner. He liked

> the [university] system's idea. If legislators could promise only limited funds to higher education, he said in a later interview, it was in their interest to encourage efficiency [42]

While Smith's support kept the bill breathing, legislators still had concerns. They worried that the higher education system's plan to save $7 million by ending payments for services such as purchasing and personnel would be a blow to state agencies. They also didn't like the 119-page bill's complexity, which required modification in more than 240 statutes, many to change the name of the university system to the Oregon Public University System or OPUS. University officials produced a slimmed-down version of the bill in late January that scrapped the name change and phased out service payments over more than two years.

Still, key leaders had doubts. Representative Carolyn Oakley (Republican from Albany), chair of the Ways and Means education subcommittee, worried about its impact on the state budget, and Kitzhaber couldn't support it because, as one of his advisers said, its request for "total exemption from a large body of statutes goes too far." Oakley proposed a watered-down compromise that would give the state's universities more control over purchasing, contracting, personnel, and printing. On the day before the legislature adjourned, it passed the twelve-page Efficiency Act.[43]

MORE HEARINGS

OHSU's SB 2, by contrast, received sustained and serious consideration by legislators in the Senate Committee on Education, which met again on February 28 and March 2, a total of eight hours, before sending it to the Joint Ways and Means Committee. The Ways and Means education subcommittee then dug into the bill on April 5, 12, 13, and 17; and the full Ways and Means Committee took up the bill just once, on April 21.

Governor Kitzhaber, other state leaders, educators, business and private hospital leaders, union representatives, students, even other legislators spoke in favor of the bill. No one spoke against it. At the Senate Education Committee's February 28 meeting, Kitzhaber testified that converting OHSU to a public corporation was compelling for two reasons: it would not be able to thrive without the change, and it would be more efficient and cost-effective with it, which was what the public wanted to see in government.

"I've heard nothing either inside or outside the legislature that suggests this is a bad idea," he said.[44]

He said the conversion would not undermine the state university system, but allow OHSU to carry out its multiple missions of education, research, and care to the indigent. Then he again surprised Kohler and his team. He said as a public corporation, OHSU could fulfill its mission without more state money.

"The intent is over the next several years to try to move the state funding component on down to zero where the school at one point will be self-sufficient," he said.[45]

Kohler and his team were stunned. That idea had never been part of the plan. Kohler's team had argued its goal was to give OHSU the flexibility to be more successful at competing for private revenue to supplement—not replace—its public funding.[46] Section 13 of SB 2 explicitly stated the university was to submit a funding request to the state Department of Administrative Services by September 1 of each even-numbered year. Administrative services was then to submit a request on behalf of OHSU "to the Legislative Assembly as part of the governor's biennial budget."[47]

Kohler, Davis, and Billups huddled in the back of the hearing room and discussed how to respond. They did not want to let the governor's statement stand on the record. On the other hand, they did not want to alienate one of their key supporters by directly challenging him in front of the committee. In the end, they decided to soft-pedal it. When a committee member asked Kohler if the university could completely divest itself of state appropriations over time, the president responded that would be possible only if the state or another entity were to provide OHSU with a $2 billion endowment to fund general operations. Otherwise, he said, the university would survive, but it would have to reduce the scope of services the state subsidizes such as education and health care for indigent patients.[48]

After the committee adjourned, Kohler, Davis, and Billups talked to individual committee members and staff to clarify that the medical university had never proposed becoming fully self-sufficient. The OHSU administrators explained they had, in fact, considered a fully private model and rejected it, as did their advisory committee, primarily because it could jeopardize their public mission, but also because they didn't believe it would work. Even as its hospital and clinical revenues increased, OHSU would be hard-pressed to support its research and its medical school and other educational programs without state revenue. Private donors would not give money to the university to sustain its operations; they wanted to support new buildings or research initiatives.[49]

In retrospect, it was a major mistake not to more directly, if politely, challenge Kitzhaber on the record, Davis said. As the years passed, the governor's statement was used by OHSU critics to fuel the myth that the university had promised to move away from state funding over time. Kitzhaber insists that Kohler had clearly stated OHSU "would not be a burden on the general fund anymore."[50] By that, Kohler said, he meant the university could live with flat funding for the next biennium, but he did not ever suggest the health center could operate with no state money. The university still relied on the state to help it cover its public missions of educating doctors, dentists, and nurses and providing health care to the poor.

Other leaders had come to believe that OHSU could operate with less state money. As a result, Kohler and his team wrangled for years with Ways and Means members and staff in the early to mid-2000s for state money and never got enough.[51] Today, with less than 2 percent of its operating budget coming from the state, OHSU has nearly become self-sufficient.

GRILLED BY LAWMAKERS

During the legislative committee hearings on SB 2, lawmakers did not question whether OHSU should become a public corporation, but rather what features and powers it should have once it made the shift. They questioned whether it would pose unfair competitive advantages as a public corporation or become too disconnected from other state universities. They wrestled with whether OHSU deserved exemptions from the public records and open meetings laws, how much bonding power it should have, how much authority the legislature should retain, who should be on its board, how the conversion would affect minority hiring and enrollment, and whether OHSU should have full control over its land.

The discourse was civil and, occasionally, humorous. For example, as Billups took the Senate Education Committee through the bill in its second session, she came to section 62, which creates the office of Demonstrator of Anatomy. "It is a person who has a certain amount of authority over the use of the remains of a deceased person," she explained.

"Is that the best term to use, 'Demonstrator of Anatomy?'" asked Senator Hartung, as the hearing room burst into laughter.

"Well, it's certainly an entertaining term," said Billups. "I don't know its historical background, but it's been . . ."

"Is that the term that is currently used?" asked Hartung.

"Yes it is," Billups said. "We didn't change the name."

The name emerged in medical schools of the thirteenth and fourteenth centuries. At the University of Paris, for example, medical students would gather around a human cadaver with two anatomists. One would read from an anatomical writing about a part of the body while the other showed, or "demonstrated," where the part was. Hence, the second anatomist was called the "Demonstrator of Anatomy." Today, the OHSU Demonstrator of Anatomy, a member of the faculty, handles body donations. Funeral homes provide the Demonstrator unclaimed indigent bodies for the medical school. The state also sometimes makes the bodies of children who die under its guardianship available to the Demonstrator of Anatomy.

Hartung and other Senate Education Committee members questioned what other Oregon hospitals, particularly those in the Portland area, thought about OHSU's conversion to a public corporation and whether the change would give the University Hospital an unfair competitive advantage. Timms told the committee he had the same questions and met with six representatives of "the bigger hospitals" in the Portland area.

"Nobody had any complaints," he said. "They were not afraid we were creating something that would have a competitive advantage; if anything, they thought they could work together better."[52]

Ed Patterson, a representative of the Oregon Association of Hospitals, said that the group's board voted unanimously to support SB 2 after hearing a presentation from Goldfarb and Billups. Some members had a major concern about whether OHSU would be competing with them on a "level playing field," Patterson said, but those concerns were offset by the advantage of having access to a high-quality academic health center capable of providing specialty care.

"They also view the university as a resource not only for the patients that they see, but a resource for all patients in the state," he said.[53]

Committee member Senator Marylin Shannon, a socially conservative Republican from a small town near Salem, still questioned whether OHSU might have an unfair advantage because of its state support. OHSU doctors, she said, "can charge less than any other tertiary physician in Portland or the surrounding area because they are [part of] a public corporation and they are subsidized with tax monies." She cited an example of a Portland ophthalmologist who claimed OHSU's Casey Eye Institute could undercut him with much lower charges. Kohler replied Casey got less state money than it needed just to cover its teaching costs. In addition, he said, it provided a disproportionate share of indigent care that more than offset the small amount of money it was getting from the state.

"So I guess when I hear questions about the playing field being even or not even, I would say it's not even," he said. "We're still on the downside rather than the upside with regard to these kinds of competitive bids."[54]

Some legislators again questioned whether OHSU would become too disconnected from the state's other seven universities if it were cut loose.

Trow (Democrat from Corvallis), the historian, expressed concern that if OHSU had its own board as a public corporation, it would lose touch with the State Board of Higher Education. The two boards should have some interconnection, he said.

"Having some direct participation of the Chancellor in what's going on in your operation is important, not that the Chancellor should run it by any stretch," he said. Kohler replied that Hallick would continue to meet with the Academic Council for the state university system and that he would do the same with the Council of Presidents. Trow wanted it in the bill.

"It is in there," said Hallick. She pointed to Section 12 of SB 2, which stated OHSU would submit any proposals to change, add, merge, or close any academic degree or certificate programs or other academic policies to the state board for approval.[55]

Senator Hartung raised the same concern with Goldschmidt when he came before the committee to testify.

"We want to keep a handle on [OHSU]," Hartung said, "like when one of your kids are ready to break away and want to leave home. You know you must do it, but also you want to keep up a meaningful connection."

Goldschmidt replied that faculty members would stay connected with colleagues at other universities as long as their work is supported. They don't make those connections, he said, "because our state system of higher education commands us to do it; it isn't because the Legislature somehow commands us to do it." He also noted that if OHSU became a public corporation, the legislature would still have authority over it by controlling the money flowing to the university, and the state board would have one or two of its members on the OHSU board.

"Our choices here are to grow or die," Goldschmidt said, "because the economics are brutal, and I don't mean your economics. I mean the health care economics."[56]

He also explained why the Public Corporation Advisory Committee that he chaired recommended amending SB 2 so OHSU would be exempt from some features of the state public records and meetings law. One exemption would allow the university to keep its search process for a new president secret. Hiring a new president for OHSU as a public corporation would be akin to hiring a "chief executive officer to manage a multi-million dollar corporation," he said. Fred Buckman—president and CEO of PacifiCorp, an electrical utility, and a member of Goldschmidt's committee—joined Kohler at the table to explain that recruiting for senior levels in a competitive corporation usually meant going after people already employed.

"They may very well wish to explore [the job] without the whole world knowing about it until they have at least made some commitment that this is an attractive next step," he said. "The open meetings law is one that makes it very difficult for you to explore and attract the very best people at the top of an organization that is in a competitive environment the way I see Oregon Health Sciences University."[57]

The Goldschmidt committee also recommended the university be exempt from the public records law in disclosing "sensitive business records" and business dealings with potential partners. Goldschmidt told the committee, "I will not be surprised, and in fact would be shocked, if the newspaper publishers haven't already showed up to tell you why it's a bad idea."[58]

Later during the same committee meeting, Gail Ryder, lobbyist for the Oregon Newpaper Publishers Association, did show up to challenge the proposed exemptions, arguing they could do damage to Oregon's public records and meetings laws.

"We believe that the business of government should be done in the public with proper notice and proper records," she said. OHSU should not be exempt from that, she said, just because it becomes semi-public.

On the business exemption, she noted, "Oregon law already conditionally exempts the trade secrets of businesses in Oregon Revised Statutes (ORS) 192, which states an exemption for trade secrets" that may include "any formula, plan, pattern, process, tool, mechanism, compound, procedure, production data or compilation of information." The Uniform Trade Secrets Act is even broader, she said.

"These two provisions provide more than enough protection of the records of businesses potentially entering into partnerships with Oregon Health Sciences University," she said. "What is meant by sensitive business records beyond what is already provided in the statutes?"

As for presidential searches, she continued, the law already allowed public agencies to deliberate on candidates for top posts in executive sessions, which in Oregon are closed to the public but open to journalists who agree not to report on what occurs. The law puts reporters in an awkward position of having to sit on potential news, but it also allows them to keep government bodies honest. While there is little public interest in unsuccessful candidates, Ryder said, the public is interested in finalists and the process leading to a selection of president and has a right to know about it.

"The interest of the public in selection of a chief executive officer for a public agency does not change just because the status of that entity has become semi-independent," she said.[59]

The proposed amendments came up again in the Senate Education Committee's third meeting on March 3. Mark Dodson, Portland attorney and state board chair when Kohler was hired, noted the amendments would keep the search for a new president secret, but "the successful candidate would be hired in public." He said the amendment to keep sensitive business information secret would protect OHSU in business dealings with private companies that would be reluctant to do business under "the chilling effect" of the public records law. The committee then voted to adopt both amendments. SB 2 would add to exemptions under Oregon's public records and meetings laws:[60]

- Sensitive business records or financial or commercial information of the Oregon Health Sciences University that is not customarily provided to business competitors.
- Records of the Oregon Health Sciences University regarding candidates for the position of university president.

The bill also adds to those meetings from which reporters are barred, even in executive session, "meetings of the Oregon Health Sciences University Board of Directors or its designated committee regarding candidates for the position of president."[61]

A QUESTION OF POWER

Lawmakers reviewing SB 2 also struggled over how much bonding authority to give to OHSU versus the legislature in allowing the university to become a public corporation. In the Senate Education Committee's second session, committee member Sen. Cliff Trow questioned whether OHSU could sink so deep in debt it would damage the rest of the state's bonding capacity. John Woodward, the San Francisco health finance expert, said OHSU's capacity for debt would be limited by the market. Douglas Goe, the Portland attorney who helped Billups address bonds in SB 2, added that if OHSU were a public corporation, the debt market "would rely on its own authority to issue debt rather than looking at the state." In short, he said, "this is not going to be state debt." But Goe also said OHSU would like to have access to some measure of state general obligation bond authority, which had been its primary capital funding source in the past. Trow was not satisfied.

"There needs to be some kind of checks and balances," he said.

Goe responded that without the flexibility to raise money based on its own revenue as opposed to tax revenue, OHSU would be strapped. Randall Edwards, executive assistant to the state treasurer who would later serve eight years as state treasurer, told the committee that his department also worried about allowing OHSU too much freedom with state debt. So, he explained, the treasury department and OHSU agreed to amend the bill to bar the university from using general obligation bonds backed by state tax money. The university would have to handle its own debt through the private market or certificates of participation, state tax-exempt bonds that the university would have to pay back with its own revenue.[62]

Kohler told the committee that the university president should be fired if he or she did not handle the university's debt properly. "I can assure you," he said, "as long as I am president, I do not intend for us to get out on a limb financially."[63]

At the Senate Education Committee's third and final meeting on March 2, Bill Nestle of the Department of Justice testified that OHSU, the higher education system, and the state treasurer had agreed that OHSU would not only have no authority to issue state general obligation bonds, but also would agree to handle its existing debt of about $110 million and to notify the state if it ever were unable to make payments on it. The committee approved that agreement in bill amendments. Senator Ken Baker (Republican from Clackamas) and Trow said the bill should also require OHSU to pay off its existing debt before incurring more. Baker proposed giving it a deadline. Hartung agreed to make that suggestion in a note to the Joint Ways and Means Committee, but no deadline made it into the bill.

The Ways and Means subcommittee on education also looked for ways to protect legislative control over a more independent OHSU. The House Republican caucus expressed concern that the legislature was "giving you this bill and basically not having the authority," said Representative Carolyn Oakley, of Albany, chairwoman of the subcommittee. "They would like to see it in writing. . . . We need some way to feel as if we still have some control over what you folks are doing, and if we are not pleased, we would like to know how to pull in the reins."

Billups assured the committee that "what the Legislature creates, the Legislature can essentially uncreate." But explicitly stating in the bill that the legislature has authority to revoke OHSU's public corporation status would make the conversion appear less stable, which could jeopardize the university's ability to borrow money in the private market, Billups explained. The university must go to the legislature every two years for money, she noted. "In reality," she said, "and in fact, you have the authority over us that you really need to have."[64]

She proposed addressing the lawmakers' concerns in a budget note that would state the legislature retains authority over OHSU. But another committee member, Representative Cedric Hayden, a conservative Republican from Lyons, proposed amending the bill by adding the following statements:[65] "The public corporation is the creation of the Legislative Assembly and shall be financially and programmatically accountable to the Legislative Assembly. The Legislative Assembly retains the authority to amend, alter or change the form and structure of the public corporation."[66]

Billups said it would be risky to put that language even in a budget note. "I fear that it will put at risk the university's ability to access the financial market," she said. Al Kowalski, manager of the Municipal Securities Group at Pacific Crest Securities in Portland, stepped up in support of Billups to say even a budget note could spook financial lenders.

"It could easily be read in today's market as a sign that something's amiss, that we're not going forward as fully supportive and as committed to this," he said, "and investors are looking for every opportunity they can to not invest and not provide the best opportunity for academic health centers to enter the market."

Representative Kevin Mannix (Democrat from Salem) then launched an exchange that sounded like something from *Alice's Adventures in Wonderland.* He observed lawmakers were asked not to speak the plain meaning about their authority because even mentioning it creates greater meaning than it has.

"So it's best to follow the Chinese method of negotiation where a wink or a nod will do," he said. "The wink or the nod is the record we've already made because of all of this being recorded and videotaped. . . . All we have to do is repeal the damn statute and it's gone, but if we say that, somebody will think we're thinking about doing it."

"Exactly," replied Kowalski.

Peggy Archer, a legislative staff member, then asked, "If you say this, aren't you implying, since you already have this authority, aren't you implying that you don't have it elsewhere unless you say it?"[67]

Hayden withdrew his amendment, but asked Archer to read it aloud so there was a "historical record of it." Archer read the amendment. He proposed adding to the budget note only the second part of his amendment, which said the university would keep records on its spending and make those available for legislative audits. Representative Gail Shibley, (Democrat from Portland), objected.

"It is unnecessary, restrictive, and the language that's in paragraph 2 of the proposed budget note is unnecessary," she said.[68]

In the end, the committee gave up on an amendment or budget note, sparing OHSU from entering the private debt market with words defining the legislative authority looming over it.

OHSU'S GOVERNING BOARD

The composition and size of the new governing board for OHSU as a public corporation also commanded attention from lawmakers scrutinizing SB 2. The advisory committee led by Goldschmidt recommended the board be small enough to act quickly and structured more like a corporate board with the president as a voting member. In Billups' original version of SB 2, the board would have nine members, including two who were also members of the State Board of Higher Education, one student member, the president, and five representatives appointed by the governor who "have experience in areas related to the university missions."

Robert Noose, executive director of the Oregon Student Lobby, representing students in all of the state's public universities, proposed a change in that plan in his testimony before the Senate Education Committee. He argued the board should have two student members serving staggered terms so every new student member on the board would have a senior student member to teach them the ropes.

Hartung wasn't sympathetic to that argument. He said even state board members have to be quick studies. "It is really incumbent on whoever the member is to get up to speed fast," he said. "We can't serve as a training ground."

Others proposed suggestions for the board's composition. The American Federation of State, County and Municipal Employees Local 328 requested a seat on the board. Timms introduced an amendment to reduce the state board representation to one member of the OHSU board. Trow said the chancellor or the state university system should be a nonvoting member of the board "to help with that interconnectedness we talked about."

Kohler recommended the board be limited in size and composed mostly of governor appointees. "If we get too many [positions] that have to be filled by various categories, I'm just concerned that we're not going to be able to move as we will need to in the future with regard to the decisions that are going to be important to this institution," he said.

The committee also debated whether the president should be on the board. Trow said the president "should work for the board, not be a member of the board." Kohler said putting the president on the board would "provide a certain continuity," but added, "this is not something that I asked for from the advisory committee at all."

Legislators were undecided. "You have to think you might make a CEO with great power and authority if he is on the board as well," said Hartung, "and maybe that's good and maybe it's not."

The committee voted down the students' request to have two members on the board, but allowed one.[69] It resumed its debate on whether the president should be on the board at its third meeting. Baker expressed deep reservations.

"In deference to Dr. Kohler here," he said, "if you make the president of the university a member of this board, you could set up a situation in which the president of the university could be the chairman of the board, and you start to collapse an awful lot of power into that individual, and we're creating kind of a new animal here. . . . I am more comfortable with the model in which you don't have that bizarre position."

Hartung countered that the advisory committee recommended OHSU adopt the structure of a private company. "If we are going to make this public corporation as competitive as it possibly can be, it is well to have the president and CEO a member of the board," he said.

Senator Shirley Gold (Democrat from Portland), agreed with Baker. "We should take a step at a time in this and maybe two years from now, after we see it all at work, maybe we'll come to a different conclusion," she said. "I'm nervous enough about doing this at all much less taking more extreme steps."

In the end, the committee voted in favor of a seven-member board comprising a student, a member of the state board, and five governor appointees. The president would not be on the board.[70]

The Ways and Means education subcommittee spent little time on the board composition. Ronda Trotman Reese, the young mother studying to become a dentist and member of the state board, testified in support of OHSU's conversion to a public corporation and said she was comfortable with having only one student member on the board.[71]

Buckman, the PacifiCorp CEO, reminded the lawmakers that the Public Corporation Advisory Committee concluded the OHSU president should be on its board.[72]

"That is something that would be expected of a private corporation," he said, "and I think that it would be unfair in an environment where we are asking Oregon Health Sciences University to compete with private enterprise for it to be shackled in its ability to compete on an equal basis."

But the issue did not come up again until the next day when Timms told the committee that the Senate Committee on Education had reconsidered and wanted Kohler on the board.

"They have re-thought their thinking," he said. "It was one of those kind of snap decisions that are made without really thinking it through. It doesn't make a lot of sense I think to have the CEO not on the board."[73]

Without comment, the committee approved the change and had no other discussion on the board's makeup and size. So in its final version, SB 2 establishes a seven-member board that includes the president, one student, one state board member, and four members appointed by the governor.[74]

WHO CONTROLS THE LAND?

In the Ways and Means education subcommittee's second session on SB 2, Representative Hayden, the conservative Republican from Lyons, dropped a bombshell that could mortally wound the public corporation by destroying its capacity to raise private money. Hayden said the House Republican caucus was supportive of allowing OHSU to become a public corporation provided the legislature would have the option to sell the state land OHSU was built on.[75]

"If Oregon Health Sciences University has the opportunity to transfer or obligate the property then of course that would preempt our ability to recover the property and sell it in 10 or 20 years if we got in a real fiscal bind," Hayden said, "so I would like to have that cleared up before I make a decision on my vote."

Kohler and his team saw trouble. OHSU would have to be able to show potential investors that it had guaranteed unfettered use of the land. Without exclusive care, custody, and control of the land, it could not borrow money. And one of the chief reasons for becoming a public corporation was to gain access to capital.

Legislative Counsel Tom Clifford, who had no political or partisan interests in the bills his office handled, tried to explain this to Hayden and the committee. The university needed the land to issue bonds, he said.

Giving the legislature the option of taking the land back to sell "may be to impair beyond repair the prospect for this Oregon Health Sciences University to proceed."[76]

But Hayden insisted there must be a way.

"We're giving them the property with the debts, and we should be able to say that we retain the option of retaking the property with the debts," he said. "In that case the debts would be covered by the security of the state, the full faith and credit of the state, and I would think anyone wouldn't hesitate to issue bonds with that kind of backing."[77]

Billups stepped up to the table and calmly tried to reason with Hayden. She said OHSU was seeking a long-term lease.

"The university really has to be in a position of being able to represent to the financial market that we have the same rights to use this property for a long period of time as any other lessor has the right to use property, and in that role we are simply a tenant," she said. "The state affirming in the statute that at any time the state could transfer or otherwise dispose of the property would really impair beyond repair the ability that we might have to access any type of financial market."[78]

But Hayden wouldn't budge. OHSU's proposal to become a public corporation was a "grand experiment," he said, and "not a final culmination of events."

"We want it in the bill so there is clear understanding that if at some future time the state would say we really need a billion dollars, and we have it in surplus property, and here it is, and we're going to give you five years notice, and we're going to sell it to Legacy, Sisters or Providence [hospitals], whomever. I would like to see that option, and I think that's fiscally prudent to do."[79]

Billups assured Hayden that the state does have authority to change the statute. But, she added, "to put that sort of language in the statute is a different matter because it sends a message to the market that we're not trusted."

She suggested a compromise. OHSU could negotiate a ground lease with appropriate state agencies and "set out what the rights and obligations of both parties are with respect to future use, sale or other transfer of property." Billups called up the experts, Doug Goe, the bond lawyer, and Al Kowalski, a higher education financial expert. Goe assured Hayden OHSU could not sell the land. "It is clear, and it's always been the deal that the title to real property and buildings remains with the state," Goe said. However, he added, OHSU was giving up its access to state-backed bonds to become independent. So it had to be able to raise money in the private market, and to do that, it had to have control of its lands and buildings so it can generate money to pay back what it borrows. He again made the case that Clifford and Billups had made.

"So if you put language in the bill that suggests that the state can come back and take those land and buildings away, those sources generating the revenues to repay the investors, you're going to cut off the public corporation at the knees to start," he said.[80]

Kowalski said bond insurers and ratings agencies would have problems with OHSU not having control of its facilities. Investors were edgy about lending money to academic health centers because they "are under the gun all across the country," Kowalski said.[81] Timms explained the university was seeking authority to sell revenue bonds, which would be paid back with OHSU earnings, rather than general obligation bonds, which are paid off with taxes.

"If we handicap the Oregon Health Sciences University by requiring certain things that affect their bonding," he said, "we could hurt what we are trying to do, and that is to allow them to operate with a little bit more freedom, and that's what we're talking about in the system, to do a better job for the patients and research and teaching."

Oakley the committee chair, asked Billups if there was a way to tighten the language in the bill to appease Hayden. Billups said she could. She proposed saying that state property under the care and control of OHSU "shall not be sold by the university and shall only be obligated in accordance with state law."

Hayden accepted the wording. "It is allowing the university to use this property, to bond this property, but not to sell this property," he said, "and future legislators may in fact elect to return control of this property to the state."[82]

Kohler and his leadership team felt like they had narrowly avoided getting washed over a financial cliff. Billups' language survived in the final version of SB 2.

A SOLUTION

In the Ways and Means education subcommittee's final meeting, Kohler said that OHSU faced a 16 percent reduction in state support in the coming biennium, which without change would have "devastating consequences" for the university. SB 2, though, would enable the university to reduce the impact and avoid closing major services and programs.

> The Legislature must deal in the realities of the revenues it has before it today, and so must we. SB 2 represents an opportunity to reinvent and streamline government, to show we are willing to do things differently, and to set OHSU on a course to realize its potential as a world-class academic health sciences center and an economic engine for the state. When this new approach proves to be the enormous success story I know it will be, it will represent a significant point of pride for all of us—the Legislature, the governor, the state, and OHSU.

This was Kohler's major selling point. Rather than ask for more money, he proposed a solution, a way for OHSU to raise money for itself.[83]

The bill reached the full Joint Ways and Means Committee on April 21, and the panel devoted most of its short time on the bill to how much money to give OHSU as a public corporation. Timms introduced the bill to the committee and noted it would give the university about $100 million plus another $3.8 million in lottery money over the 1995–97 biennium as recommended by the governor.[84] Most of the state money, $62 million, was allocated to the university's educational and general services, $28 million to support the hospital and clinics and $10 million to the Child Development and Rehabilitation Center. The lottery money was also divided three ways: $134,000 for the university's physician assistants program, $1.7 million to the AHECs, and $2 million to nursing education.[85]

OHSU would be getting 16 percent, or $19.5 million, less from the state than it was receiving in its current biennium.[86] As Kitzhaber had whispered to Kohler at the news conference earlier in the year, OHSU would get no more in the 1997–99 biennium. It would be on its own to grow.

Legislators pored over SB 2 in their committees for about sixteen hours in total, and probed many other issues. Billups took them through every section of the thirty-four-page bill. They wanted assurances the legislation would comply with state and federal requirements for its disabled workers, and that it would continue to press for more minority representation in its workforce and student body. They looked at how the conversion to a public corporation might affect research and OHSU's commitment to its traditional education and indigent care missions. They examined OHSU security, student fees, employee rights, audits, retirement plans, the university's freedom to invest in stocks, its transition plans, and more. Nearly all of them showed respect, and sometimes admiration, for the university and what it was trying to do—a far cry from those days in the early 1980s when legislators looked at the university and its struggling hospital with disdain and even considered shutting it down.

During one session of the Ways and Means education subcommittee, Representative Larry Wells, a Republican from the small town of Jefferson near Salem, stepped back and asked Fred Buckman, the PacifiCorp president, "if you could put in a few words, the argument I could use if I was out with an average constituent, out on someone's farm or whatever, and he asked me why I should support this or why I supported this bill. . . . In just a few short words, why is this good for the state?"[87]

Buckman used a lot of words in his first attempt. "Oregon Health Sciences University is unique in that it has a public responsibility over and above the public responsibility that private hospitals have, both from an educational perspective and from a perspective of providing services in rural areas and to the indigent." He went on to explain its competitive challenges.

"You think the average guy on the street really understands what you're saying there?" replied Wells.[88]

Buckman took another shot.

> The average guy on the street understands that Oregon Health Sciences University provides services in rural areas and St. Vincent's [hospital] doesn't have to, and that Oregon Health Sciences University had a higher percentage of people who cannot pay their bills than other hospitals do. If you are asking it to do those extraordinary things, at the same time you can't make it more cumbersome for the hospital to deal with the things it needs to deal with in order to do its business.[89]

In the final hearing before the full Joint Ways and Means Committee, Representative Mannix took a turn at explaining the purpose of SB 2.

> We need to understand that when we talk about a public corporation it's sort of like sending your child off to school. You still maintain contact although the child becomes somewhat independent, and you are still a parent although you get nervous sometimes about your responsibilities. There is still a link here. . . . Oregon Health Sciences University is a different kind of creature in government, and we recognize that with this bill . . . We have a one size fits all Department of Administrative Service system for payroll, for benefits, for salaries, and that size is being stretched way out of whack sometimes to accommodate some functions. Oregon Health Sciences University with its grants and its special programs is a different kind of creature, and we have really stretched the fabric of the state government trying to cover it in terms of con-

> tracting personnel, purchases, all of that stuff. This bill recognizes that we are really better off giving it a new suit of clothes rather than trying to stretch the state suit of clothes.[90]

Senator Mae Yih, a conservative Democrat from Albany and longtime critic of OHSU, was the only person on the Joint Ways and Means Committee, or in all of the public hearings and work sessions of all the legislative committees, to oppose SB 2 and speak against it.

> I just want to say that I am not convinced that state agencies should become public corporations to avoid some regulations. We all live under regulations of different state agencies. The farmer must live under DEQ [state Department of Environmental Quality], LCDC [state Land Conservation and Development Commission], OSHA [federal Occupational Safety and Health Administration], and they would like to get away from regulations too, but there is no way for them to become a public corporation. I think that we need to work with agencies to reduce unnecessary regulations, but becoming a public corporation I do not believe is the way to do it. They are still going away with our land, state buildings, state equipment. I just don't think that's the way to go.[91]

With only Yih objecting, the Joint Ways and Means Committee on April 21 referred SB 2 to the Senate floor with a "do pass" recommendation. That gave Kohler's team only a matter of days to shore up support before the Senate voted. Davis counted votes, focusing particularly on some of the less-than-enthusiastic liberal Democrats. One of those was Trow, the history professor from Corvallis. Davis had long had a good working relationship with Trow, but lately he had been dodging her. When she finally caught up with him in a capitol hallway, she asked him if he had concerns about SB 2.

"He said, 'Look, I don't know if I can vote for it because I'm very worried that the university won't continue to carry out its public missions.'"[92]

Trow ultimately said he would support the bill, but with reluctance.

Senator Richard Springer (Democrat from Portland), also seemed to be on the fence, though OHSU was in the district he represented. Davis had a page deliver a note to him on the Senate floor during session one day, asking him to come to the lobby between votes to talk to her. Springer told Davis he would probably vote for the bill, but wasn't sure. He didn't like the idea of an essential public service such as OHSU operating more like a private business. He worried OHSU would start turning away poor patients as some private hospitals were rumored to do. He trusted the current leadership, he said, but was concerned about what could happen down the road when others were in charge. Davis made the best case she could for SB 2, but as Springer walked back into the Senate Chamber, she could count him only as "probably."[93]

Davis was confident OHSU had the votes it needed when the bill came up for a vote on the Senate floor on April 27. Senator Timms carried the bill to the floor and spoke eloquently on its behalf. No one spoke against the bill. The Senate then voted, approving the measure 24-3. Three Democrats opposed the bill. They were Yih and two liberals from Portland, Senators Bill McCoy and Randy Leonard. Hartung, a supporter, was away on legislative business and did not vote. Neither did Republican Senators Randy Miller and Marylin Shannon, supporters who had been excused from the session for other reasons.

Davis was not surprised that McCoy opposed the bill. A veteran legislator and former chair of the Human Resources Committee, he was a staunch advocate for the poor, and it was predictable he would worry about how the poor would fare under a corporate model for OHSU. Leonard, a first-term senator who would later become a member of the Portland City Council, was a complete surprise. He had at no point expressed any concerns about the bill. He would later tell Davis that Springer had convinced him to vote against the measure, even though Springer ended up supporting it. Springer said he had not explicitly told Leonard to vote "no," but had been critical of the bill in a conversation with Leonard.[94] In a 2016 interview, Leonard said he was not opposed to the public corporation concept, but he didn't want to see OHSU or any other government entity so free from government oversight. OHSU wanted to retain the benefits of its government status, such as a cap on tort claims, yet wanted to be free from government accountability, he said.[95]

"I don't regret the vote," he said. "If they could be a public corporation while at the same time having some process where the Legislature looks at their budget, I would support it."[96]

The House unanimously approved SB 2 on May 15, with three of the sixty members excused for other business.[97] Gordon Smith, the Senate president, signed the bill on May 19 as did Speaker of the House Beverly Clarno (Republican from Redmond). Five days later, Governor Kitzhaber signed the bill into law.

As Davis' favorite line in her four-page legislative white paper said, "OHSU had been unleashed to succeed."

Kohler spoke at Kitzhaber's bill signing ceremony on May 24, calling the legislation "dramatic change":

> SB 2 is a remarkable achievement, one that is already being looked at with envy by academic medical centers around the country. While others have made their hospitals independent, we are first in the nation to spin off the academic and research programs along with the hospital. There is no question that SB 2 will serve as a model for others around the country.[98]

On July 1, OHSU officially became a public corporation.

Two months later, its major employee union went on strike.

Notes

1 Public Advisory Committee, *Final Report*, Jan. 20, 1995, pp. 2, 3.

2 Ibid., p. 2.

3 Ibid., pp. 4, 5.
4 Ibid., p. 5.
5 Ibid., pp. 5, 6.
6 Sura Rubenstein, "Cutting Loose," *The Oregonian*, Jan. 23, 1995. p. B01.
7 Ibid.
8 Ibid.
9 Lois Davis, interview, Oct. 3, 2014, her office at Portland State University.
10 Lesley Hallick, provost and vice president for academic affairs, letter to Rep. Carolyn Oakley, chair of Ways and Means Education Subcomittee, April 4, 1995, and attached "Impact of Oregon's state rural health programs" and "Oregon Area Health Education Centers Program: A Sample of AHEC Accomplishments, 1990 to Present." Contained in Legislative History of SB2, a compilation of documents, OHSU legal office.
11 Senate Committee on Education Minutes, Public Hearing on Senate Bill 2, Tape 39A, Feb. 28, 1995, transcript, Oregon State Archives, p. 2.
12 Portland Mayor Vera Katz to the Senate Committee on Education and its members, letter, Feb. 17, 1995.
13 Lois Davis, unpublished account of her work on Senate Bill 2 called "Politics and Policy," Oct. 12, 2013, p. 13. In an interview on Feb. 12, 2016, Kitzhaber confirmed that he had told Kohler at the news conference to expect a flat budget. He said President Peter Kohler had "promised me that they were not going to need much general fund money. . . . I know I had run into Peter several times on the amount of money he wanted to get from the general fund, and I clearly remember him saying the amount of money OHSU was going to need from the general fund was going to decline."
14 President Peter O. Kohler was apparently unaware that the Oregon State Board of Higher Education at its December, 1994, meeting had stipulated that if OHSU was to become a public corporation, state money for OHSU's instructional programs would flow through the state board as a line item, and the amount would be fixed at the 1995–97 levels through 1997–99, after which state support would be scaled down.
15 OHSU, "From State Agency to Public Corporation," 1995.
16 Ibid.
17 Davis, interview, Oct. 3, 2014.
18 Janet Billups, interview in her office at Oregon Health & Sciences University, Oct. 6, 2014. Billups said, "No one monopolized the conversation, and we were pretty efficient, very focused. It was a really good group. There was a lot of laughter. There were very intense meetings, but never intense toward one another. . . . It was an extraordinary exception to the teams that I had seen before and after."
19 Jim Walker, telephone interview, Sept. 29, 2014.
20 Janet Billups, in written, unpublished 2014 account of her work in OHSU's conversion to a public corporation.
21 Ibid.

22 Senate Committee on Education Minutes, Public Hearing on Senate Bill 2, Tape 39A, Feb. 23, 1995, transcript, Oregon State Archives.
23 Peter O. Kohler's prepared testimony before the Oregon State Senate Education Committee, Feb. 23, 1995, a document in compiled Legislative History of Senate Bill 2, OHSU legal office.
24 Ibid.
25 Ibid.
26 Ibid.
27 Senate Committee on Education Minutes, Public Hearing on Senate Bill 2, Tape 40A, Feb. 23, 1995, transcript, Oregon State Archives.
28 Ibid., Tape 39B.
29 Ibid., Tape 40A.
30 Ibid.
31 Ibid., Tape 39B.
32 Senate Committee on Education Minutes, Public Hearing on Senate Bill 2, Tape 44A, Feb. 28, 1995, transcript, Oregon State Archives.
33 Senate Committee on Education Minutes, Public Hearing on Senate Bill 2, Tape 40B, Feb. 23, 1995. transcript, Oregon State Archives.
34 Senate Committee on Education Minutes, Public Hearing on Senate Bill 2, Tape 39A. Feb. 28, 1995, transcript, Oregon State Archives.
35 Peter O. Kohler, MD, "Oregon Higher Education and OHSU Today: Foundation of Tomorrow's Economy," Feb. 10, 1995. Peter Kohler collection, OHSU Archives. Video of speech online at: https://www.youtube.com/watch?v=lQA53RVjdeY.
36 Kohler was in the car with the vice chancellor of the University of Oklahoma en route to the OU Medical Center in central Oklahoma City when they saw smoke rising above the city after Timothy McVeigh blew up the federal building. The dinner was canceled, and Kohler and the vice chancellor spent the day visiting emergency rooms and studying the city's impressive emergency response system.
37 Kit Lively, "Autonomy Comes at a Price for Oregon's Public Colleges," *The Chronicle of Higher Education,* July 14, 1995.
38 Joye Mercer, "N.J. Governor's Plan to Eliminate Higher-Education Department Gets Mixed Reviews From College and State Officials," *The Chronicle of Higher Education,* April 6, 1994, p. A44.
39 Robert J. O'Neill Jr., "Local Governments' Enduring Reinvention Imperative," *Governing,* Oct. 30, 2013. Online at: http://www.governing.com/columns/smart-mgmt/col-reinventing-government-book-osborne-gaebler-impact-local-innovation-principles.html.
40 Lively, July 14, 1995.
41 Ibid.
42 Ibid.
43 Ibid.
44 Senate Committee on Education, Hearing on Senate Bill 2, Tape 43A, Feb. 28,

1995, transcript, Oregon State Archives.

45 Governor John Kitzhaber (interview, Feb. 1, 2016) said there may have been some "miscommunication" between him and President Peter Kohler and that he would not have intentionally blindsided Kohler. "I swear to God," he said, "one of the pitches he made to me is, 'We are not going to be a burden on the general fund anymore . . .' .What I heard him say, and I think this is one of the arguments I made to sell this to people who didn't like it, not the least of which was the university system, is that it is going to free up general fund money long term because they are going to be self-sufficient."

46 Lois Davis, unpublished 2013 written account of OHSU's conversion to a public corporation, p. 16.

47 Enrolled Senate Bill 2, page 6, section 13(1).

48 Lois Davis, unpublished 2014 written account of OHSU's conversion to a public corporation, p. 16.

49 Ibid., pp. 16, 17.

50 John Kitzhaber (former governor), interview, Feb. 12, 2016, downtown Portland.

51 Lois Davis, unpublished 2014 written account of OHSU's conversion to a public corporation, p. 17.

52 Senate Committee on Education Minutes, Hearing on Senate Bill 2, Tape 39A, Feb. 28, 1995, transcript, Oregon State Archives.

53 Senate Committee on Education Minutes, Hearing on Senate Bill 2, Tape 44B, Feb. 28, 1995, transcript, Oregon State Archives.

54 Senate Committee on Education Minutes, Hearing on Senate Bill 2, Tape 49A, March 2, 1995, transcript, Oregon State Archives.

55 Senate Committee on Education Minutes, Hearing on Senate Bill 2, Tape 42A, Feb. 28, 1995, transcript, Oregon State Archives.

56 Ibid, Tape 41B.

57 Ibid.

58 Ibid.

59 Ibid., Tape 43B.

60 Senate Committee on Education Minutes, Hearing on Senate Bill 2, Tape 48B, March 2, 1995, transcript, Oregon State Archives.

61 SB 2 (enrolled), 68th Legis. Assemb., Reg. Sess. (Oregon 1995), § 62a, 19 and 20; 62b, 1, 62c, 1; pp. 18, 19.

62 Senate Committee on Education Minutes, Hearing on Senate Bill 2, Tape 42B, Feb. 28, 1995, transcript, Oregon State Archives.

63 Ibid., Tape 43A

64 Joint Ways and Means Education Committee, Hearing on Senate Bill 2, Tape 79B, April 13, 1995, transcript, Oregon State Archives.

65 Ibid., Tape 81A.

66 Proposed Amendments to A-Engrossed Senate Bill 2, SB 2-A22, April 10, 1995. Contained in Legislative History of SB2, a compilation of documents, OHSU legal

office.

67 Joint Ways and Means Education Committee, Hearing on Senate Bill 2, Tape 81A, April 13, 1995, transcript, Oregon State Archives.

68 Ibid.

69 Senate Committee on Education, Hearing on Senate Bill 2, Tapes 43B, 44B, Feb. 28, 1995, transcript, Oregon State Archives.

70 Senate Committee on Education, Hearing on Senate Bill 2, Tapes 49A, 48B, March 2, 1995, transcript, Oregon State Archives.

71 Joint Ways and Means Education Committee, Hearing on Senate Bill 2, Tape 78B, April 12, 1995, transcript, Oregon State Archives.

72 Ibid., Tape 79A.

73 Joint Ways and Means Education Committee, Hearing on Senate Bill 2, Tape 81A, April 13, 1995, transcript, Oregon State Archives.

74 In 2001, with OHSU's merger with the Oregon Graduate Institute of Science and Technology, the OHSU Board of Directors was expanded to 10 members. The board in 2016 included Joe Robertson, the president; Suzy Funkhouser, a medical student; Ken Allen, executive director of the Oregon branches of the American Federation of State, County and Municipal Employees; and David Yaden, who was also a member of the Oregon State Board of Higher Education at the time of his appointment in 2009. Since Yaden joined the OHSU board, however, the State Board of Higher Education has been dismantled and replaced by a new 14-member body called the Oregon Higher Education Coordinating Commission.

75 Joint Ways and Means Education Committee, Hearing on Senate Bill 2, Tape 79B, April 13, 1995, transcript, Oregon State Archives.

76 Ibid.

77 Ibid.

78 Ibid.

79 Ibid.

80 Joint Ways and Means Education Committee, Hearing on Senate Bill 2, Tape 80B, April 13, 1995, transcript, Oregon State Archives.

81 Al Kowalski, higher education financial expert, told the committee that "from discussions we've had in New York as recently as a month ago, it would mean that bond insurance would not be available to Oregon Health Sciences University, and that would be a very dire consequence. It would also probably mean significant rating consequences."

82 Joint Ways and Means Education Committee, Hearing on Senate Bill 2, Tape 79B, April 13, 1995, transcript, Oregon State Archives.

83 Peter O. Kohler, "Opening Remarks for Works Session on S.B. 2", April 17, 1995, presidential papers, OHSU archives.

84 Joint Ways and Means Committee, Hearing on Senate Bill 2, Tape 9B, April 21, 1995, transcript, Oregon State Archives.

85 Proposed Amendment to Senate Bill 2, Sections 91 and 92, A-engrossed bill, p. 37.

86 Joint Ways and Means Committee, Hearing on Senate Bill 2, Tape 9B, April 21, 1995, transcript, Oregon State Archives.
87 Joint Ways and Means Committee, Hearing on Senate Bill 2, Tape 80A, April 12, 1995, transcript, Oregon State Archives.
88 Ibid.
89 Ibid.
90 Joint Ways and Means Committee, Hearing on Senate Bill 2, Tape 9B, April 21, 1995, transcript, Oregon State Archives.
91 Ibid.
92 Davis, interview.
93 Davis unpublished account, 2014.
94 Ibid.
95 Randy Leonard (former state senator from Portland and city commissioner for Portland), interview, July 17, 2016.
96 Ibid.
97 Representatives Tom Brian (Republican, Tigard); Tony Corcoran (Democrat, Cottage Grove); and Denny Jones (Republican, Ontario), were not present for the vote.
98 Peter O. Kohler, *Talking Points for Bill Signing Ceremony*, May 24, 1995, OHSU archives.

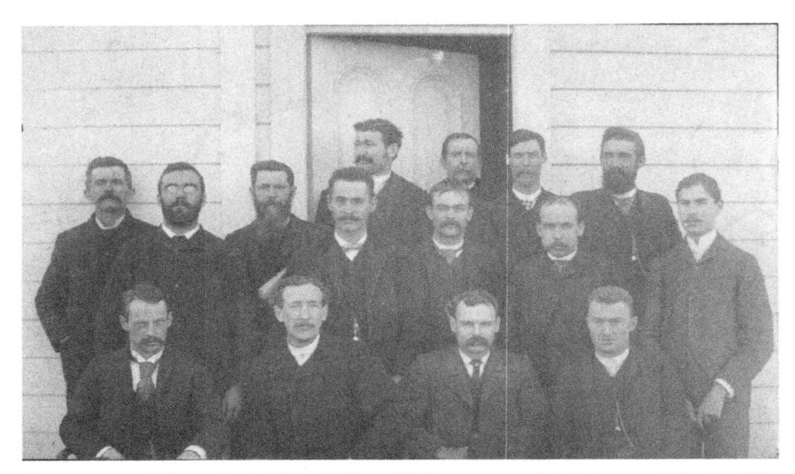

The University of Oregon Medical School's Class of 1889 poses somewhere in downtown Portland. The University of Oregon chartered the medical school in 1887 at the request of eight physicians, including four who broke away from a Willamette University medical school. The original University of Oregon school occupied two rooms of a former two-story grocery store at NW Twenty-Third Avenue and Marshall Street in Portland. The school moved in 1919 onto Marquam Hill and into a new medical school building, Mackenzie Hall, named after Dr. Kenneth A.J. Mackenzie. The men in this photo from the OHSU Archives are not named and may include some faculty members. *Courtesy of OHSU Historical Collections & Archives.*

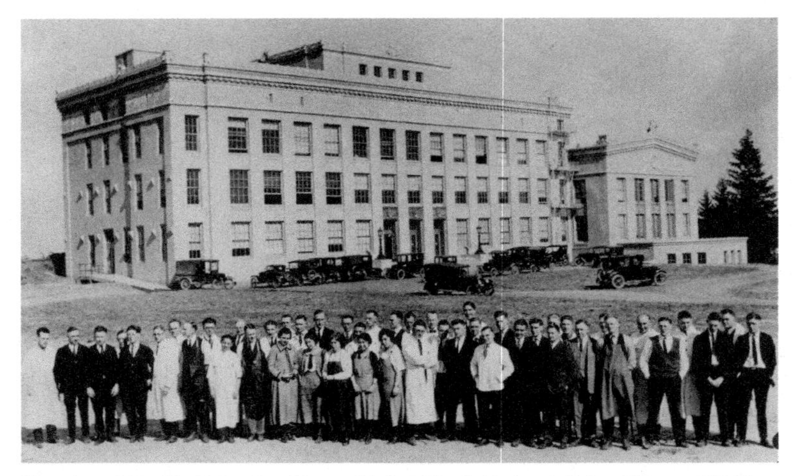

Photo from 1925 of the University of Oregon Medical School's Mackenzie Hall on Marquam Hill. The school's first building was completed in 1919 and named after its second dean, A. J. Mackenzie, MD, who persuaded the Oregon-Washington Railroad and Navigation Company to donate 20 acres on the hill to the school. *Courtesy of OHSU Historical Collections & Archives.*

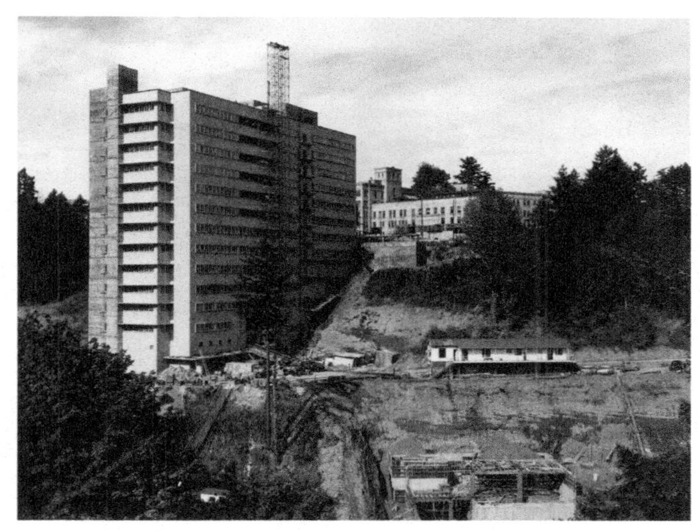

Under the leadership of David W. Baird, dean of the University of Oregon Medical School, and with federal funds secured by US Sen. Mark Hatfield, the university in 1956 constructs a teaching hospital, today's OHSU Hospital, on Marquam Hill. *Courtesy of OHSU Historical Collections & Archives.*

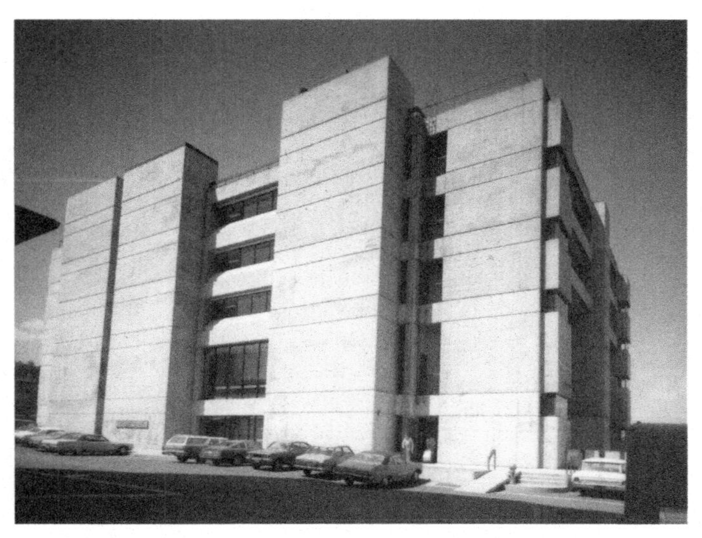

OHSU's eight-story Basic Science Building, now known as the Richard T. Jones Hall for Basic Medical Sciences, shown here in 1974, three years after it was completed. The building was designed by Campbell Yost Partners, an architectural firm known for its exposed concrete styles. The building has features of an architectural style called Brutalism with its angular, heavy cement exterior and windows framed and divided by thick bands of steel. The Brutalism style expressed strength and functionality and was popular among universities in the 1960s and 1970s. *Courtesy of OHSU Historical Collections & Archives.*

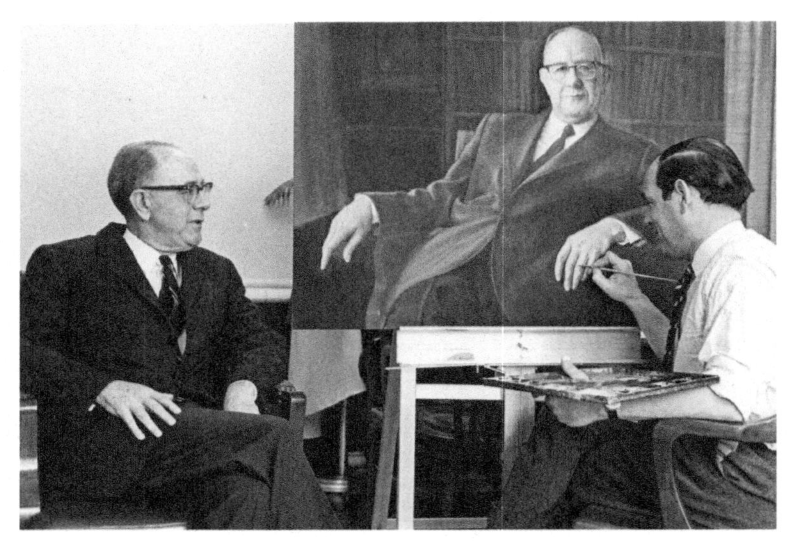

Dr. David W. Baird poses for a portrait in 1968 during his final year as dean of the University of Oregon medical school. He became dean in 1943 and led the school through a major expansion, including construction of University Hospital, and a new building for basic science and administration that is named after him. During his 25 years as dean, the medical school's fulltime faculty grew from 26 to 276 and the number of departments doubled to 39. He was a friend and adviser to Oregon's US Sen. Mark Hatfield. *Courtesy of OHSU Historical Collections & Archives.*

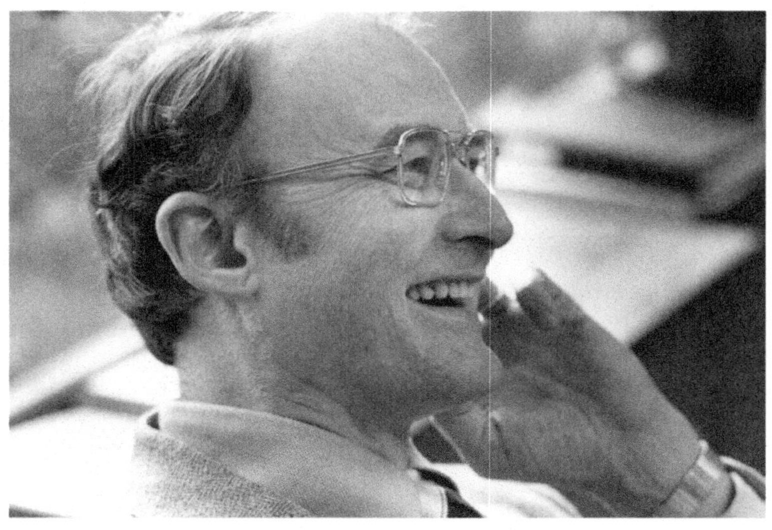

Dr. Lewis William (Bill) Bluemle, a nephrologist, served as the first president of the University of Oregon Health Sciences Center after it was created in 1974. He was tall and distinguished with a charming demeanor and sharp mind. He helped organize the university as an academic health center independent of the University of Oregon. But he found Oregon too parochial and left after less than three years. *Courtesy of OHSU Historical Collections & Archives.*

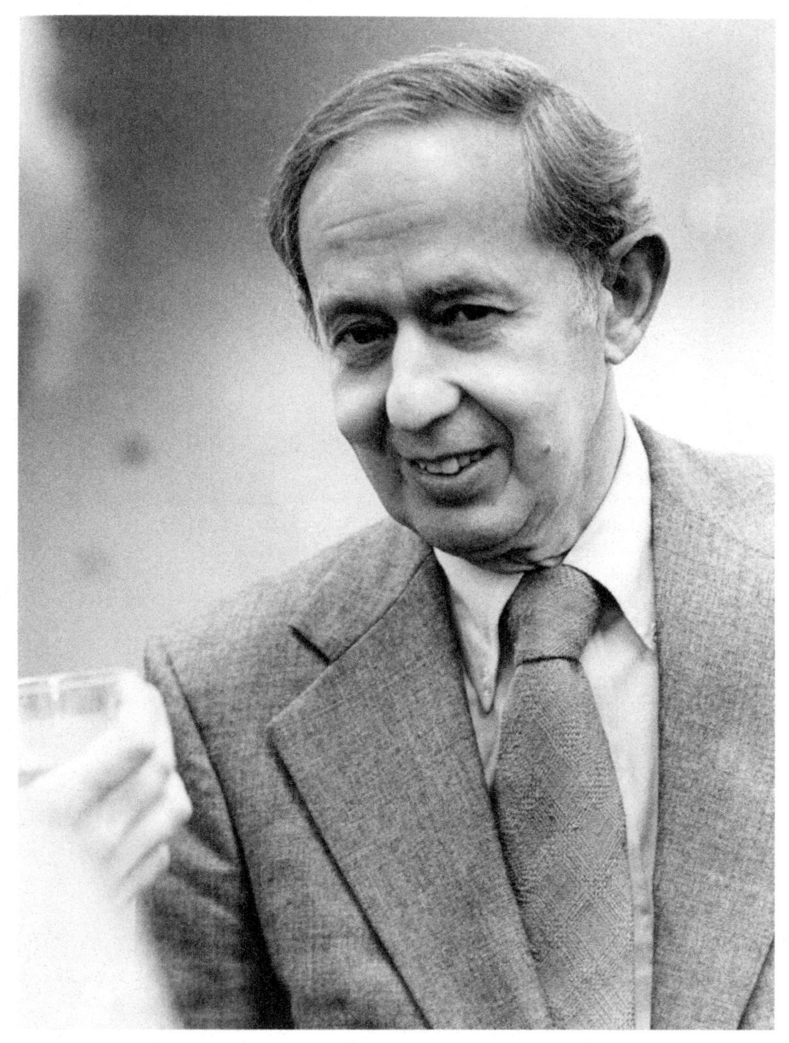

Dr. Robert Stone, a pathologist, was hired by Dr. Lewis William (Bill) Bluemle, as dean of the University of Oregon Health Sciences Center medical school. Stone, who served two years as director of the National Institutes of Health under President Richard Nixon, was an effective and tough dean. But he developed a reputation for also being mechanical and impersonal and at odds with many of the school's leaders, including Bluemle. *Courtesy of OHSU Historical Collections & Archives.*

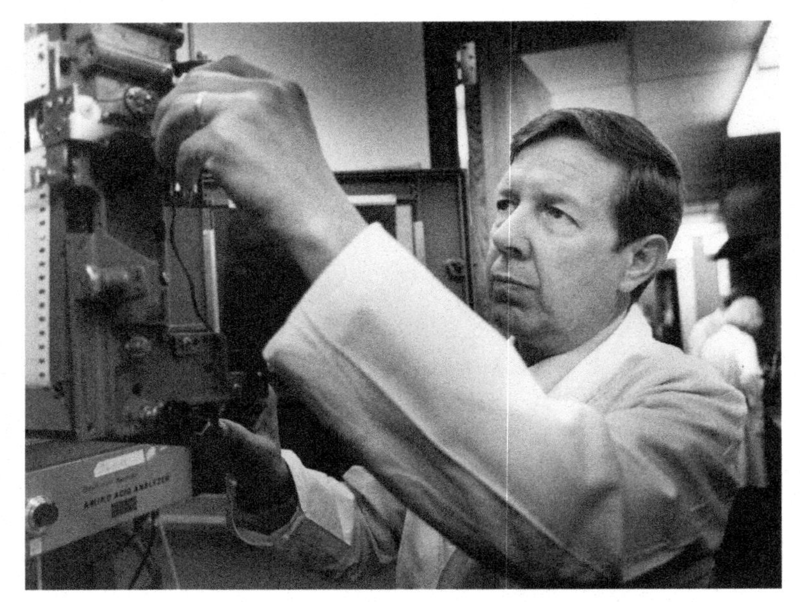

Dr. Richard Jones works in his laboratory. He chaired the biochemistry department in 1977 when he was appointed interim president after the University of Oregon Health Sciences Center's first president, Lewis William Bluemle, departed. Jones served as president 14 months until Leonard Laster was hired as the academic health center's second president in 1978. *Courtesy of OHSU Historical Collections & Archives.*

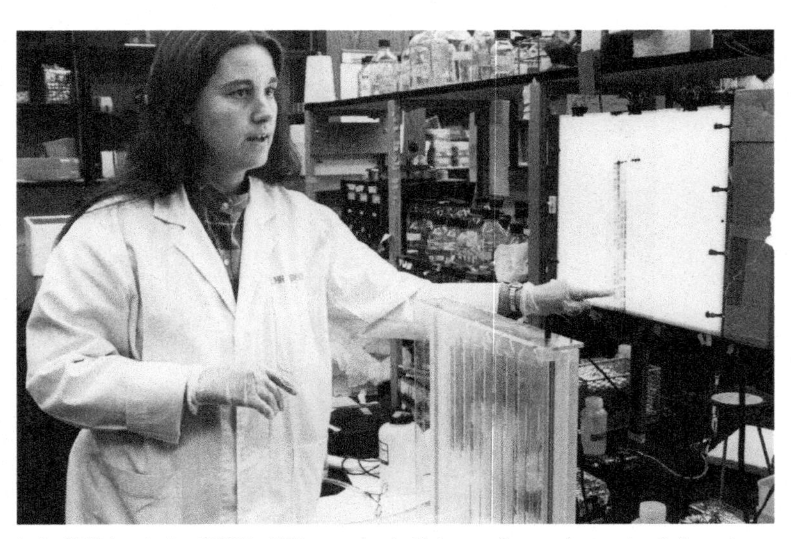

Lesley Hallick arrived at OHSU in 1977 as a molecular biology professor and researcher. In her early years at OHSU, she became a sounding board for President Leonard Laster. She said this photo was taken about 1987 or 1988. *Courtesy of OHSU Historical Collections & Archives.*

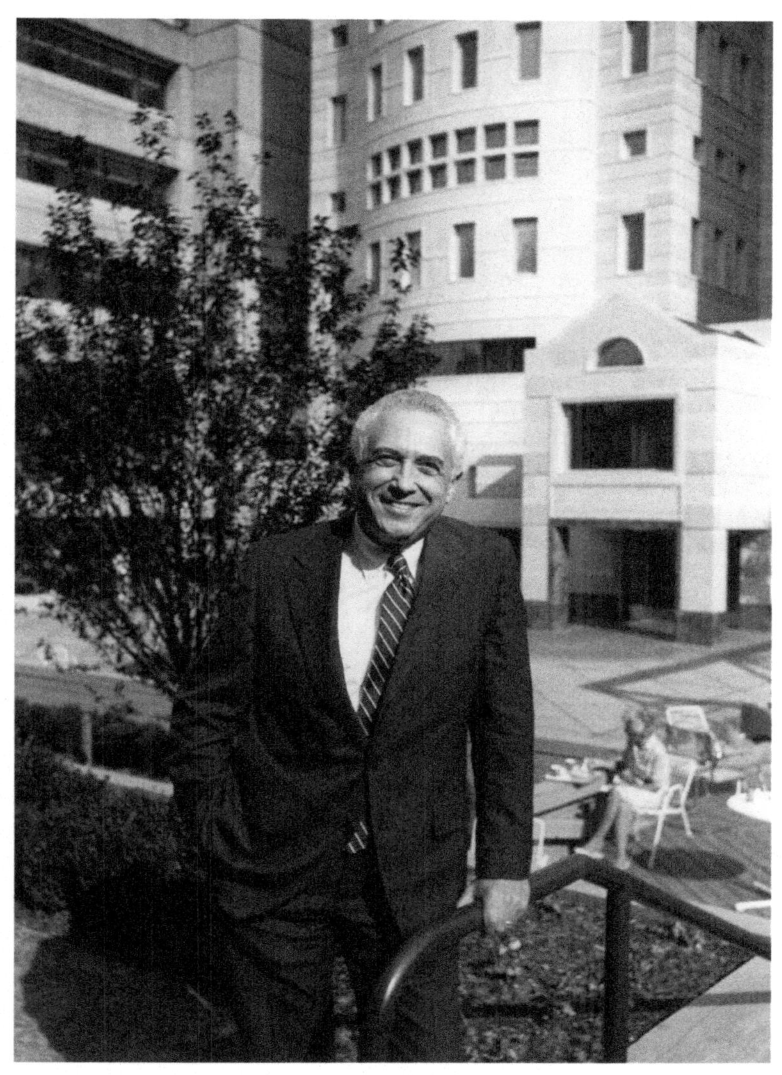

Dr. Leonard Laster, OHSU's second president, stands outside the newly completed building for the Vollum Institute for Advanced Biomedical Research in 1987. During his nine years at OHSU, the bright, charming gastroenterologist launched numerous expansion projects like the Vollum that set the stage for his successor, President Peter Kohler. Of the Vollum building, he said that what matters is not the cost and square feet, but rather the people who work inside. *Courtesy of OHSU Historical Collections & Archives.*

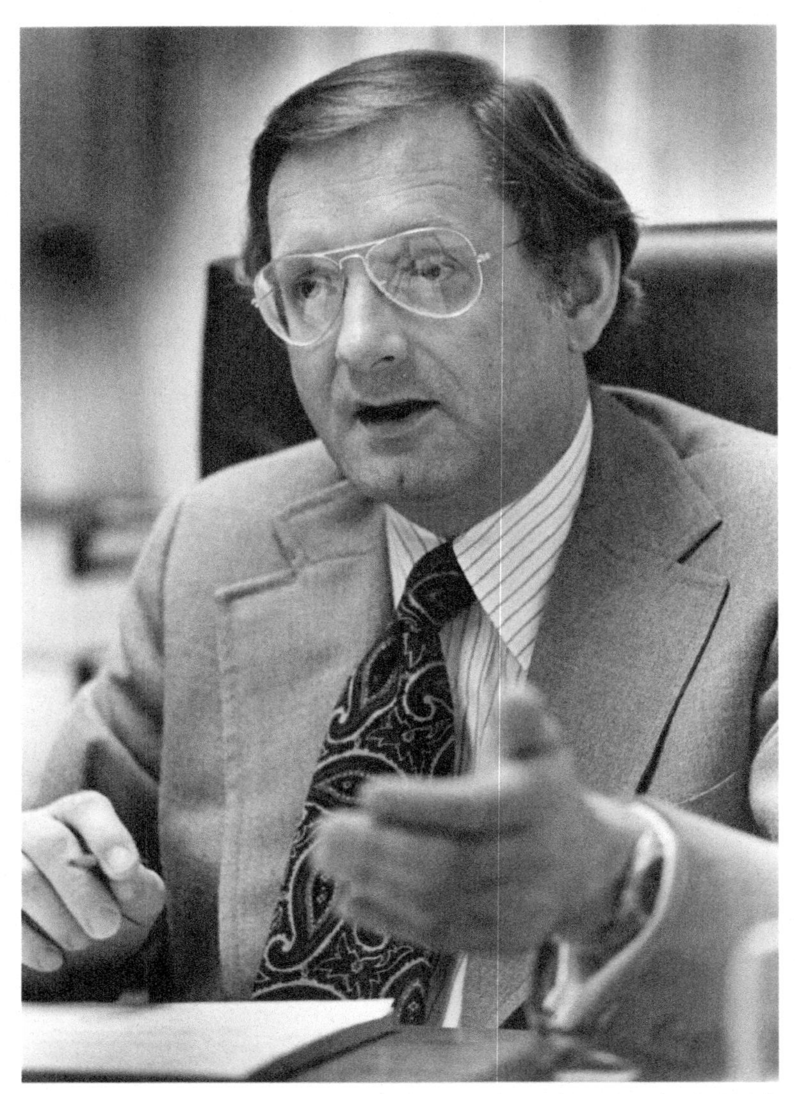

Dr. Donald Kassebaum, hired by President Lewis William Bluemle, served as vice president for OHSU's hospital services and director of the University Hospital under President Leonard Laster. Kassebaum initially liked Laster, but over the years, their relationship grew strained, coming to a head in 1986 when they agreed on a mutual parting. *Courtesy of OHSU Historical Collections & Archives.*

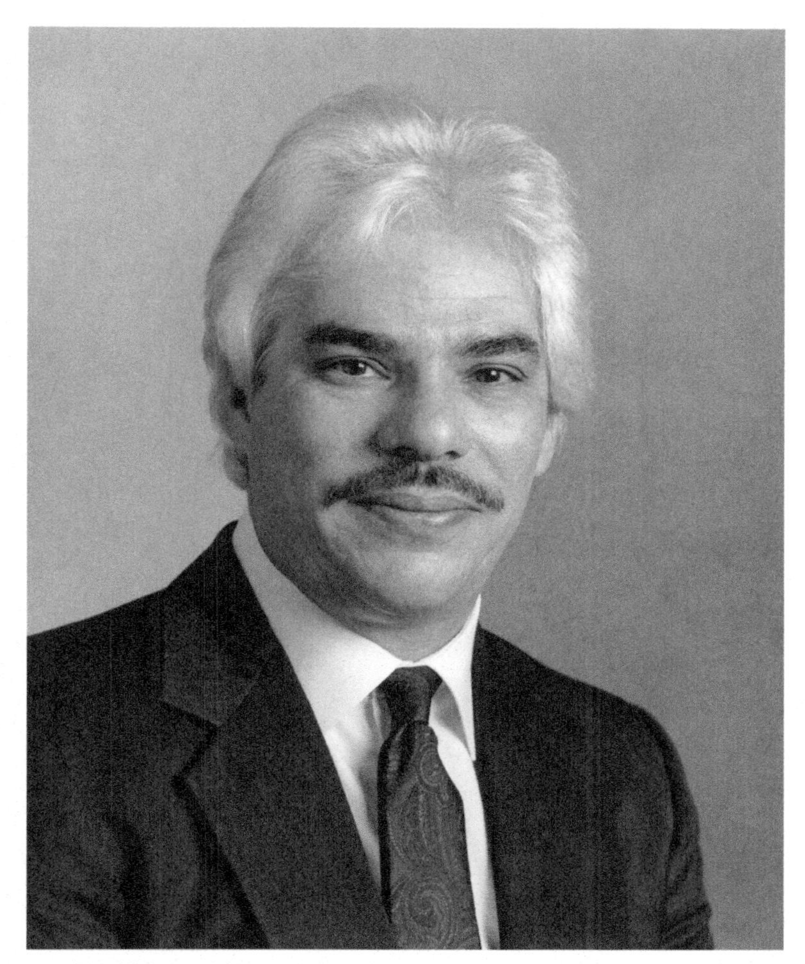

Timothy Goldfarb, pictured here in the late 1980s, joined OHSU in 1984 as an associate administrator of University Hospital and eventually became part of President Peter Kohler's leadership team in charge of all of the university's hospitals and clinics. He found OHSU so dysfunctional when he arrived that he tried to warn newly-hired James Walker, hospital chief finance officer, not to come. *Courtesy of OHSU Historical Collections & Archives.*

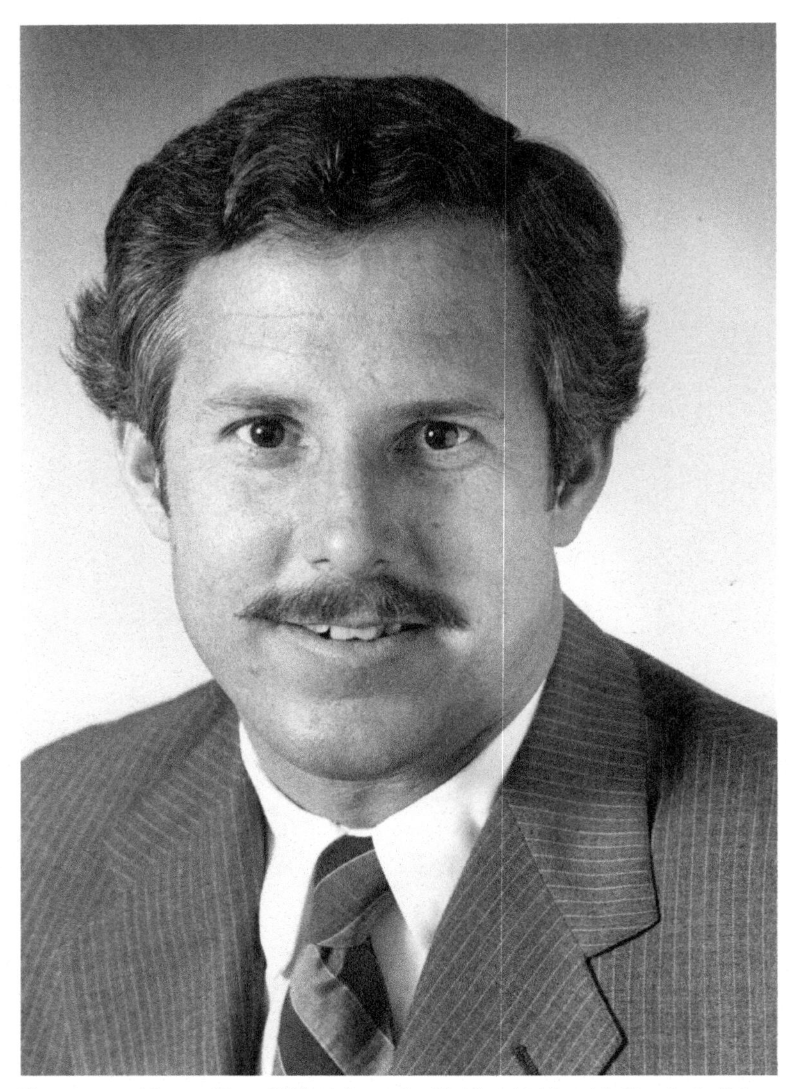

The young, good-humored James Walker left a comfortable job as chief financial officer for the University of New Mexico Hospital in 1983 to fill the same position at OHSU Hospital, though others warned him not to take the job. President Peter Kohler made him part of his core leadership team, and Walker played a key role in leading OHSU through its transition to a public corporation. *Courtesy of OHSU Historical Collections & Archives.*

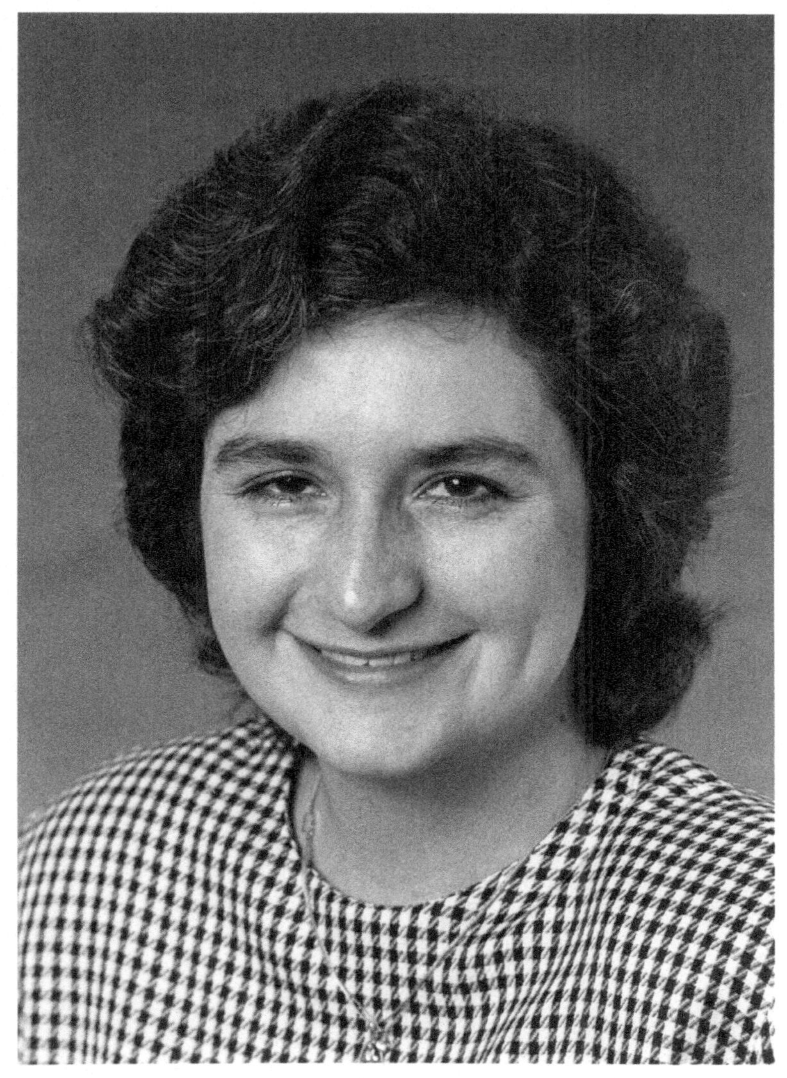

A young Lois Davis, chief of staff for US Representative Ron Wyden of Oregon, dropped by OHSU for an informational interview with President Leonard Laster in 1986, and the same day he offered her a job as lobbyist and liaison to the faculty. While he left OHSU eight months later, Davis stayed for 23 years. *Courtesy of OHSU Historical Collections & Archives.*

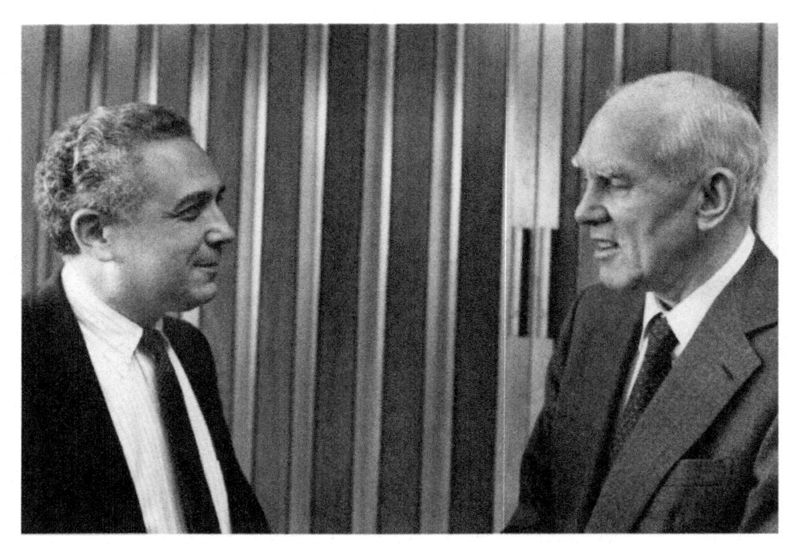

Dr. Leonard Laster, left, with friend and Tektronix founder Howard Vollum, who contributed $30 million to a building and endowment for the Vollum Institute for Advanced Biomedical Research, a major leap forward for research at OHSU. Laster called Vollum "one of the most brilliant people I've ever known." *Courtesy of OHSU Historical Collections & Archives.*

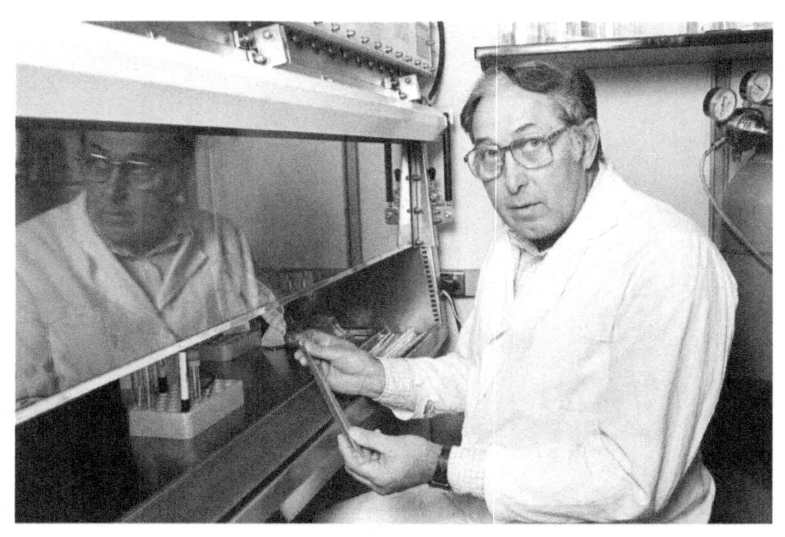

Edward Herbert, a top-notch molecular biologist at the University of Oregon, turned down a job at Harvard University to become founding director in 1983 of the Vollum Institute for Advanced Biomedical Research, specializing in the study of the molecular basis of the nervous system. President Leonard Laster said Herbert gave the institute "soul." Herbert died tragically of pancreatic cancer early in 1987, months before the institute could move into its new building. *Courtesy of OHSU Historical Collections & Archives.*

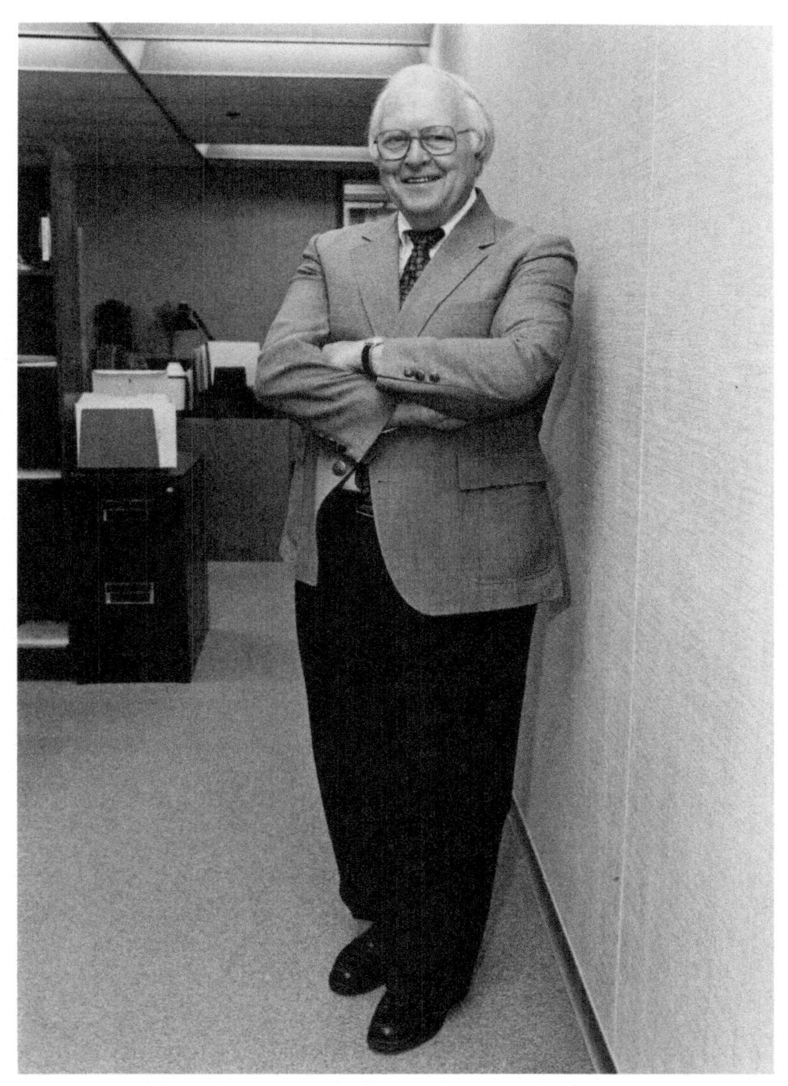

Dr. Julian S. "Dutch" Reinschmidt, joined the University of Oregon Medical School in 1970 as director of its Regional Medical Program and later of its continuing education program. President Peter Kohler put Reinschmidt in charge of leading OHSU's rural programs and Area Health Education Centers, which Provost Lesley Hallick called a key decision. "Dutch was beloved," she said. "He immediately had credibility across the state." *Courtesy of OHSU Historical Collections & Archives.*

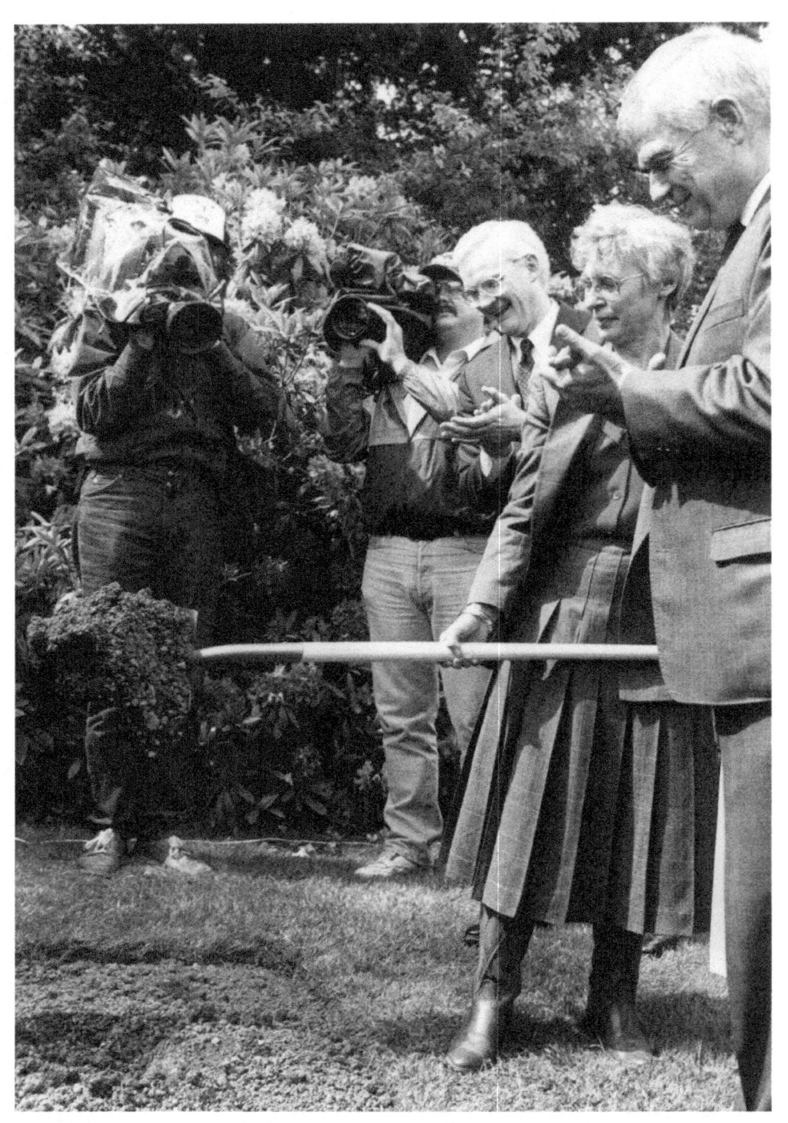

OHSU President Peter Kohler (left) and US Sen. Mark Hatfield applaud as Carol Lindeman, dean of the School of Nursing, breaks ground in 1990 on a $14 million building for the school. Lindeman led the effort to complete the building, which received federal support secured by Hatfield. The building was completed in 1992. *Courtesy of OHSU Historical Collections & Archives.*

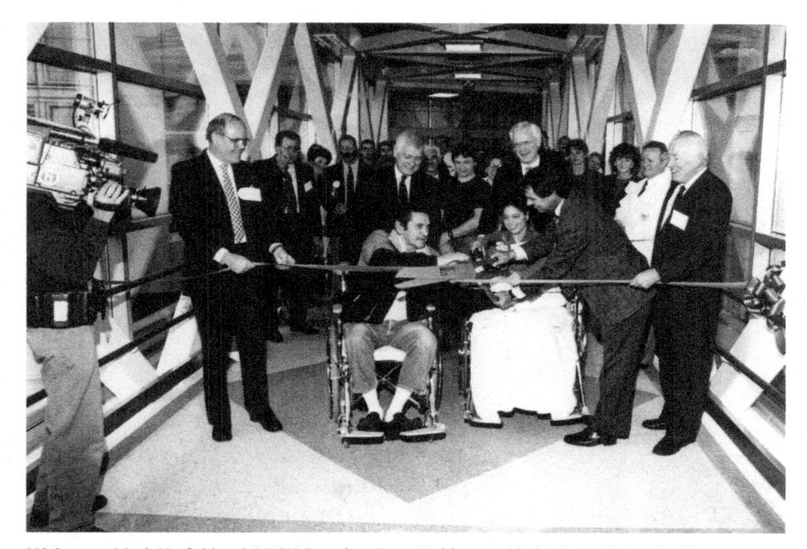

US Senator Mark Hatfield and OHSU President Peter Kohler stand behind people in wheelchairs as Barry Bell, director of the Veterans Affairs Medical Center, cuts the ribbon for the 1992 opening of the 660-foot-long bridge connecting OHSU Hospital to the VA Medical Center. Smiling at the far right is Dr. John W. Kendall, an endocrinologist, researcher and dean of OHSU's medical school from 1983 to 1992. Hatfield and former OHSU President Leonard Laster initiated the bridge project, but Kendall led it through to its completion. He also helped the medical school overhaul its curriculum in the early 1990s into a forward-thinking approach that reduced lectures and increased hands-on learning, drawing top students and national attention. He argued OHSU missed an opportunity to grow when it failed to go after research money during the rapid expansion of the National Institutes of Health during the 1950s and 1960s. *Courtesy of OHSU Historical Collections & Archives.*

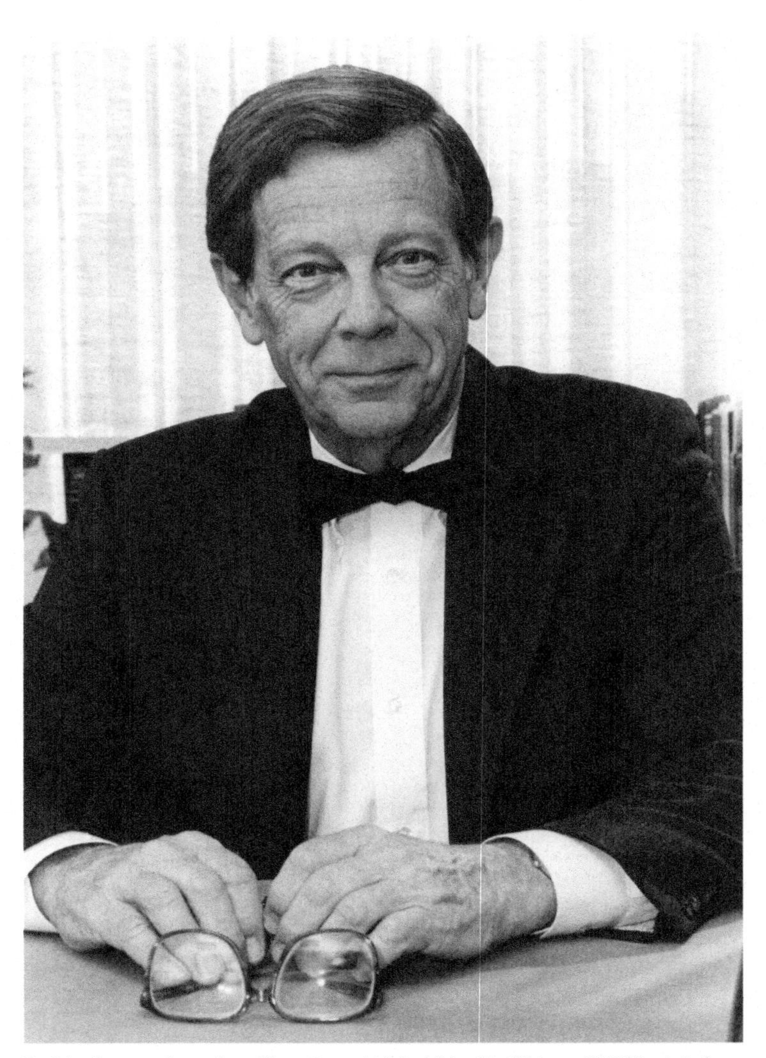

Dr. John Benson, who graduated from Harvard Medical School in 1946, was OHSU faculty's first full-time gastroenterologist and later dean of the medical school from 1991 to 1992, when the school's curriculum was overhauled. He joined OHSU as a professor and head of the Division of Gastroenterology in 1959, joined the board of the American Board of Internal Medicine in 1961 and became its president in 1975. He was one of one of OHSU's most nationally prominent physicians. *Courtesy of OHSU Historical Collections & Archives.*

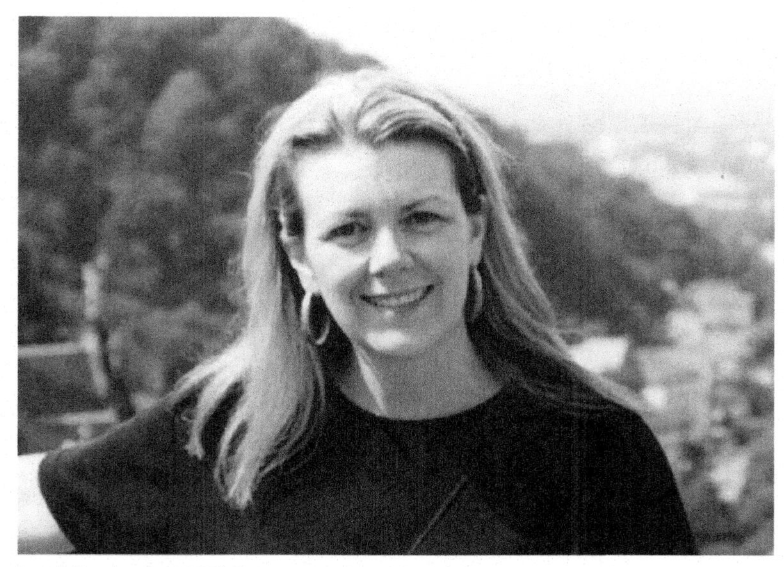

Janet Billups became OHSU's first attorney when Kohler hired her in 1992, made her part of his leadership team, and gave her the monumental challenge of drafting Senate Bill 2, the legislative and legal framework for OHSU's conversion to a public corporation. She continues to head OHSU's legal department. *Courtesy of Janet Billups.*

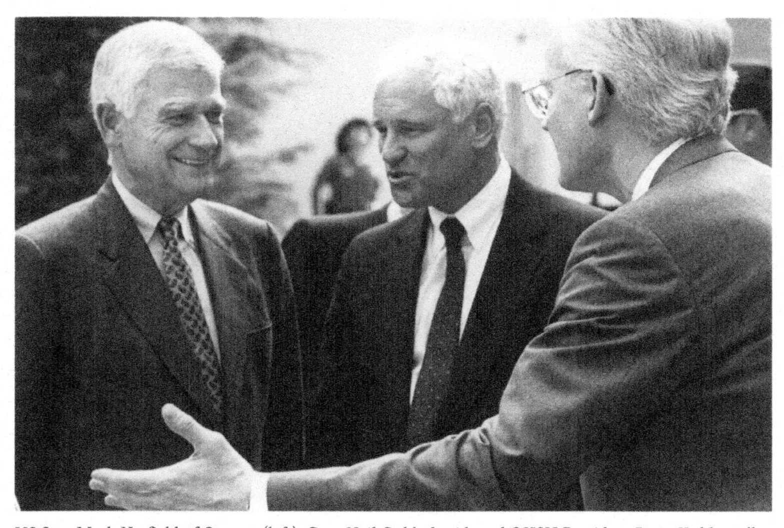

US Sen. Mark Hatfield of Oregon (left), Gov. Neil Goldschmidt and OHSU President Peter Kohler talk at a ground breaking event in 1990 for the Center for Research on Occupational and Environmental Toxicology (CROET). Hatfield and Goldschmidt proved strong supporters of OHSU's conversion to a public corporation and its subsequent expansion. *Courtesy of OHSU Historical Collections & Archives.*

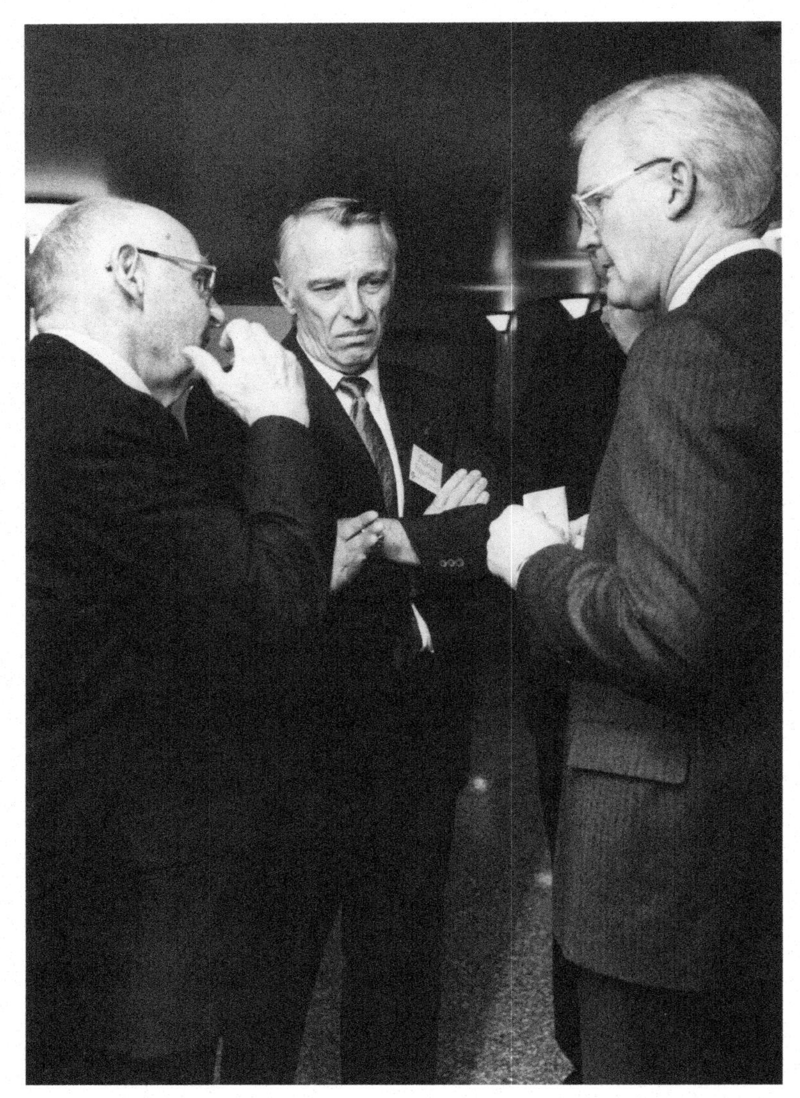

President Peter Kohler talks sometime around 1990 with Dr. Kenneth Swan (left), an ophthalmologist who built OHSU's Department of Ophthalmology into one of the nation's best, and Dr. Frederick Fraunfelder (center), who led efforts to build the privately-funded Casey Eye Institute, which opened in 1991. *Courtesy of OHSU Historical Collections & Archives.*

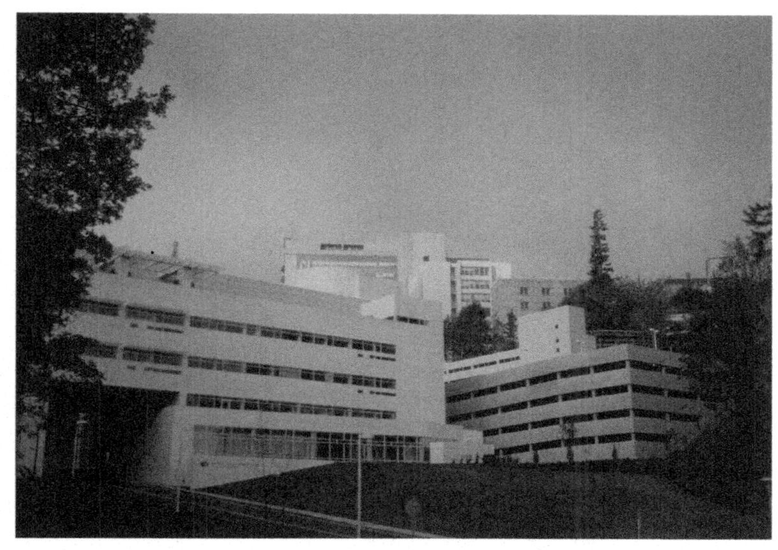

The Casey Eye Institute perches on the east side of the OHSU campus shortly after the building's completion. The privately-funded, $23 million building, which opened in 1991, provides a striking, elegant gateway to the OHSU campus. GBD architects, a Portland firm, designed the five-story building with clean lateral lines and ever-changing light. The 82,000-square-foot building, with an adjoining 320-car garage, includes the nation's largest glass floor designed by New York artist James Carpenter. The institute was named after contributors James Casey, founder of United Parcel Service, and his brother, George Casey. *Courtesy of OHSU Historical Collections & Archives.*

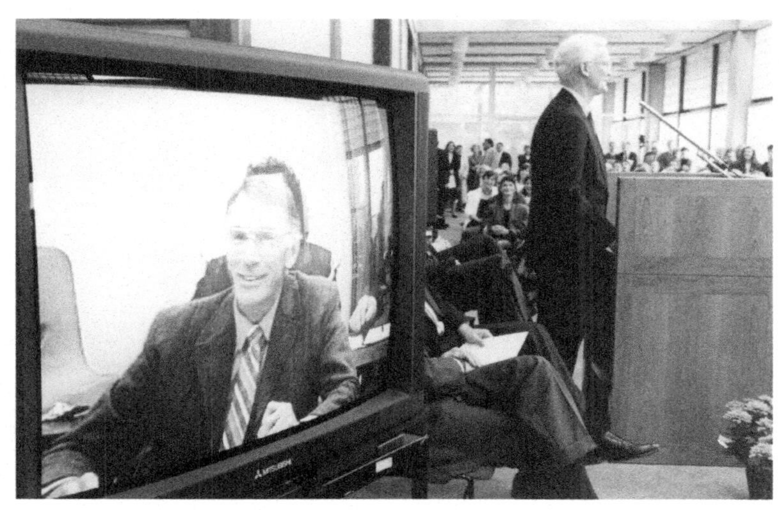

OHSU President Peter Kohler speaks at the 1991 opening of the Biomedical Information Communication Center, a high-tech medical library near the hospital on the university's Marquam Hill campus. *Courtesy of OHSU Historical Collections & Archives.*

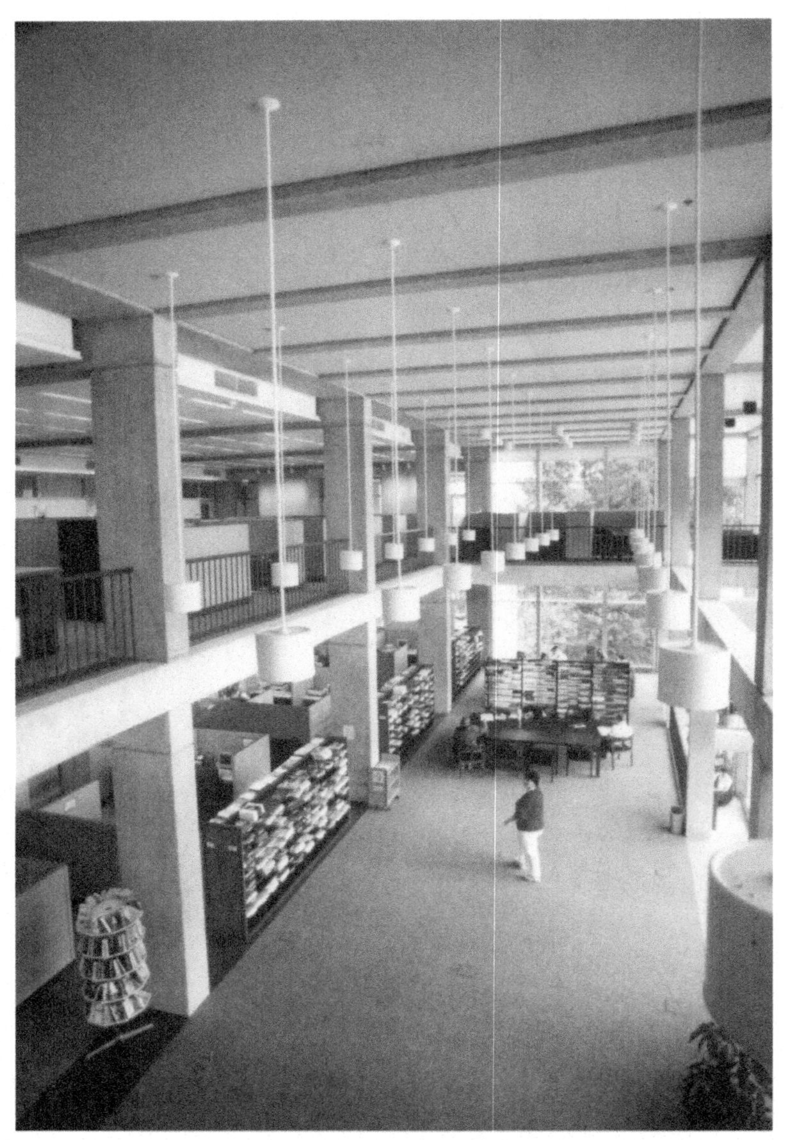

The elegant open interior of the $13 million Biomedical Information Communication Center fills with light. The "library of the 21st Century," which opened in 1991, allows distance learning and teleconferencing between rural doctors and OHSU specialists and remains one of the most sophisticated electronic medical libraries in the world. *Courtesy of OHSU Historical Collections & Archives.*

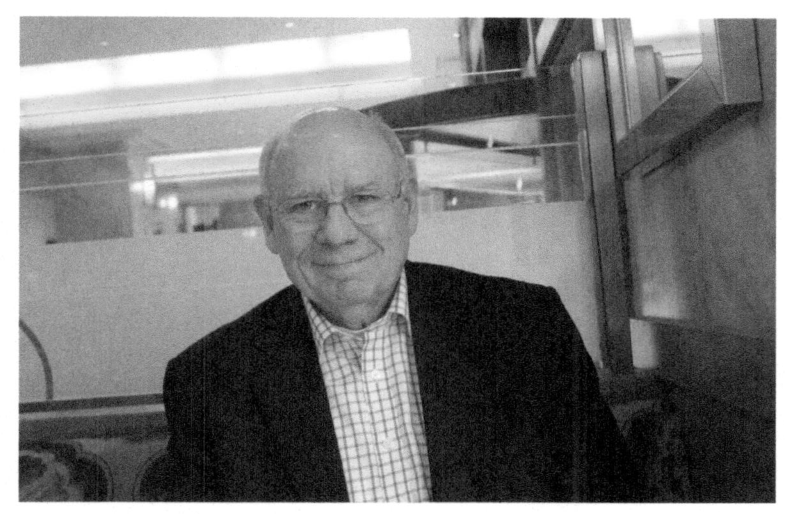

Dr. Grover Bagby, an expert and researcher on blood disorders, was a top research grant winner for OHSU, which is one reason President Peter Kohler made him director of OHSU's Oregon Cancer Center. In that role, Bagby recruited Dr. Brian Druker, who became one of the university's most renowned researchers for his discovery of a compound that has essentially cured a rare form of leukemia. *Image credit: William Graves.*

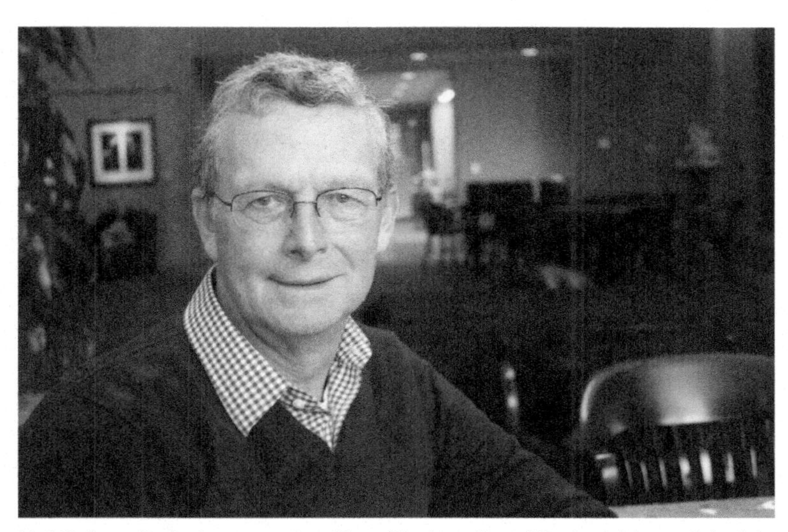

Mark Dodson, a Portland attorney and president of Northwest Natural Gas, headed the search that led to the hiring of Peter Kohler as president of OHSU in 1988. At the time of the search, Dodson was chair of both the State Board of Higher Education and the board's search committee and pushed hard for the selection of Kohler over other candidates. He served as the first OHSU board's unofficial secretary and remained heavily involved in OHSU's early years as a public corporation. *Image credit: William Graves.*

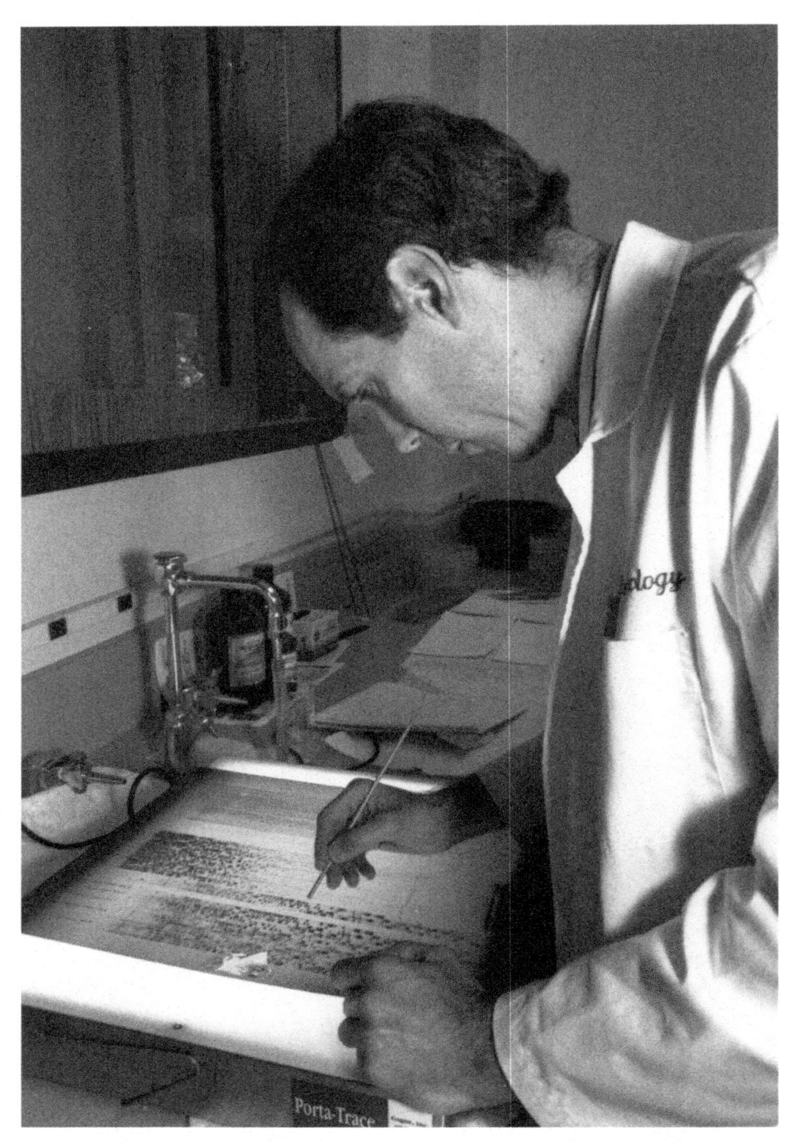

Dr. Brian Druker works in his laboratory where he discovered the power of a compound that was later named Gleevec in treating people with chronic myelogenous leukemia. Tens of thousands of CML patients are alive because they take a simple Gleevec pill daily. Druker epitomized the kind of researcher OHSU liked to go after—bright, ambitious and on the rising arc of a promising career trajectory. OHSU's Lois Davis said Druker's success "cast a sort of halo over the whole institution." *Courtesy of OHSU Historical Collections & Archives.*

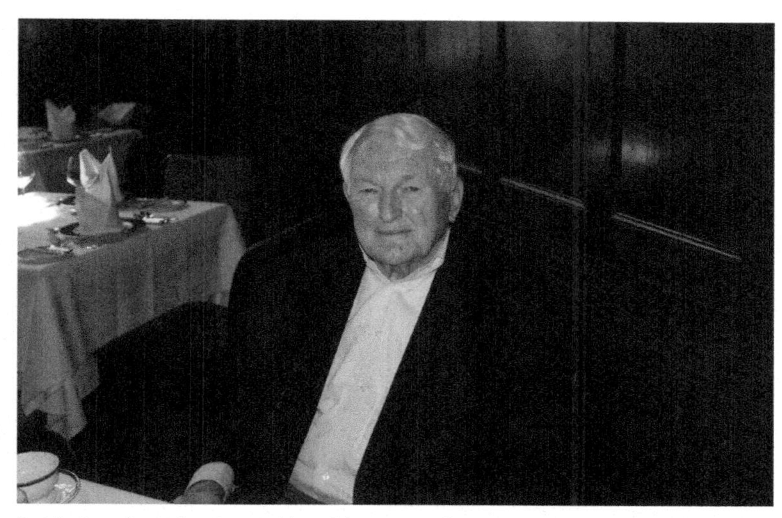

Paul Bradgon, former longtime president of the private and prestigious Reed College in Portland, was hired in the early 1990s to head the Oregon Medical Research Foundation, which funded research and operated the Oregon Regional Primate Center. Bragdon helped organize the merger of the Oregon Medical Research Foundation with the OHSU Foundation. He also helped with the merger of OHSU and the Oregon Graduate Institute of Science and Technology. *Image credit: William Graves.*

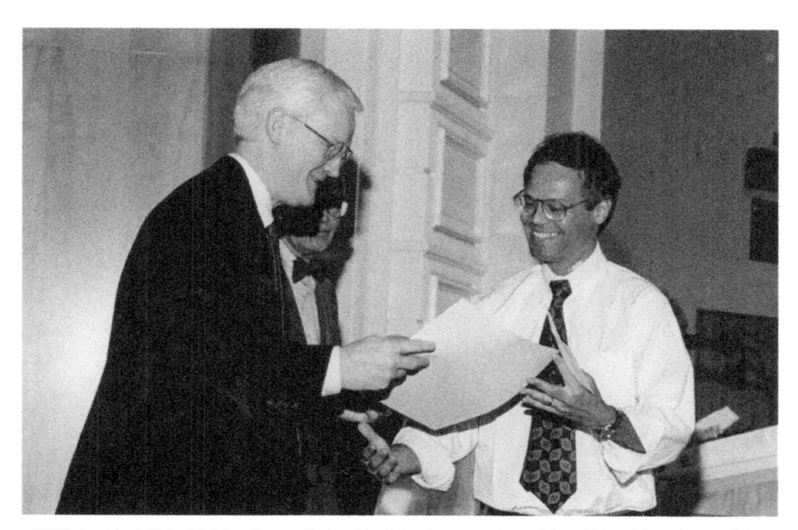

OHSU President Peter Kohler gives a distinguished faculty award in 1994 to Richard Goodman, a biochemist and molecular biologist who served as director of the Vollum Institute for Advanced Biomedical Research from 1990 to 2016. Kohler considered Goodman his first important recruitment. Goodman lured many nationally prominent scientists to Vollum and helped the institute gain a respected national profile. *Courtesy of OHSU Historical Collections & Archives.*

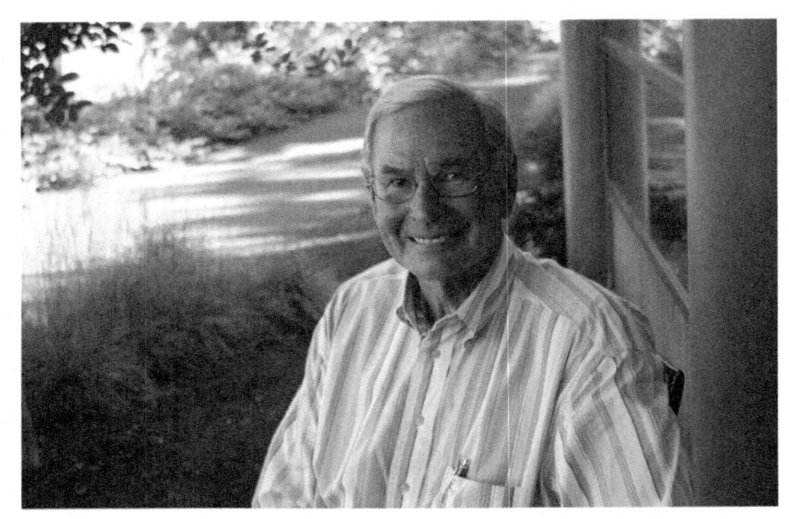

Mike Thorne, a plain-speaking Pendleton rancher and former state senator, helped OHSU President Peter Kohler expand health services in rural Oregon and was a strong supporter of the university's conversion to a public corporation. *Image credit: William Graves.*

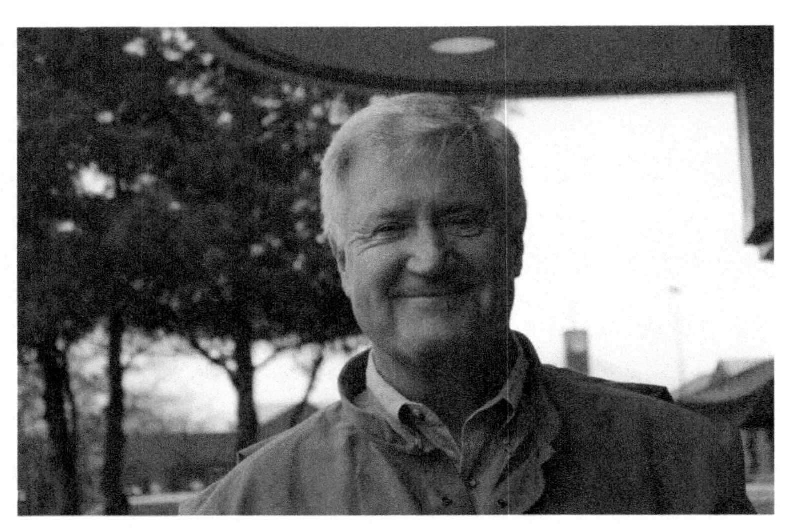

Fred Buckman, former president and chief executive officer of PacificCorp, served on the committee that recommended OHSU become a public corporation and chaired the university's first board of directors. The six-foot-four-inch, low-key executive saw OHSU through much of its explosive expansion on Marquam Hill and Portland's South Waterfront. *Image credit: William Graves.*

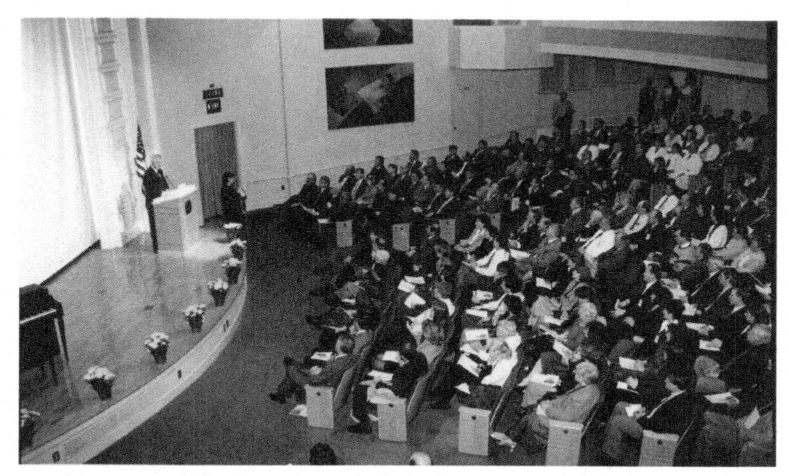

US Sen. Mark Hatfield speaks at the February, 1998, opening of the new OHSU research building named after him, the fourteen-story Mark Hatfield Research Center. *Courtesy of OHSU Historical Collections & Archives.*

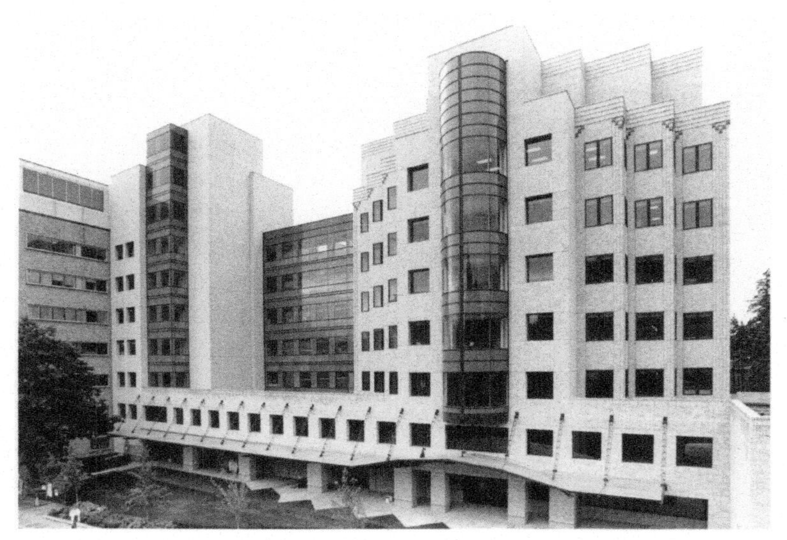

This view of the west face of the $60 million, 266,000-square-foot Mark Hatfield Research Center shows it attached to OHSU Hospital to the left. The research center was constructed in three phases between the library and hospital with both private and federal money. It provides space for a variety of research enterprises and an emergency room. *Courtesy of OHSU Historical Collections & Archives.*

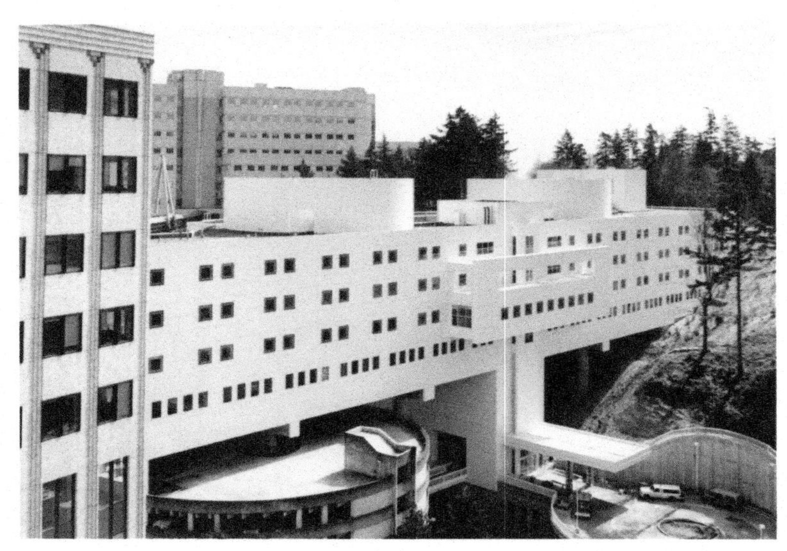

The state-of-the-art Doernbecher Children's Hospital spans a canyon on the Marquam Hill campus. The $73 million, four-story hospital, opened in 1998. An *Oregonian* reporter called the hospital, built with university bonds and $35 million in donations, "the most visible triumph for OHSU since it freed itself from state control in 1995." *Courtesy of OHSU Historical Collections & Archives.*

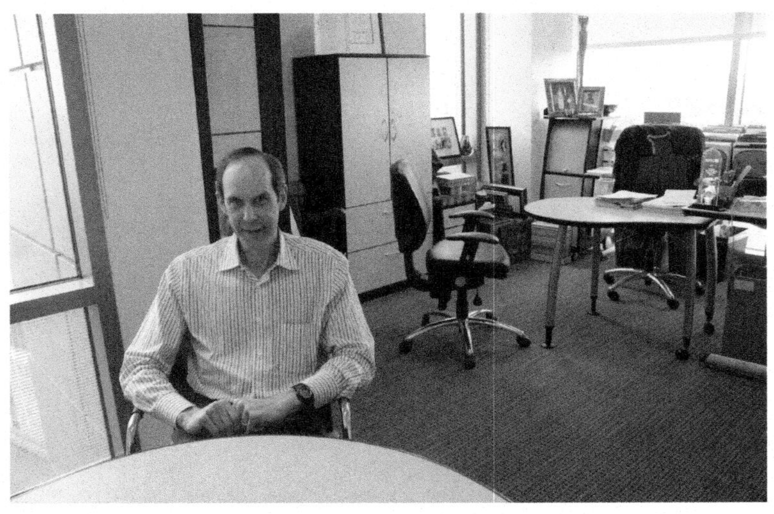

Dr. Brian Druker, now director of OHSU's Knight Cancer Institute, commands a plate glass corner office on the fifth floor of the Hildegard Lamfrom Biomedical Research Building with perfect views of the wilderness he loves: Mount St. Helens to the north and Mount Hood to the east. *Image credit: William Graves.*

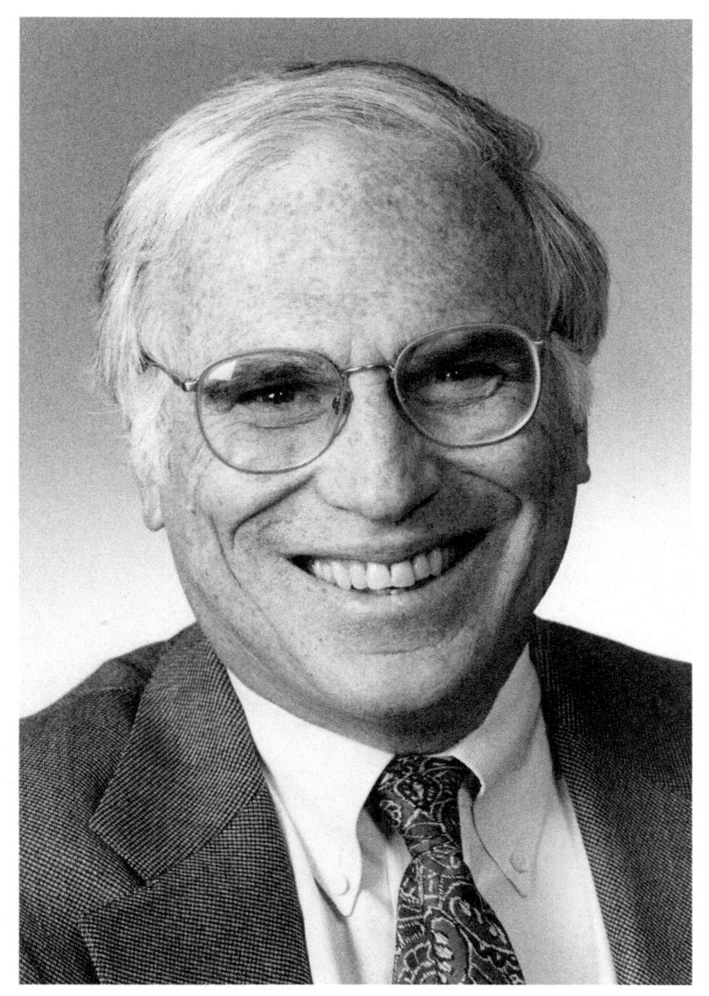

Dr. Joseph Bloom served as chairman of the OHSU Department of Psychiatry under OHSU President Leonard Laster and later became dean of the medical school under Peter Kohler from 1994 to 2001. He called Laster a bull in a china shop. He was strongly supportive of keeping the entire OHSU medical center whole under its transformation to a public corporation. Like Kohler, he feared spinning off just the hospital, as other academic health centers had done, would create political and financial conflicts between the hospital and the university. Bloom, who earned his psychiatrist degree at Harvard Medical School, headed the Alaska Native Health Service before joining OHSU in 1977. He's considered an expert on the legal sanity defense. *Courtesy of OHSU Historical Collections & Archives.*

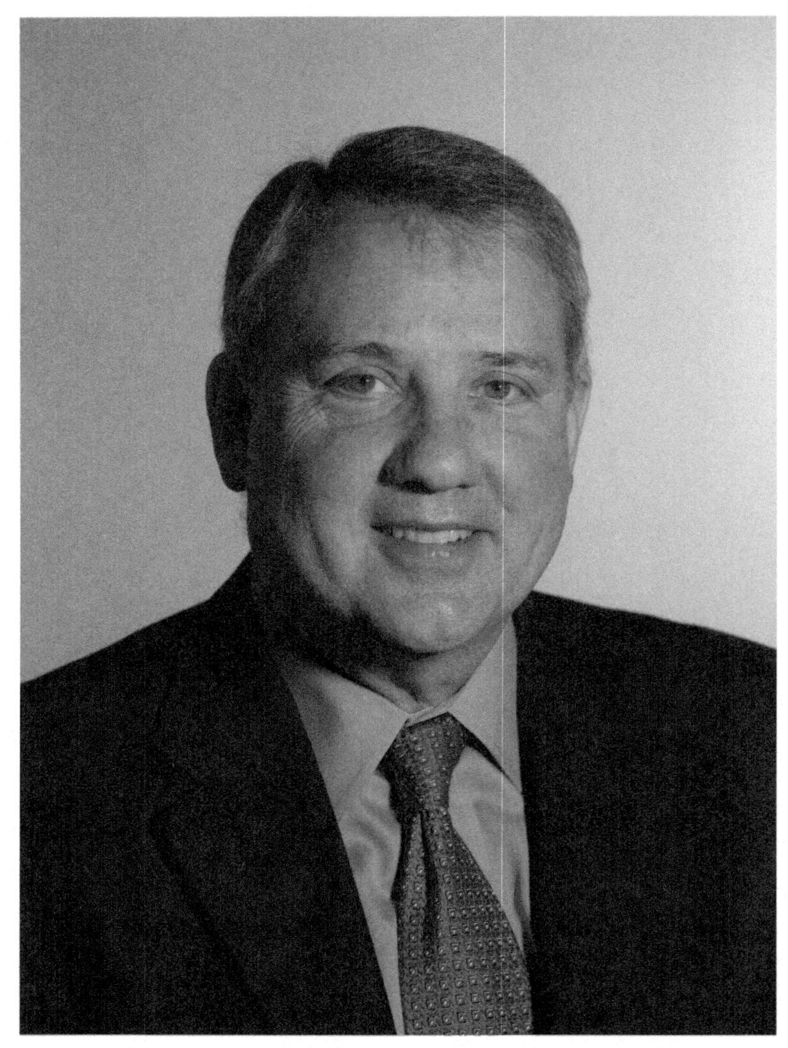

Dr. Joseph (Joe) Robertson Jr., OHSU president since 2006, works in the same Baird Hall office that Peter Kohler occupied. Robertson, an ophthalmologist, has led OHSU through continuous expansion in keeping with Kohler's vision. *Image courtesy of OHSU.*

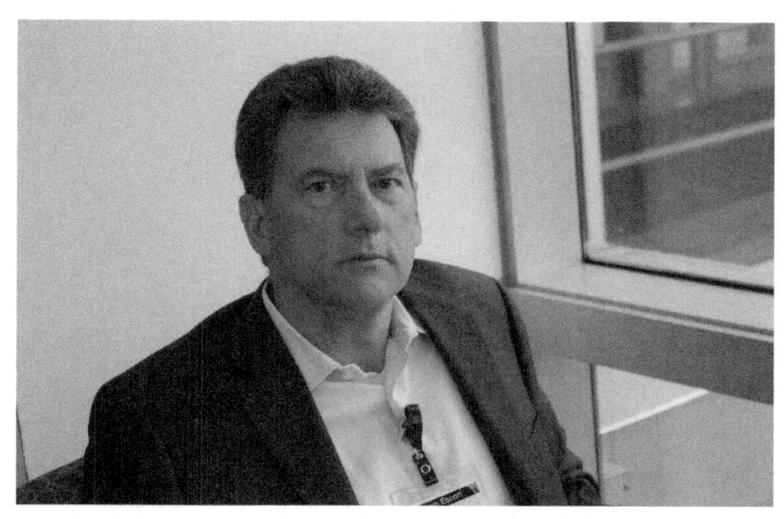

Attorney Steve Stadum, a legal expert on real estate, worked for OHSU in various administrative positions for seventeen years. He helped the university secure a critical lease on its land and later expand on Portland's South Waterfront. He was eventually promoted to OHSU's chief administrative officer and then executive vice president. He left the university in 2016 to be executive vice president and chief operating officer for the Fred Hutchinson Cancer Research Center in Seattle. *Image credit: William Graves.*

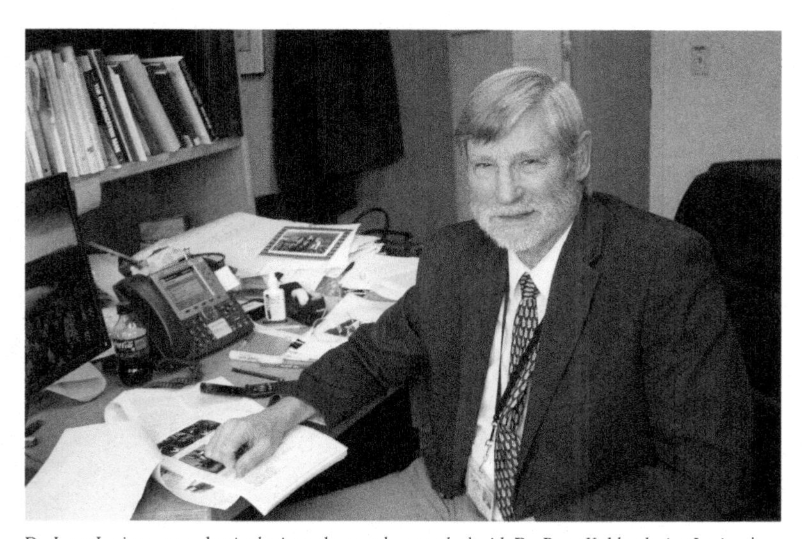

Dr. Lynn Loriaux, an endocrinologist and researcher, worked with Dr. Peter Kohler during Loriaux's 20 years at the National Institutes of Health and later joined Kohler at OHSU in 1990 as head of the Division of Endocrinology, Diabetes and Clinical Nutrition. In 1994, he became chair of the Department of Medicine, a post he held until 2013, after which he returned to head the endocrinology division. Under his leadership the department grew from 52 faculty members to 260. Loriaux supported OHSU's move to a public corporation, but he's concerned that more recent flows of big donations into specialty centers are undercutting the university's education and research missions. *Image credit: William Graves.*

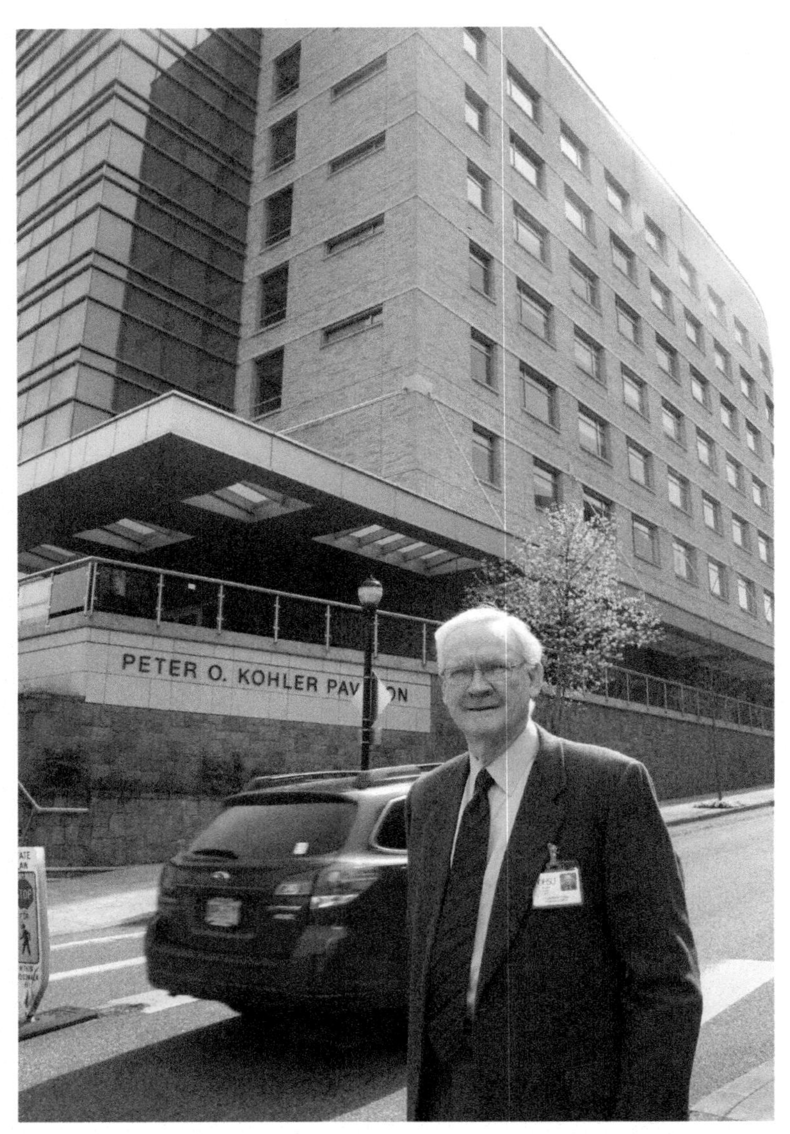

Peter Kohler stands before the OHSU patient care building named after him when it opened in 2006. Kohler still has an office—and a parking pass—on campus, which he visits every month or two, often in connection with meetings as a member of the Pacific University Board of Directors. *Image credit: William Graves.*

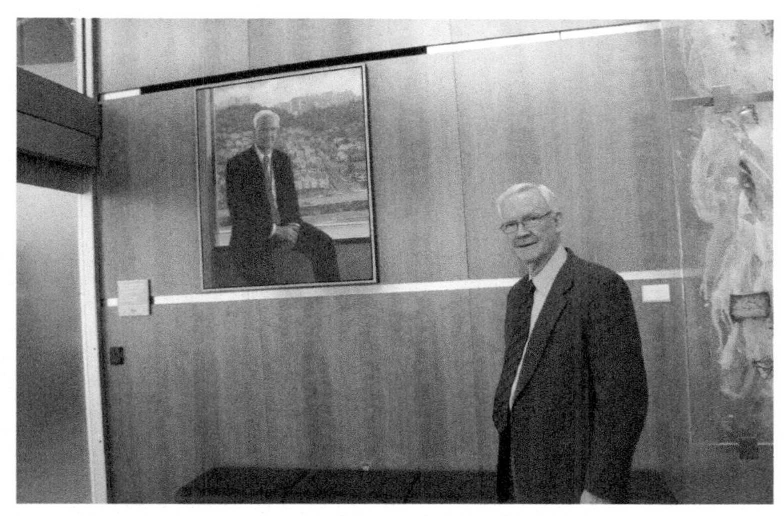

Peter Kohler poses next to his portrait, which hangs in the lobby of the Peter O. Kohler Pavilion. After leaving OHSU, Kohler returned to Arkansas, where some of his children live, to serve as vice chancellor at the University of Arkansas for Medical Sciences. He helped establish satellite medical programs in northwest Arkansas and has led a major effort to reduce obesity and diabetes among a large migrant population from the Marshall Islands. He moved into semi-retirement in the summer of 2016. *Image credit: William Graves.*

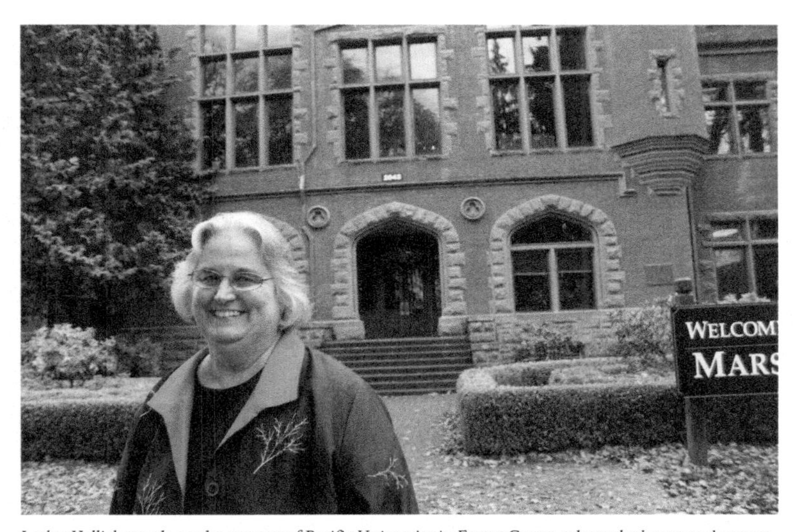

Lesley Hallick stands on the campus of Pacific University in Forest Grove, where she has served as president since 2009. Prior to that she worked 32 years at OHSU, initially as a molecular biology professor and researcher and later as President Peter Kohler's vice president of academic affairs, or provost. She helped persuade faculty and legislators to support OHSU's conversion to a public corporation and then helped lead it through its transformation. *Image credit: William Graves.*

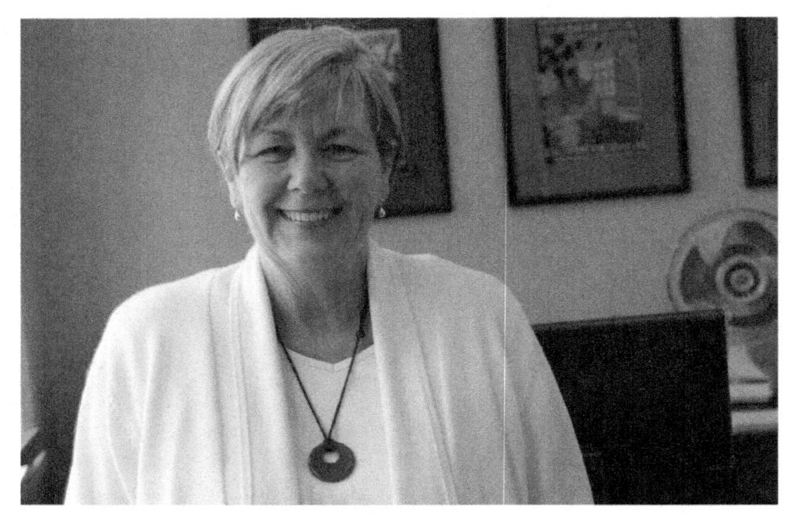

Janet Billups is the only member of former President Peter Kohler's leadership team still working at OHSU. She leads the university's legal office as General Counsel, a post she has held most of the two decades OHSU has been a public corporation. She oversees seven in-house and multiple outside lawyers. *Image credit: William Graves.*

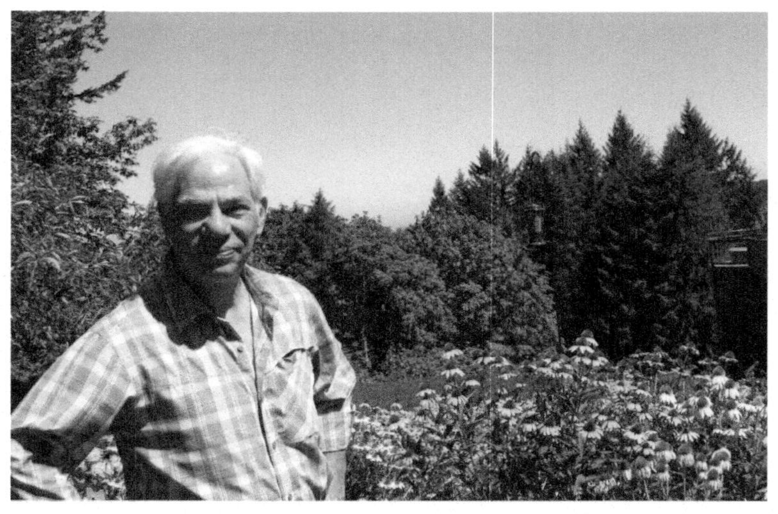

Timothy Goldfarb stands outside his home in Washington County west of Portland in 2015. After leaving OHSU, where he was in charge of hospitals and clinics, he became in 2001 chief executive officer of Shands HealthCare, a health care system affiliated with the University of Florida Health Science Center. He retired in 2015. *Image credit: William Graves.*

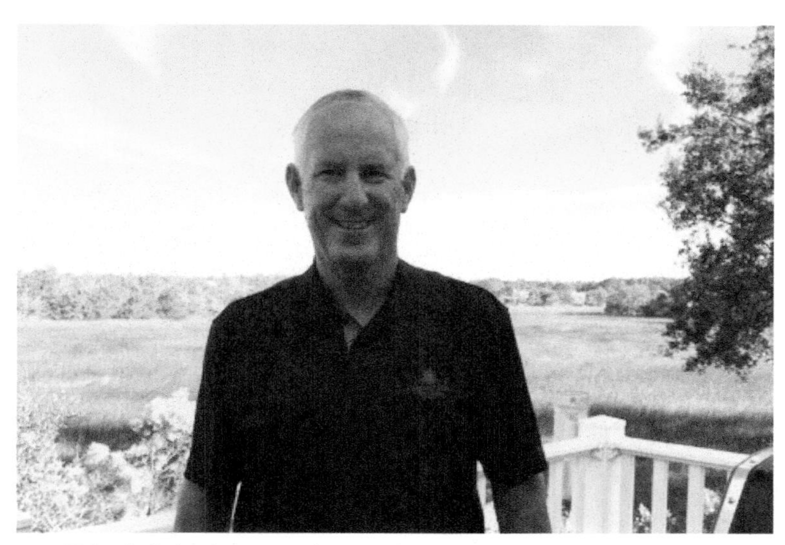

James Walker finally found retirement after several failed attempts. He left OHSU in 2003, but then two months later stepped in for two years to help Lewis & Clark College in Portland recover from a financial scandal. He retired to St. Simons Island, Georgia, but OHSU called him back for nine months in 2009 to help it weather the Great Recession. He settled in 2016 where his career began—in Albuquerque, New Mexico. *Image courtesy of Jim Walker.*

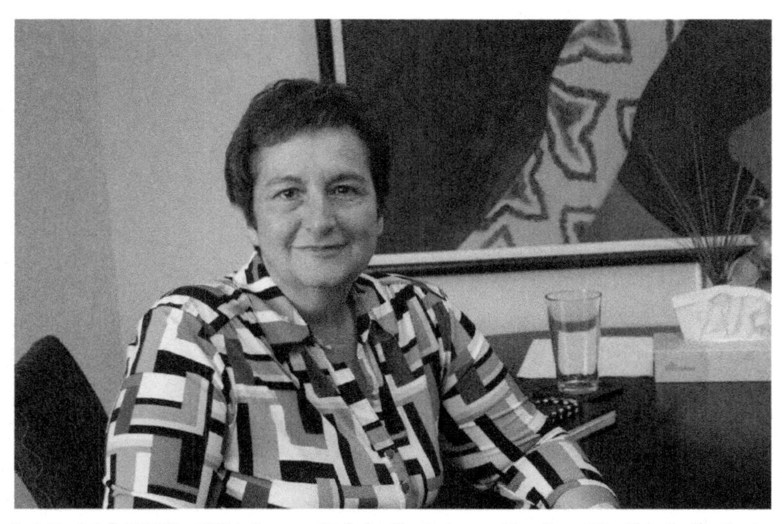

Lois Davis left OHSU in 2009 to become chief of staff and vice president for public affairs for Portland State University. OHSU, where she had worked as vice president for public affairs and marketing, had reached healthy stability, she said, and she needed a new challenge. *Image credit: William Graves.*

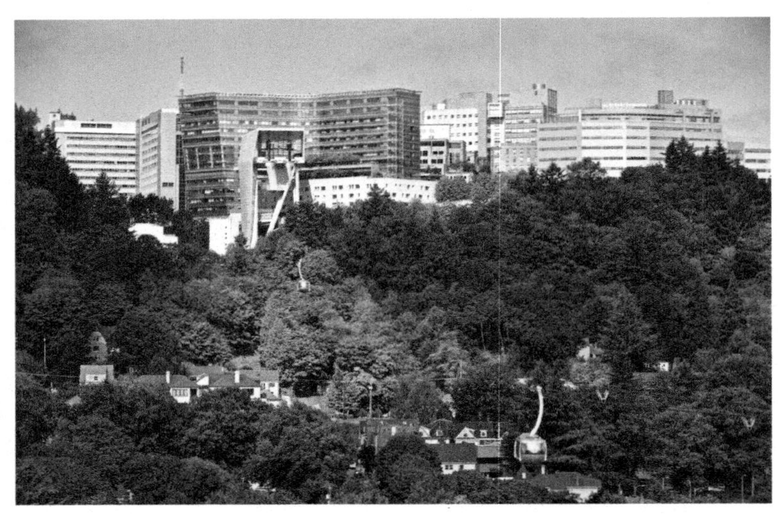

Two silver, bullet-shaped tram pods float above the Corbett-Terwilliger-Lair Hill neighborhood along S.W. Gibbs Street in Southwest Portland on their journeys to and from the Peter O. Kohler Pavilion and OHSU's complex campus sprawling over Marquam Hill. *Image credit: Mark Graves.*

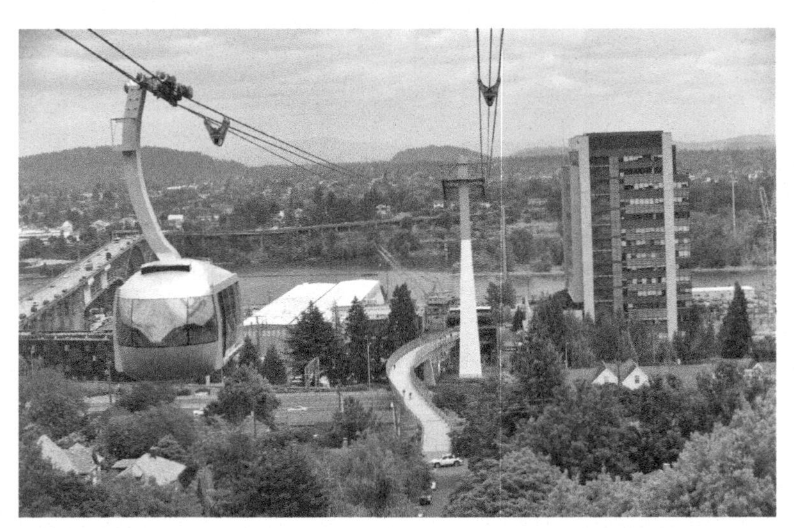

The tram descends toward its docking station next to the Center for Health & Healing on Portland's South Waterfront near the Willamette River. The sixteen-story center opened in 2006 and gave the university another 400,000 square feet of space for surgery, research, clinics, classrooms and a fitness center with pools, spas, weight rooms, and lab facilities. *Image credit: Mark Graves.*

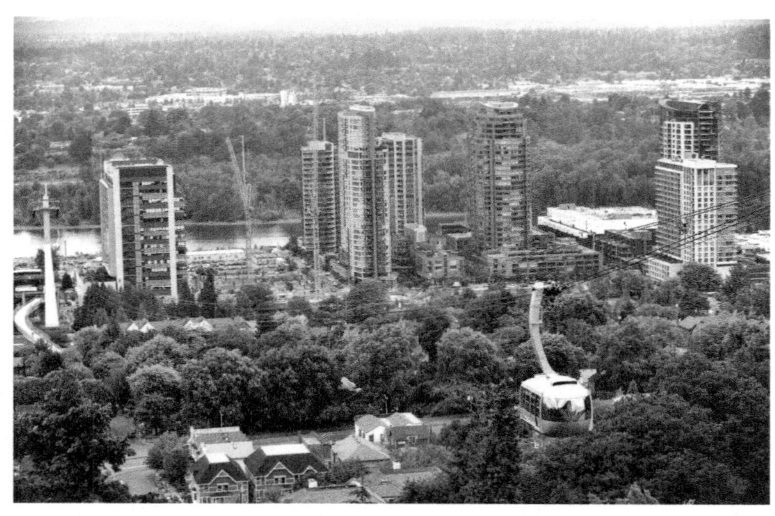

A small city of sleek, thin, glass-and-steel apartment and condominium skyscrapers tower on the south flank of the OHSU health center along with other apartment buildings, shops, and restaurants, all served by the Portland Streetcar. This development on Portland's South Waterfront continues to unfold. *Image credit: Mark Graves.*

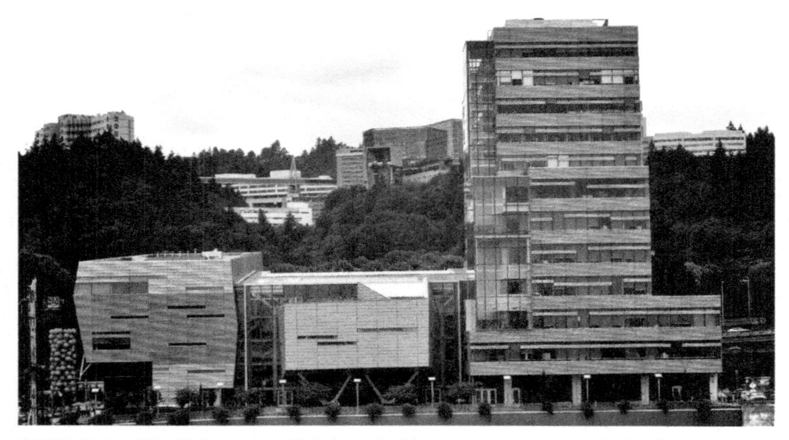

OHSU's $160 million Collaborative Life Sciences Building, a joint venture with Portland State University and Oregon State University, opened in 2014 on a once barren brownfield on the South Waterfront. The building provides space for biomedical research, for medical, nursing, and pharmacy school classrooms, and for the OSHU/PSU School of Public Health. Adjoining it is the $135 million Skourtes Tower for the School of Dentistry. *Image credit: Mark Graves.*

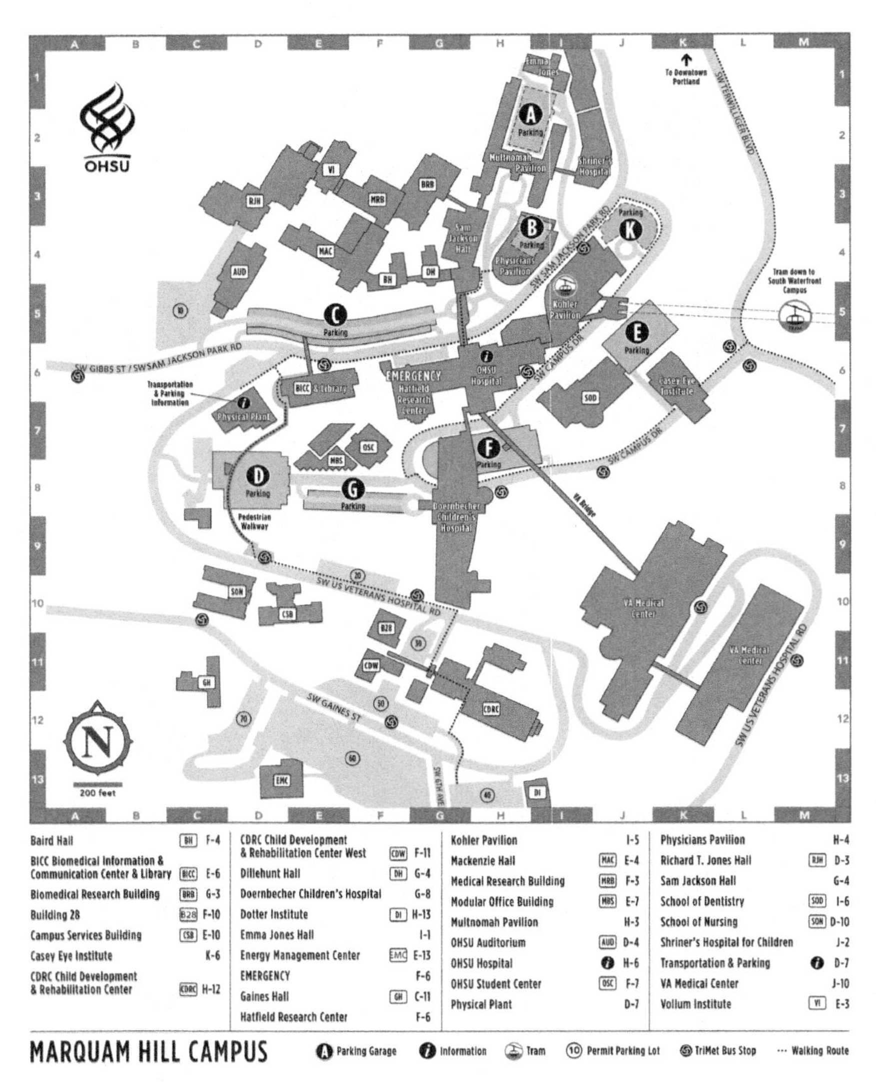

Courtesy of OHSU.

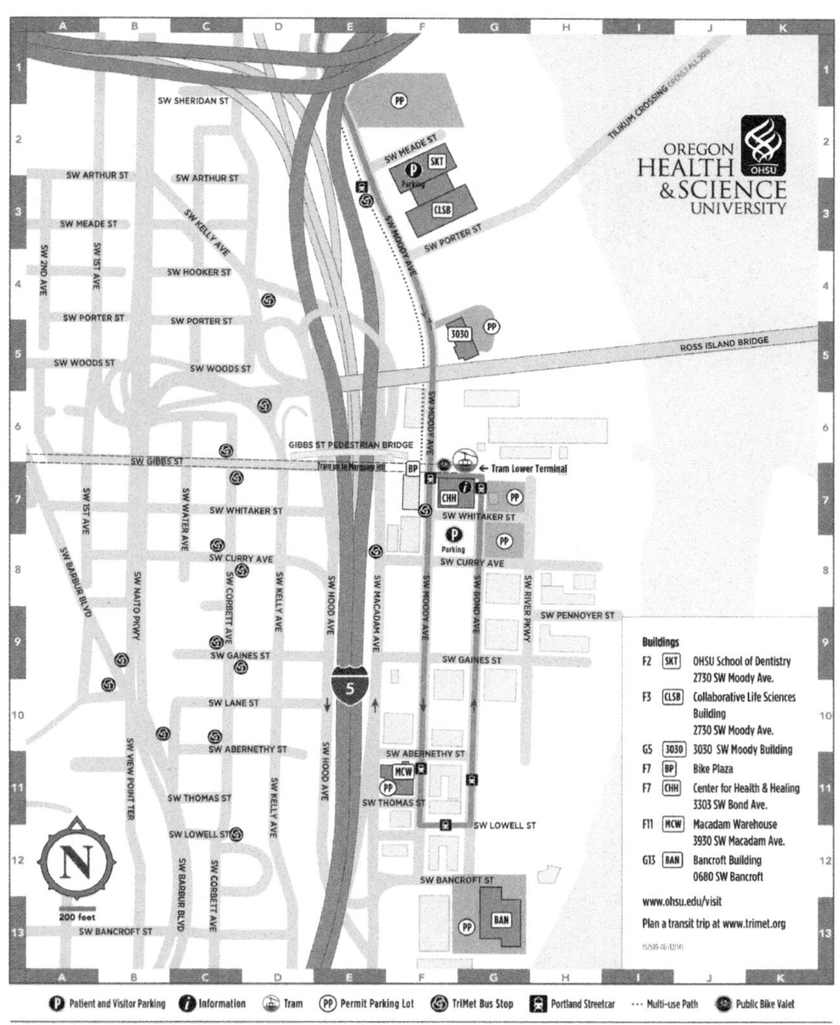

SOUTH WATERFRONT CAMPUS

Courtesy of OHSU.

Chapter Five

Transition: The First Year

With their victorious passage of SB 2, Peter Kohler and his administrative team were immediately slammed with an array of tasks and deadlines for transforming their institution. There was no time to savor their win with a victory lap or party. Billups, Davis, and Hallick have vague memories of leaving work thirty minutes early, one smoggy June afternoon shortly after Governor Kitzhaber signed the bill, for a quick celebratory drink on the outside deck of one of the restaurants along the Willamette River below OHSU.[1] Hallick said sentiment among the team could be summed up as: "Whew, two minute pause! Now we had better get on with the work in front of us."[2]

OHSU's hard-won new independence came at the cost of new responsibilities, and that meant work. Even with its new public corporation authority, the staff of OHSU could have chosen to stay with the more comfortable status quo or risk only incremental change, said Fred Buckman, the PacificCorp leader who would chair OHSU's first board.

"The willingness of the staff to accept the challenge to be transformational is what made this a real success," he said.[3]

Kohler's top priority was to get more money to address the university's severe deferred maintenance needs.

"The first thing we looked at was how do we get sufficient funds to fix the bad problems on the campus and then begin to look at what we can do to move forward," he said. "We had a lot of aspirations for building out the research productivity of the campus."[4]

Even before SB 2 passed, Kohler created a transition team headed by Jim Walker, by then promoted to vice president for finance and administration. For Walker, the new task meant only more pressure.

"We knew if this transition failed, it would cast doubt on the whole management team and its public corporation model," said Walker. "It would also be very public and would erode our ability to access debt on Wall Street."[5]

During their long drive to sell SB 2, Kohler's team had learned the enormous value of clear communication, both on and off campus. One big reason the team won so much support for change was that it kept talking to everyone. So when Kohler and his team turned to the transition in that summer of 1995, they made sure they communicated frequently and clearly about what the institution's transformation to a public corporation would mean. One way Kohler did that was to launch a newsletter called *Transition News,* which was distributed across campus every two weeks.

"Superior customer service, to our patients and to one another, will be our hallmark as we move forward," wrote Kohler in the first issue of *Transition News* on May 30, six days after Kitzhaber signed SB 2. "Our commitment to quality education, cutting edge biomedical research, the highest standard of patient care as well as a productive work environment will guide the transition priorities."[6]

To operate independently as a public corporation, the academic health center would have to organize procedures, rules, and staff for seven members of its new board of directors appointed by the governor. It would need to lease land from the state, assume new liability risks, create new purchasing plans, rethink retirement programs, and establish a larger legal department, an independent accounting system, a payroll department, and a human resources office. University officials also would have to make presentations to rating agencies and bond insurers as the university independently assumed responsibility for its $109 million in outstanding debt.

What's more, Kohler's team started hearing that some leaders within the state higher education system and other state agencies were angry about OHSU's success and would cut it no slack. The state vice chancellor of finance, for example, didn't want to lose control of OHSU's budget or the fees it paid to help support the state university system infrastructure, Hallick said.

"We thought that we would have two years to put in place all the information systems, etc., required to be independent of the Oregon State System of Higher Education, but in the 'anger' phase, we suddenly had only one year," she said.[7]

So Kohler led OHSU in a race to transform the university into a functioning, independent public corporation in one year. In an August 1 editorial titled "OHSU's Sea Change," *The Oregonian* said the success of OHSU's bold experiment should be measured by how well it cut costs, continued quality care for the indigent, produced general practitioners, upgraded its specialty programs, attracted research money, won patents, and collaborated with other hospitals.

"The health care seas are rough. This experiment will show whether OHSU can make it to the top."[8]

By these measures, OHSU would make it to the top.

WORKERS STRIKE

But that wasn't apparent in September, when OHSU administrators faced the more immediate problem of a full-blown strike by the American Federation of State, County and Municipal Employees (AFSCME) Local 328, the first labor strike in the medical school's history. The university's talks with its other union, the Oregon Nurses Association, also had been stalled since two days after OHSU became a public corporation. A rival union, the University Federation of Nurses, was seeking to take control of the nurses' bargaining unit, though it would not prevail.

In the early hours of Thursday, September 21, the first AFSCME strikers walked off their jobs and were greeted by 250 cheering and chanting union members outside the admitting areas to the north and south buildings of University Hospital. Picketers carried signs that said "On strike against OHSU" and chanted "People united will never be defeated."[9]

OHSU management was not caught completely off guard by the strike, Kohler said, "but we were surprised that they would think it was a good idea."[10] He had every intention of raising staff pay when the public corporation began increasing revenue, but the university could not do so immediately. Kohler wanted to go out and talk to the strikers, but Davis held him back. The university had a good relationship with the union, Davis said, but striking demonstrators can get worked up.[11]

The relationship was good, agreed Lovell, the field staff worker for the union. But OHSU administrators had been distracted by their drive to pass SB 2 in the legislature, she said, and did not seem to recognize the implications of a fact-finder's report on their negotiations, which had advanced to mediation. The fact-finder sided with the union's assertion that its members were underpaid compared to other state workers in similar jobs because of the state's payroll classification system. Its report would reveal to union members how underpaid they were, and they would demand action. But OHSU's labor relations director didn't seem to convey that reality to Kohler and his administrative team, she said.

"Nobody had bargaining on their radar because they were so preoccupied, understandably so, with the public corporation that they didn't pay attention to our union," she said.

What's more, OHSU had employed a new human resources director for its transition to a public corporation, and she aggravated the union with eleventh-hour interference. The director demanded a one-year contract, contrary to what the union was accustomed to, and she wanted to comb through the contract for other changes. Lovell said the fact-finder's report, poor communication with OHSU administrators, and the new human resources director created a "perfect storm" of discontent that led to the strike.[12]

University management rejected the fact-finder's report and made a final offer of a 3 percent across-the-board increase in wages for all AFSCME, with additional money available to increase pay scales in some categories that were substantially below market rates. The union represented 3,200 workers, which included most of those who were not doctors, researchers, or nurses, such as cooks, nursing assistants, laboratory and X-ray technicians, janitors, office workers, and phlebotomists.

The union wanted to see workers, whose salaries had been frozen for two years or more, get a 4 percent increase in pay and a bigger fund to help bring jobs up to market pay. In a statement, the hospital said that it made $18 million in profits in the previous year, but its state financing had been cut by $19 million and additional federal cuts could be coming.[13]

The workers said OHSU leaders had promised to bring their pay up to market levels after it became a public corporation. That was the plan, university officials agreed, but not in the first two months. And Kohler also wanted to improve faculty salaries, which were even further behind than those of the union members. It would take more time for the university to make the conversion and start reaping sufficient money to boost salaries. Even so, Kohler told reporters, the university as a public corporation was offering employees a better deal than it would have offered as a state institution. State employees represented by AFSCME got only a 2 percent pay increase, he noted.[14]

The hospital scaled down its services during the strike, postponing elective surgeries and diverting some patients to other hospitals. Still, on Thursday and Friday, the first two days of the strike, surgeons managed to perform two heart, one liver, and two kidney transplants. Early Friday, Governor Kitzhaber urged parties to work harder for an agreement.

"This dispute must be settled as expeditiously as possible," he said, "even if the parties must move into 24-hour bargaining to do so."[15]

By Sunday, the two sides were back at the bargaining table. Union leaders settled on a 3 percent wage increase plus a larger $740,000 fund to push wages toward market pay in thirty-three job categories. That evening, union members voted to accept the contract.

"We won," said Lovell. "It wasn't about getting a lot more money; it was about a description of how the money was to be spent."

Kohler and his team's long, trusting relationship with the union contributed to the strike being short-lived. "If there's such a thing as a friendly strike, it sort of was that," Kohler said.[16]

However, Doug Hurd, president of AFSCME, said the bargaining process had not met the union's expectations and management had not been clear about it taking several years to bring salaries to market level. And while workers waited, he noted, management had plans to bring facilities up to market standards swiftly. Management and the union had some issues to work through, he said.[17]

Kohler and his team, though, faced a bigger challenge in keeping their new public corporation afloat and thriving in the new world of managed health care. The business was already saturated in the Portland area and dominated by what *Oregonian* reporter Steve Woodward called the Big Three: Kaiser Permanente, Legacy Health System, and Providence Health System.[18] Portland health leaders said there wasn't much room for a new player.

OHSU opened some primary care clinics in Portland, but Kohler and Timothy Goldfarb, his hospitals administrator, recognized that they could not compete for acute primary care. Instead, they would focus on what the academic health center could provide better than anyone else—cutting-edge technology and extremely specialized medicine and surgery such as pediatric intensive care and transplant operations.

OHSU also had one other advantage: it was now a public corporation. The academic health center had always exploited the advantages of partnerships, such as its joint agreements with the federal Veterans Affairs Hospital that helped pay salaries for some of its faculty and researchers. But now, Kohler and his team realized, the flexibility and autonomy the university gained as a public corporation would make it easier to forge partner agreements. OHSU could enter joint ventures as a state agency, but potential partners, particularly private ones, generally were reluctant to deal with the university because of state bureaucratic barriers and delays and because they were so exposed under the open records law. Now free of the state and higher education system, OHSU struck agreements with other health providers on collaborative ventures that allowed all players to streamline operations, avoid duplication, and give OHSU more market share. In one agreement, for example, the university teamed up with Kaiser Permanente to combine some laboratory functions, saving millions of dollars on standard laboratory tests. In addition, the university joined with hospitals and physicians statewide in Health Futures, a consortium to improve care through sharing of experience and resources.

The university also formed partnerships with the Big Three to exploit its strengths in providing tertiary care. It contracted with Kaiser Permanente, for example, to offer advanced pediatric services and heart and liver transplants. *The Oregonian*'s Woodward noted that as a public corporation, OHSU was having to make some major shifts:[19]

- A strong-willed independent group of physicians had to learn to collaborate more with the business side of OHSU and one another.
- OHSU's longtime mission of serving indigent patients had to be balanced by its search for paying patients.
- A high concentration of specialists with millions in research grants had to give ground to training more primary care doctors essential for managed care systems.

THE BOARD

Kohler also had to report now to OHSU's new seven-member governing board. Kitzhaber, on Kohler's recommendations, filled the board with prominent leaders, two of whom had served on the public corporation advisory board. The board included Fred Buckman, CEO for PacifiCorp;

Neil Goldschmidt, former Portland mayor and Oregon governor; Mike Thorne, Port of Portland director and former legislator; Ronda Trotman Reese, the dental student who also had served as a student member of the state higher education board; Robert "Bob" Bailey, one of the state's leading agriculture leaders as president and CEO of Orchard View Farms in The Dalles and also a member of the state board; and Patricia "Trish" Smith, a property developer from Bend. Mark Dodson was not on the board, but the board made him its official secretary. As president, Kohler also was a board member.

The board had its first meeting as a transition team on June 6, before OHSU officially became a public corporation. Kitzhaber had recommended Buckman chair the board, and members agreed to have him run the first meeting.[20] In that first unofficial meeting, the board established some policies on meeting attendance, conflicts of interest, committee structure, the university's bonding authority, the proper relationship of the foundation to the public corporation, retirement issues, and the need to hire a communications expert with a strong corporate ethos. Kohler also wanted to be delegated clear authority on what he could act on without board approval. He told the board he would err on the side of bringing it issues early.

"One of Peter's gifts is his 'no-surprises' approach to business," said Goldschmidt. "If he continues that approach, we should be fine. The team he has put together is the key. Our goal is to make sure the board isn't an impediment to acceleration. . . . Velocity is going to be a critical issue at some point."[21]

Buckman added that he wanted "to know things are being 'managed well.'" He said, "I am more interested in how, as a board, we can add value. There are two principle ways we add value. Simply by being here, we have empowered you to become a public corporation. Second is that we come from diverse backgrounds and can give advice."[22]

Jim Walker told the board that the Paine Webber financial firm had assured OHSU it has "the strength to issue bonds." Among other things, he said, the university wanted to issue $30 million in bonds for the first phase of the project to build a new Doernbecher Children's Hospital, for which the university had already raised $30 million in donations. He said the university wanted to break ground within the next two months, depending on how quickly it could find a lender on Wall Street.[23]

The board agreed to have its first official meeting on July 1, the day OHSU became a public corporation. The 10:30 a.m. meeting was conducted through a telephone conference call with Buckman, Bailey, and Goldschmidt absent. It lasted only ten minutes. The board took two actions: it elected Buckman chair, and it delegated authority to Kohler to act on the university's behalf in daily operations.[24]

Buckman said the board's initial priority in its early days was to define "our relationship with the state" as a public corporation.[25] The full board assembled again at 1:00 p.m. July 26 on the OHSU campus for its first full, official meeting.

"We are off to the start of something very important here," Kohler said, "and there is considerable national attention focused on us, and how this might serve as a model for other academic health centers. We are breaking new ground, and we want to do it well."[26]

For the next two hours, the new board focused on a central issue for any corporation: money. Kohler noted that at least one bond insurer had given the university a triple-A bond rating, which would be key to borrowing money for deferred maintenance, the new Doernbecher Children's Hospital, and other projects he wanted to get underway. After Hallick gave the board an overview of OHSU's academic programs, the discussion quickly turned to tuition and fees. Though tuition increases would vary among the medical, nursing, and dentistry schools and other graduate programs, the university was seeking an overall $1.4 million, or 16 percent, increase in tuition revenue for the 1995–96 fiscal year. In subsequent years, just as students feared when OHSU proposed becoming a public corporation, university leaders could not resist raising tuition to help ease the financial pressures they were always under. The school's tuition already was relatively high and it would soon become one of the highest among the nation's public medical schools, but it would not surpass private medical schools.[27]

In this first year as a public corporation, tuition would help the university offset a 17 percent drop in state revenue. The state gave OHSU $52 million, about $10 million less than the previous year. The university expected to earn more money and save more with the increased flexibility and efficiencies that came with its transition to a public corporation.[28] But the change also brought new costs, such as hiring the university's first human resources director. And the hospital and clinical operations included new expenses associated with new outpatient clinics in Portland to help OHSU compete for managed care patients. Walker told the board he still expected to see the health services stay in the black, and the university would sustain sufficient revenue to operate on a half-billion dollar budget. Board members wanted to track finances closely. They agreed to meet monthly for the first year and would be looking for budget updates at every meeting.[29]

"When a budget comes up with increased expenses and reduced revenue, it sends up a big red flag," Buckman said.[30]

Never before had OHSU had such focused oversight.

"We knew right from the beginning this would not be a hands-off board," said Walker. "They challenged all of us and were not reserved in their criticism."[31]

The board organized to focus on OHSU's new corporate structure. On October 5, Buckman formed two subcommittees: one on strategic planning and another on competition and competitive strategy. At that meeting, the board also approved a resolution authorizing OHSU to proceed with the pricing and purchase of bonds. But there was still one obstacle to getting the bonds, a hurdle that was demanding the time and patience of Kohler, Walker, and Billups. The university needed control of the land it stood upon. It needed control of Pill Hill.

LEASE WAR

To enter the bond market, OHSU had to have possession of its land, which it aimed to secure through some kind of lease with the state. But the Department of Justice—led then by Attorney General Ted Kulongoski, who had opposed OHSU's conversion to a public corporation—was arguing the new law created by SB 2 did not require the state to negotiate the lease. As Billups and others had explained to legislators during hearings on the bill, without the lease, bond lenders would not have the necessary assurance that OHSU controlled the land on which it operated its hospitals and clinics, its primary source of money to pay back loans.

"No decent investor is going to buy bonds when you don't own the land you are building on," Billups said.[32]

Walker was edgy. He wanted to move fast to borrow money and start upgrading OHSU's buildings, break ground for the children's hospital, and launch other projects, but the lack of a land lease stopped him cold. It also put in doubt whether the university had a positive relationship with the state, another red flag for lenders, said Walker.[33] Without a land lease, Kohler's vision, his whole plan for expanding OHSU, would crumble.

OHSU's new board of directors, though, wasn't so worried about the lease, recalled Buckman. The directors knew Kulongoski opposed the public corporation and saw his dragging his feet as a statement that "I have no intention of helping you guys out." But the board was confident he would relent sooner or later.[34]

Kulongoski said in a 2016 interview "I had no involvement with the lease," though his office debated it with OHSU. He also said that while he opposed the public corporation, he never publicly campaigned against it at Governor Kitzhaber's request. Kitzhaber "sat me down and said he wants this to happen," Kulongoski said.[35]

Billups had hired Doug Goe, the bond attorney at Ater Wynne in Portland, to help. In the face of the attorney general's resistance, Goe turned to Steve Stadum, a managing partner at Ater Wynne and an expert on land deals.[36]

Stadum soon learned the Attorney General's Office was concerned about language in SB 2 that stated title to OHSU's land would remain with the state, but "the university shall have the exclusive care, custody and control of such real property and facilities." Stadum agreed the language was unusual and unclear. The university's interest in the real estate was not stated as a title or leasehold interest or easement.

"I think it was intended to mean everything but legal title, but frankly I think there may have been a little hostility or resistance to the concept of Senate Bill 2 and public corporation," Stadum said. "Kulongoski did not like it, and I think that trickled down to the AG office, and I think that they latched onto this as something that was a problem."[37]

Stadum concluded that what OHSU was really looking for and should seek was a perpetual ground lease, a ninety-nine-year automatically renewable lease for a dollar. "Then you have an interest in real estate that the legal counsel for the underwriter can recognize," he explained. Walker, Billups, and Goe agreed to Stadum's proposal. He then met in Salem with state attorneys, including Suzanne Townsend of the Attorney General's Office and Harvey Rogers, the state's bond lawyer. They responded that the state had no authority to enter into a ground lease. There were some more exchanges, but the state was not budging.

As negotiations continued, Stadum commissioned a title search on all of OHSU's property to ensure there were no covenants or disputes that could complicate a lease. The search turned up no problems, though it did reveal some parcels of land were donated to the state with the stipulation they be used for buildings devoted to health and research. It also showed that the VA Hospital was on land owned by the federal government.

At its September meeting, the State Board of Higher Education asked the university system's vice chancellor for finance to help OHSU negotiate a lease with the state Department of Administrative Services (DAS). But

Kulongski's office told the vice chancellor that DAS lacked the authority to enter such a lease.[38]

OHSU's negotiations with the state seemed deadlocked. Walker was restless. Stadum was worried. Rogers then suggested a possible path to an agreement. If Stadum could get the governor and leadership of the legislature to say a lease was what they intended with the language in SB 2, the state might be willing to negotiate a deal. "Somebody needs to tell these guys to sign a ground lease," Stadum told Kohler.[39]

Kohler and Davis enlisted the help of Kitzhaber, Senate President Gordon Smith and Representative Beverly Clarno, a Republican and Speaker of the House from Redmond in Central Oregon. Billups composed a letter that clarified the legislature's intent to lease the state land to OHSU.

"OHSU has accepted considerable responsibility and liability in return for this bond authority and exclusive, long-term use of its property," said the letter, dated October 3, 1995. It explained that OHSU was assuming responsibility for more than $100 million in debt and $200 million worth of deferred maintenance on its buildings—unlike four other academic health centers that spun off their hospitals in Arizona, Colorado, Florida, and West Virginia. Those states gave their institutions either a long-term lease or outright transfer of land. The letter also said:

> We understand that for OHSU to succeed, it needs to be able to participate effectively in the bond market as anticipated by SB 2. The best way to carry out the purpose of SB 2 is to implement the language that provides OHSU with exclusive use of its property by a long-term ground lease that can be terminated only if the state pays the debt through bond sales, appropriations or other financing strategies.[40]

The letter was signed by Smith, Clarno, and Kitzhaber, the state's three top government leaders. But justice department lawyers said the letter provided no legal reasons for them to change their position, recalled

Billups. They appeared to be trying to fulfill Kulongoski's desire to stop OHSU from becoming a public corporation, though Kulongoski did say he was not involved with the lease negotiations.[41] The Attorney General's Office refused to issue the necessary opinions or complete the documentation, she said.

"I didn't live inside their heads," said Billups, but they "engaged in the most difficult, ultra-conservative, protracted negotiations that we had all ever seen or that Steve [Stadum] had seen."[42]

DAS then proposed to the higher education board that the board retain title to the property on behalf of the state, strike a lease with OHSU and allow DAS to manage it since the department could not by law hold property that is not occupied by a state agency. Kulongoski reluctantly accepted this deal, but only under certain conditions. The state board would have to get consent for the lease from a credit corporation that would allow the board to hold the deed in trust. And OHSU, DAS, and the state board were to write agreements spelling out their various outstanding obligations in the event of any default by OHSU on its loans.

Even then, Kulongoski implied in comments to the State Board of Higher Education on November 17 that the land lease posed possible pitfalls for the board and state:

> It doesn't matter what Oregon Health Sciences University calls itself; it still has a relationship with the state as a public entity. People sometimes give things titles and try to imply that they are something else, but they are still an instrumentality of the state. . . . What we have tried to do, as I have said, is to draft a lease that provides the least risk to the state system. . . . Ultimately, from my perspective, somebody in the State of Oregon is going to be held responsible if there is a default.[43]

Townsend of Kulongoski's office explained that the legislature may have overstepped its bounds in SB 2 by giving OHSU "exclusive care, custody and control" of property owned by the state. She suggested the state may not have authority to grant the lease and makes that clear in the lease agreement.[44] Despite all the cautions and conditions from the Attorney General's Office, the state board adopted a resolution to approve a fifty-year lease agreement, which was signed in December. Finally, OHSU was free to go to Wall Street after a loan.

Even after the lease was signed, Stadum was troubled that it wasn't for longer. Fifty years was short enough to create borrowing problems. Two or three decades into the lease, OHSU would face the dilemma of trying to get long-term loans that extended beyond the life of the lease. Four years later, Stadum was looking to start his own law practice when Walker invited him to apply for the general counsel post in OHSU's legal office. Billups had traded the job for part-time legal counsel so she could spend time with her new daughter. The opening drew many applicants, but Stadum won the job. In that role, he soon persuaded legislators to modify SB 2 to give OHSU a perpetual ninety-nine-year revolving lease on the land for $99. The amended lease was signed by Kohler and state officials on August 5, 1999.[45] Stadum later became chief operating officer of the Knight Cancer Institute at OHSU and left in 2016 to be executive vice president and chief operating officer for the Fred Hutchinson Cancer Research Center in Seattle.

BONDS AND OPPORTUNITIES

Long before the lease agreement was struck, Walker, Kohler, and John Woodward, the San Francisco public debt banker and consultant to OHSU, had been meeting with Wall Street rating agencies and bond insurers. With the lease nailed down, they began making formal pitches for money. On one trip, Kohler and Walker made three presentations in one day at 9:00 a.m., 11:00 a.m., and 3:00 p.m. to three rating agencies, including Standard and Poor's and Moody's. Walker and his staff had spent months preparing hundreds of pages of information.

"These were big guys," Walker said. "They wanted answers to questions on a lot of things. . . . It was very stressful. We knew if we got turned down by Wall Street or were not able to access debt at reasonable rates, the public corporation could not happen."[46]

In January, just six months after becoming a public corporation, OHSU successfully issued a $215 million bond package backed solely by the good faith and credit of the institution. As a state agency, it would have taken the health center years to win approval for a bond sale of that magnitude if it could be done at all. Because the bonds were sold at favorable rates and OHSU had authority to shape the financing package to its needs, the deal raised the university's annual debt payments only slightly.

The health center also received $30 million from the OHSU Foundation. It applied $59 million of the financing to its old debt. About $100 million was allocated to replace Doernbecher Children's Hospital, upgrade University Hospital's patient care units and expand adult and pediatric critical care capacities. Another $20 million was used to upgrade laboratories and classrooms. The public corporation was in business. This was the largest capital infusion in OHSU's history, but just the beginning of the academic health center's dramatic transformation.[47]

As the capital began to flow, Kohler looked for a way to bring more coherence to the university. OHSU's many institutions and centers, such as the Casey and Vollum institutes, operated so independently that many people assumed they were separate organizations clustered near OHSU. The academic health center has historically "operated as a confederacy," Kohler told the board in November of 1995. As a public corporation, it would be developing clearer linear relationships for accountability and responsibility, and it would be giving more attention to communication and marketing.[48] He had appointed Davis the university's corporate communications director, in charge of telling OHSU's story to the people of Oregon. This was a priority of the board's too. It wanted the university to sharpen its brand and market itself.

"Prior to the conversion, we had done very little marketing at all, in part because we weren't allowed to as a state agency," Davis said.[49]

But once Davis became corporate communications director, "I was both being trotted out to meet with Nike folks [in nearby Beaverton] about their marketing program and being told that I should go to various conferences and meet with people that were doing corporate marketing."[50]

Davis and her staff concluded they were selling a service, not a commodity, and looked for a way to distinguish OHSU from its health care competitors. One distinction was that in addition to health care, the institution educated doctors and other health professionals and engaged heavily in research. How could OHSU turn that into some kind of slogan? Kohler came back with a suggestion after attending a meeting of the Association of Academic Health Centers (AAHC), where he and his counterparts were discussing the same idea. The group of AAHC presidents had concluded that the way they commonly portrayed their institutions as being built on the three-legged stool of teaching, caring for patients, and doing research didn't carry much "marketing buzz," Kohler said.[51]

> So we were sitting there trying to think of better ways to describe it. And everybody was throwing out options. And one of the options our group particularly liked was 'Why don't we instead of patient care call it healing. Instead of calling it teaching, call it learning. And instead of research, call it discovery. So let's think of a slogan that would be something related to healing, discovery and learning.'[52]

Kohler brought the idea back to Davis and his executive group. Administrators liked the words healing and discovery, but wanted to stick with teaching instead of learning. So they settled on a slogan that OHSU continues to use today: "Where health, teaching and discovery come together." The university wanted to convey to patients that they "were going to get the advantage of the best and brightest minds, people on the cutting edge of research," Davis said. That was a truth that she experienced first-hand when she was treated at OHSU for breast cancer. A whole team of doctors attended not only to her disease, but to the psychological effects that come with it, she said. At one point, the medical team faced a question about which of several possible medical protocols it should follow.

"My oncologist picked up the phone and called colleagues at eight of the top cancer institutions in the country and asked, 'What should I do?'" she said. "We ended up doing what six of the eight said to do. He had access because he was in research and understood it. So that's what we [her marketing team] sold."

By the end of the year, with the completion of the new labor and delivery floors in the C-Wing of OHSU Hospital, they could start selling OHSU as a good place for mothers to deliver their babies.

"We also had to convince people that we were no longer the county hospital where you delivered your baby in the hallway and shared a bathroom with four women," she said. "One of our first ads was this wonderful television ad about the mother-baby unit."[53]

The ad featured a woman rocking her baby in a beautiful, warm modern suite. "It has all these warm, soft feelings around it that people didn't necessarily associate with OHSU," she said.

OHSU was turning the old iconic image of its struggles with the state, of its pre-public corporation days, into a symbol of its rebirth as a modern health care organization with new facilities and top-notch doctors. The run-down former county hospital labor and delivery unit that the state would not let it fix, the grim labor and delivery unit described in Susan Stanley's book, *Maternity Ward,* the place where poor mothers with no other choice crowded in small rooms or even hallways to deliver their babies, had been replaced. Now mothers would find spacious, private, well-equipped, warmly decorated delivery and recovery suites with spa tubs and rocking chairs, and they would be served by teams of doctors who often not only were familiar with the latest research but were actually doing it. Davis and her staff played the ad to the OHSU board's marketing subcommittee, led by Goldschmidt.

"Well, I really don't like it," he said after watching the ad.

The room, filled mostly with women, was dead silent. Goldschmidt looked around and could see the women loved the ad.

"Oh yeah," he said. "I guess I'm not your target audience, am I?"

Davis and her staff went ahead and placed the ad in local media. There was no way to be sure how effective it was, Davis said, but OHSU began attracting more women to deliver their babies. Some still were poor, but a growing number were insured women who paid.[54]

As Davis worked to polish OHSU's new image, Kohler wrestled with a host of other matters he needed to handle during the course of OHSU's first year as a public corporation. The Joint Commission on Accreditation of Healthcare Organizations was conducting a site visit of University Hospital.[55] The new Doernbecher Children's Hospital design and construction plan needed to be approved and carried out. After OHSU settled with the American Federation of State, County and Municipal Employees in the fall, the Oregon Nurses Association in the spring seriously considered going on strike over issues related to job security and the scope of their authority within the institution.[56] In another development, Senator Hatfield asked Kohler to testify on April 11, 1996, in OHSU's Old Library Auditorium on the merits of federal investment in biomedical research. He wanted Kohler to speak in support of the Clinical Research Enhancement Act of 1996, legislation that would stabilize funding for clinical research.[57]

Kohler also was getting more attention as OHSU's national profile began to rise. The university was drawing interest not only because of its radical move to become a public corporation, but also because of real improvements in its health care, hospital finances, research growth, and overhauled medical school curriculum. *US News and World Report*, in its spring 1996 review of medical schools, ranked OHSU medical school third best among primary care schools and it ranked its Department of Family Medicine fourth best. The NIH listed OHSU at sixtieth for research funding among the nation's 2,000 research institutions, which put it in the top 3 percent.

These improvements in OHSU's stature led to accolades for Kohler. The National Special Events Advisory Board of the Jewish National Fund of America, for example, offered him its Tree of Life Award for his "contributions to the people of Oregon."[58] He also received the Gold Medallion for Humanitarianism from the American Lung Association of Oregon. But what mattered more to Kohler was getting on various corporate boards where he could learn more about private business since he was trying to apply corporate practices to OHSU.[59] He joined, for example, the Portland Mayor's Business Roundtable and Standard Insurance Company's board of directors, where he would serve more than two decades. He also was invited onto the boards of HealthChoice Inc., First Interstate Bank of Oregon, and the Portland branch of the Federal Reserve Bank of San Francisco.

Other academic health center leaders across the country were aware of the university's conversion to a public corporation and many of them wanted to know more. In July of 1995, David J. Ramsay, president of the University of Maryland at Baltimore, with the fifth-oldest medical school in the nation, asked to visit. Ramsay wrote Kohler that the health center's hospital had become independent ten years earlier with positive results.

"It has changed from a disastrous money-losing enterprise with a poor physical plant into a successful operation, with a new building and healthy reserves," he wrote. "I have seen firsthand the advantages of operating outside the state bureaucracy."[60]

Ramsay said he had organized a group to explore whether to privatize the entire university, including its schools of law, medicine, nursing, pharmacy, dentistry, and social work. Ramsay visited OHSU on October 12 and 13 and had interviews with Kohler, Billups, Hallick, Walker, Goldfarb, Davis, and others. He was concerned, Kohler recalled, that while the hospital was prospering, its independent board sometimes was at odds with the university's board and its academic and research aspirations. Kohler said Ramsay was exploring whether he could make the entire academic health center independent as OHSU had done and bring the university and hospital under the oversight of a single board. Whatever Ramsay's group concluded, the University of Maryland at Baltimore remains a public university and one of the nation's top academic health centers.

A group of four executives from the Medical College of the Virginia Commonwealth University Medical Center in Richmond visited OHSU in the spring of 1996. The medical school was getting about 13 percent of its funding from the state, leaving it heavily dependent on hospital and clinical revenue. Carl Fischer, associate vice president for health services, wrote Kohler that OHSU's "responses to the emerging health care market are of extreme interest to us."[61] Later in the year, David Blumenthal and Dr. Paul Griner of the Association of American Medical Colleges asked to visit OHSU because they were studying changes in structure at academic health centers that foster "strategic decision making in response to the many challenges these centers face."[62]

But it was early for people to be making a case study out of OHSU. As visitors arrived to see how the university had transformed itself, Kohler and his team were still racing to carry out the change.

NEW DUTIES; NEW WORKERS

After the land lease was finally secured, Billups turned to other legal tasks connected with the conversion. She needed to transfer the liability risk from the state to the university and establish full legal services for the medical center since it was no longer a state agency entitled to representation by the Attorney General's Office. She and the DAS Division of Risk Management drew up an agreement to handle the first task. The deal would transfer risk management from the state to the university over a short time, which meant OHSU had to get more insurance coverage. The university recruited a professional risk manager to build its program. The agreement also included the transfer of medical malpractice lawsuits that were being handled by the Department of Justice. Now Billups' office would handle them. The university recruited Rod Norton, a lawyer who handled medical malpractice suits for the Department of Justice, to help, and the transition was smooth.

The Attorney General's Office also gave OHSU all of its files related to legal work it had done for the university. As the university took full control of its own legal services, it hired more lawyers to round out its first legal department. It hired, for example, Jim Mattis, a generalist at the Department of Justice, and Carey Critchlow, a lawyer in private practice, to handle employment law services. Now with its own lawyers, its own risk management program and its own legal department, OHSU was fully independent of the state Department of Justice.[63]

The academic health center had one year under the public corporation law to assume full control of various functions that the Oregon State System of Higher Education had been handling for it, in many cases through its offices at the University of Oregon in Eugene and Oregon State University in Corvallis. These functions included the general ledger, accounting, payroll, purchasing and accounts payable, cash management, supply logistics, human resources, pensions, and communications. In the past, OHSU had offices that gathered information for these functions and sent it to the state system or other state agencies to be processed. The university, for example, forwarded information from its campus for the general ledger and sent it to the state system. OHSU had never run checks for payables or payroll and did not have bank accounts for a cash management function. Its human resources office had just gathered information and sent it to the state university system administration.[64]

Most workers at OHSU did not notice much change in their jobs after the university became a public corporation. But managers responsible for establishing new functions did, and that kept Walker up at night.

> To be really honest, when we first started, in the first 90 days, I was having a hard time sleeping. Here was this thing that we pushed for two years to get—it became a big issue statewide, and

> we pushed for it with the governor and the State Board of Higher Ed. If we fall on our face in payroll, finance and general ledger, it's going to be really tough. Talk about being on the hot seat—if we couldn't get the infrastructure [in place] it was going to fall apart. If we couldn't get the debt structure to work, we would have to go back to [state higher education leaders] hat in hand.[65]

Walker soon discovered many of his management workers could not handle the rapid shift from a state to corporate culture. They could supply information for payroll, purchasing, accounting, and other functions, but they couldn't process that information into balance sheets, purchases, checks, and other practical services that the university would now have to handle. Walker needed people who could move fast, make decisions on their own and work sixty to seventy hours a week at times if that's what it took to carry out the changes on time. Many of his managers, Walker realized, would have to go or the public corporation would fail. He had plenty of experience firing people when they didn't measure up, but he had never had to cut smart, hard-working people. He had to demote or fire nearly all of his management staff because they "couldn't change fast enough," he said.

"This was a radical change in a very short time," Walker said. "The transition of replacing many of the management positions in these areas started by the late summer of [1995]. This was a very difficult period for all, including myself."[66]

If Walker had not had experience working for a private construction company and an independent university hospital, he would not have been able to handle the change either, he said. "They would have had to get rid of me."[67]

During OHSU's first months as a public corporation, Hallick also was juggling multiple duties. In addition to her jobs as provost, research overseer, and transition team member, she was interim director of the Biomedical Information Communication Center, the high-tech library initiated by former OHSU President Laster with help from Senator Hatfield. On top of that, she and Walker had concluded they needed to integrate the hospital and the university's financial and computer systems if the health center was going to be able to handle all of its new functions, such as payroll and purchasing, and be competitive. They had to create a single system that everyone could use.[68]

At the time the hospital and university were using different internet technologies. The hospital used the Token ring local area network while the university used Ethernet networking. Hospital and university leaders resisted the proposal to integrate as a single network. Hospital administrators were convinced adding the university to their network would drag them down with inefficiencies they could not afford in their race to become more competitive. University staff, on the other hand, feared that integrating would mean patients would always get first priority and they would not be able to meet their needs for research and teaching.

Still, Walker and Hallick proceeded with creating a unified system. Everyone would have access to parts of the system, such as the library, but other parts, such as financial or patient information, would be restricted to appropriate groups who would have passwords and security codes for access. The unified system also would have to accommodate Microsoft personal computers and Apple Mac computers, a blend requiring various kinds of Band-Aids, Hallick said. In addition, the network had to accommodate two cultures. The hospital operated by extreme discipline and expected everyone to use its standardized system and software. University researchers, on the other hand, were explorers, eager to try new things, including building their own networks for research purposes. Hallick enlisted the help of David Robinson, a tech-savvy neuroscientist, to bridge the two cultures. He explained to researchers that IT workers had good reasons for keeping the hospital network standardized, and he explained to the IT leaders that researchers have bona fide research needs and were not trying to undermine their network with their rogue operations.

"It was just really a challenge, partly because we were right on the edge of the technology's ability to be compatible across those different kinds of systems," Hallick said, "and yet it was so critical."[69]

It would take about four years to fully integrate the hospital and university computer networks. But within eighteen months of becoming a public corporation, OHSU had converted to a single biweekly payroll system, moved to an annual budget process, and converted its accounting system to one that allowed for capitalization and depreciation in long-term budget planning.

The integration was unusual among academic health centers at that time and gave OHSU a competitive management advantage, Hallick said. Eventually, OHSU became capable even of integrating faculty and clinical salaries. For decades, faculty had collected one salary from the university and another completely separate paycheck for their medical services. Under the unified system, they got one paycheck that included money from both sources.

"It was just an amazing run," said Hallick, "getting everything into one information system, one financial system, so that we could develop a system that would make sure that we paid everybody. We did it, and we didn't miss a beat in payroll."[70]

OHSU's freedom from the state brought savings, but it also came at a price. While the state's other universities and community colleges were receiving modest state funding increases, OHSU received no more. The state gave it about $60 million in its first year as a public corporation, amounting to about 12 percent of its revenue. The university spent $24 million of that for uninsured, non-paying patients and for education support in University Hospital and the Child Development and Rehabilitation Center. Most of the rest was spent to provide other educational support.

The university was largely able to adjust to its limited state support through new opportunities and efficiencies, but by the end of its first year as a public corporation it was facing a $4 million-to-$6 million deficit. Kohler and his team decided to lay off eighty-two hospital and clinical workers, including managers and nurses, and freeze 112 positions. Leaders of OHSU worker and nurses unions said they understood why the cuts were necessary. "We want [administrators] to succeed," said Randi L. Post, representative of the Oregon Nurses Association.[71]

In its first year as a public corporation, however, OHSU made changes in the way it conducted business that would produce a growth surge far outpacing its 1996 job cuts. The academic health center had established a full-fledged human resources department that consolidated personnel, benefits, employment, and other functions previously scattered over the campus and handled through various agencies. It developed an alternative, less-expensive pension plan designed to fit its employees, who could still choose to stick with the state's Public Employees Retirement System. In addition, OHSU entered a joint project with an insurance company that allowed it to hold an equity interest, which would not have been permitted were it still a state agency.

Along with these changes, the academic health center also:

- Replaced its state risk management program with its own, lowering worker compensation costs.
- Simplified labor negotiations and moved more employees' pay toward market levels.
- Instituted a state-of-the-art telephone system, expected to save $500,000 to $800,000 a year.
- Brought faculty pay into line with competitive market rates.
- Negotiated contracts previously administered through the state, including a 20 percent reduction in the price of natural gas, saving $400,000 a year.[72]

With the university's new independence, its new board and new systems in place, and with its bond money rolling in, new buildings began to rise on campus. One of the first was a fitting symbol of OHSU's successful conversion to a new era: the modern, dramatically upgraded labor and delivery unit on the twelfth and thirteen floors of the OHSU Hospital C-Wing addition.

Notes

1 Janet Billups, email to author, Dec. 15, 2014: "I'm not sure all of us were there," wrote Billups. "It was a smoggy day and not very comfortable weather. It didn't last long."
2 Lesley Hallick, email to author, Dec. 19, 2014.
3 Fred Buckman, interview, Dec. 10, 2014, Beaverton, Oregon.
4 Peter O. Kohler, MD, interview, Dec. 5, 2014, Baird Hall, OHSU.
5 Jim Walker, "OHSU Transition to Public Corporation," unpublished account, 2013.
6 "A Message from President Kohler," *Public Corporation Transition News,* May 30, 1995, Vol. 1, No. 1.
7 Hallick, email, Dec. 19. Hallick said, "The stated reason [for the accelerated timetable] was that they were going to migrate to a new system, and it would be too much trouble to migrate us to it as well only to divorce a year later."
8 "OHSU's Sea Change," *The Oregonian,* Aug. 1, 1995, p. B06.
9 Steve Woodward, Oz Hopkins, and Cami Castellanos, "Talks Fail, 3,200 OHSU Employees go on Strike," *The Oregonian,* Sept. 21, 1995, p. A01.
10 Kohler, interview.
11 Ibid.
12 Diane Lovell, interview, Sept. 23, 2014.
13 Woodward, Hopkins, and Castellanos, Sept. 21, 1995.
14 Steve Woodward and Cami Castellanos, "OHSU is Diverting Emergency Patients as Talks Collapse," *The Oregonian,* Sept. 20, 2014, p. B01.
15 Janet Filips, "Union, University Officials Will Resume Talks," *The Oregonian,* Sept. 23, 1995, p. C01.
16 Kohler, interview.
17 OHSU Board of Directors Meeting, Nov. 2, 1995. Minutes available from OHSU Strategic Communications.
18 Steve Woodward, "OHSU braves the real world of managed care," *The Oregonian,* Sept. 24, 1995, p. A01.
19 Ibid.
20 Buckman, interview. Buckman said Governor John Kitzhaber had asked him during the legislative session if he would serve on the board. Buckman replied he didn't really have time, but if the governor wanted him on the board, he would do it. But, Buckman added, "he never asked if I was willing to be chairman. The first I knew I was chairman was when I saw the press release." In an interview on Feb. 12, 2016, Kitzhaber does not remember blindsiding Buckman and said it would not be his modus operandi to do so. "That would not be a smart thing to do," he said. "You would want your chair to be an enthusiastic chair."

21 OHSU Transition Board Meeting, minutes, June 6, 1995.
22 Ibid.
23 Ibid.
24 OHSU Board of Directors Meeting, minutes, July 1, 1995.
25 Buckman, interview.
26 OHSU Board of Directors Meeting, minutes, July 26, 1995.
27 Ibid., and document attached to minutes, "OHSU University Hospital Major Changes, Budget 95/96 Compared to Projected 94/95." Minutes available at OHSU Strategic Communications.
28 Ibid.
29 OHSU Board of Directors Meeting, minutes, July 26, 1995.
30 Ibid.
31 Walker, unpublished account of OHSU transition to a public corporation, 2013.
32 Janet Billups, interview, April 2, 2014, her Baird Hall office, OHSU.
33 Jim Walker, interview, Feb. 25, 2015.
34 Buckman, interview.
35 Ted Kulongoski (former attorney general and governor of Oregon), interview, July 18, 2016. Kulongoski said he was involved with the conversion of the State Accident Insurance Fund (SAIF), from a state agency to a public corporation in 1980. He wasn't impressed with the results for SAIF, which was the state workers' compensation insurance agency. He saw improprieties and other problems as the agency "stumbled quite a bit in the first 10 years," he said. "I didn't think it had worked very well. . . . This is not what everybody thinks it is."
36 Steve Stadum, interview, Dec. 11, 2014. Stadum recalled, "Doug came to me and said, 'We're having some problems with the AG office, and it could affect the bond issue and would you be able to help get involved with me.'"
37 Ibid.
38 Oregon State Board of Higher Education minutes, Meeting No. 647, Nov. 17, 1995, p. 492.
39 Stadum, interview, Dec. 11, 2014.
40 A copy of this letter is on file in the office of Janet Billups at OHSU.
41 Kulongoski, interview.
42 Billups, interview.
43 Oregon State Board of Higher Education minutes, Meeting No. 647, Nov. 17, 1995, pp. 494, 496. Attorney General Ted Kulongoski also said, "We have negotiated a lease that tries, to the best of our ability, to anticipate the issues and risks that are of concern to the Oregon State Board of Higher Education. Obviously, my interest is in protecting the state—that is my responsibility; that is my client."
44 Ibid., p. 496. Suzanne Townsend of the attorney general's office said, "The lease makes it quite clear in Section Three that the state is not warranting that it has authority to lease the property that is the subject of the lease. So, to reduce the risk to the state, the charges that we took an action for which we had no authority, we have

made it clear that we're not warranting that we have the authority to do it."

45 *Amended and Restated Ground Lease*, signed by Peter Kohler, OHSU, and C. David White, Oregon Department of Administrative Services, Aug. 5, 1999.

46 Walker, interview, Feb. 25, 2015.

47 Walker, unpublished account of OHSU transition to a public corporation, 2013.

48 OHSU Board of Directors Meeting, minutes, Nov. 2, 1995.

49 Lois Davis, interview, March 9, 2015, in her Portland State University office.

50 Ibid.

51 Peter O. Kohler, MD, interview, April 9, 2015, in his office in the Medical Research Building, OHSU campus.

52 Ibid.

53 Davis, interview.

54 Ibid.

55 Lesley Hallick noted that the Northwest Commission on Colleges and Universities, the nonprofit, independent regional accrediting agency recognized by the US Department of Education, was both intrigued and concerned about OHSU's conversion to a public corporation and made two visits to campus in the spring of 1995.

56 Beth Alexander, MD, Lois Davis, and Peter O. Kohler, MD, "Changing Structure to Improve Function: One Academic Health Center's Experience," *Academic Medicine* 72, no. 3, April 1997, p. 266.

57 US Senator Mark O. Hatfield, letter to Peter Kohler, March 22, 1996.

58 Leonard Kleinman, chairman, Jewish National Fund of America, letter to Peter O. Kohler, March 18, 1996.

59 Kohler, interview, April 9, 2015.

60 David J. Ramsay, DM, president of University of Maryland at Baltimore, in letter to Peter O. Kohler, July 31, 1995.

61 Carl R. Fischer, associate vice president for health services, Medical College of Virginia Medical Center of Virginia Commonwealth University, letter to Peter O. Kohler, March 14, 1996. Fischer wrote: "As I have talked with individuals around the country, I have repeatedly heard the wonderful things you are doing at Oregon Health Sciences University. . . . Your responses to the emerging health care market are of extreme interest to us. In particular, we would be interested in how you have dealt with integrating the hospital, the practice plan and the School of Medicine. We are also interested in what you have done to consolidate finances and incentivize the involved parties. The changing role of the departmental chairmen and the involvement of clinical faculty and center directors are also matters of interest to us. Finally, we would appreciate knowing your strategies with regard to primary care and networking with other physicians and hospitals."

62 Paul F. Griner, MD, Association of American Medical Colleges, letter to Peter O. Kohler, Nov. 22, 1996.

63 Janet Billups, "The Design of the Public Corporation—The Lawyer's Perspective," an unpublished account of Oregon Health & Sciences University's conversion to a

public corporation, 2013.

64 Walker, unpublished account of OHSU transition to a public corporation, 2013.

65 Dana L. Director (vice president of research operations and student affairs at OHSU), "The Impacts of Change in Governance on Faculty and Staff at Higher Education Institutions: A Case Study of OHSU" (dissertation, Portland State University, 2013), p. 95.

66 Ibid.

67 Walker, interview, Feb. 25, 2015.

68 Lesley Hallick, interview, May 27, 2014, Pacific University.

69 Ibid.

70 Ibid.

71 Steve Woodward, "OHSU staff budget goes under the knife," *The Oregonian*, June 12, 1996, p. D01.

72 Alexander, Davis, and Kohler, "Changing Structure to Improve Function," pp. 263-268.

Chapter Six

Research: Path to Prominence

In 1992, Dr. Brian Druker was a young researcher at the Dana-Farber Cancer Institute in Boston exploring tyrosine kinase, an enzyme that can function like an on and off switch in cellular functions. He suspected the enzyme was involved with chronic myelogenous leukemia (CML), a rare but deadly disease in which the bone marrow produces too many white blood cells. He was looking for a way to turn the switch off in CML patients. He had spent six years at the cancer center as an instructor, which he described as "indentured servitude between the end of your fellowship and a real faculty appointment." So he approached the head of Dana-Faber to ask for a promotion to assistant professor.

"Oh, you have a lot of publications," said the director. "Almost as many as I do."

Then he started counting the number of publications in which Druker was first author.

"Well, you only have a couple of first authors here," the director said. "I don't think you're going to make it. I don't think you have a future here."

The director did offer to let Druker run a molecular diagnostic laboratory, but when Druker listed the equipment and funding he would need, the director balked, saying "we can't afford that." Later looking back, Druker said he probably "did need a kick" to move on with his career.

"I needed somebody to say, 'Do you believe in yourself? Do you think you have what it takes to make a difference?'" he said. "I decided at that point I was going to make a difference."[1]

Druker started looking for a place committed to cancer research where he could interact with medical students and enjoy living.

"Part of it was that I wanted to find an institution where I could teach students, I could be part of a growing, developing program," he said. "The institution had to have a commitment to growing its cancer program."[2]

A friend who knew Druker was job searching told him that OHSU President Peter Kohler had just made a commitment to one of his talented researchers, Dr. Grover Bagby, to expand cancer research. Bagby, a top grant winner whom Kohler wanted to keep, was thinking about going back to Baylor College of Medicine Medical Center in Houston. To keep him, Kohler asked him to build a new Oregon Cancer Center. Druker had been collaborating on his CML project with Jim Griffin, who was friends with Dr. Bagby. Griffin put in a good word to Bagby on Druker's behalf. Druker and Bagby met at an American Society of Hematology meeting in December of 1992, and Bagby invited Druker to campus in January of 1993.

"I flew out on one of those glorious winter days where the sun was out," Druker recalled. "It must be one of, probably one of the dozen days where the sun is out in January. And I flew up and saw Mount Hood, Mount Saint Helens and just immediately fell in love with this place."[3]

That evening, Bagby took Druker out to dinner and introduced him to Senator Hatfield.

"Grover gave him background about who I was, where I was coming from," Druker said. "[Hatfield] looked me in the eye and said, 'You're exactly the kind of people I want to see moving to Oregon.'"[4]

That helped seal the deal. And Grover would prove to be the perfect boss, Druker said.

"Here was somebody who was going to put his arm around my shoulder and say, 'I believe in you. And I'm going to do what it takes to make you successful. And I'm going to help you. But I'm not going to get in your way.'"[5]

Bagby had moved to OHSU in 1985 to work in hematology and oncology at the Veterans Affairs Hospital. But he also taught at OHSU. He could see in Druker the kind of a professional OHSU liked to go after—bright, ambitious, on the rising arc of a promising career trajectory—a rising star. And Bagby knew what Druker was looking for.

"So Brian had a lot of choices about going to different places in the country," said Bagby, "but I think part of what brought him here was freedom. Nobody was going to get in his way."[6]

Druker's goal upon arriving at OHSU was to find a drug that would shut down a tyrosine kinase enzyme called Ber-Abl and move that into clinical trials for human CML patients. He had in the late 1980s helped a Boston company called Ciba-Geigy, now Novartis, set up a drug discovery program to identify inhibitors of kinases. He contacted Nick Lydon, a researcher he knew at the company, to see if the company's scientists had come up with any compounds that might shut down Ber-Abl, and they had some candidates. Being so far away, Druker was beginning to miss the "scientific environment" in Boston.

"It got me to thinking. . . . Was this the best move?" he said. "I began to wonder, 'Am I really going to be able to make it here to the level I really want to get to, despite the fact I established great collaboration with other top-notch scientists?' I began to wonder, 'Was this really going to be the place that was going to catapult my career and was this a good choice?' A couple years later, you look back, and of course, this is the right place for me."[7]

Druker arrived at OHSU in July of 1993. By August, he had six compounds from Ciba-Geigy to test. By the end of August, he identified one that killed CML cells without harming normal cells. He and Lydon began working together with academia and industry to move the compound out of the laboratory and into clinical trials. Within his first six weeks at OHSU, Druker was working on a drug that ultimately was going to revolutionize the way the medical world thinks about fighting cancer.

Because of market size, potential for toxicity, and other complications, it took five years to get the compound into clinical trials, where it proved to be remarkably effective. In 1998, the first human patient, Bud Romine, a retired railroad engineer from Tillamook, Oregon, took a pill of Imatinib, the compound that killed CML cells in the laboratory. The initial doses were so small that they had no effect. But by January of 1999, Romine and every other patient in the trial had normal blood counts. Druker and his team were seeing something many thought never was possible—eradication of cancer with a daily pill.[8] No chemotherapy or radiation therapy or surgery. Just a pill a day. Today, more than fifteen years later, tens of thousands of CML patients are alive because they take a daily pill of what was named Gleevec. For this one rare form of blood cancer, Druker found what looks like a cure. Not only that, he helped put OHSU on the national map.

"Brian Druker in and of himself was a marketing campaign" for OHSU, said Davis. "His success was so remarkable, it cast a sort of halo over the whole institution, certainly in the cancer area, but beyond that. Frankly, once you get a Brian Druker there, then you can attract other people like him in terms of leading-edge clinicians, researchers, and it kind of snowballs."[9]

A key step in this dramatic advance was creating the Oregon Cancer Center and putting Bagby in charge of it. That not only held Bagby, but also drew Druker.

"One of the key things that really led to our growth was convincing Grover Bagby to stay here instead of going to Baylor and promising we would work with him to set up a cancer center," Kohler said. "Bagby was our top grant getter, meaning he had abilities scientifically to write proposals and conduct research that was important to sustain funding. He is an ideal example of the kind of person we could build on. Then, obviously, he could build a program, which is what he did, and he recruited Druker, who was clearly a rising star, but I want to give Bagby credit for having done that."[10]

Bagby not only recruited Druker, but a whole team of researchers and National Cancer Institute support grants. Within three years, the Oregon Cancer Center was operating on a $4.2 million budget, nearly half going to provide more space and equipment. One of the center's recruits, Dr.

Craig Nichols, had helped cyclist Lance Armstrong overcome testicular cancer with treatments in 1996 at Indiana University Medical Center in Indianapolis.[11]

OHSU's cancer center grew into the Knight Cancer Institute. Druker replaced Bagby as director and now commands a plate glass corner office on the fifth floor of the Hildegard Lamfrom Biomedical Research Building with perfect views of the wilderness he loves: Mount St. Helens to the north and Mount Hood to the east. In 2014, the center received a $500 million fund-raising challenge from Phil Knight, cofounder of Nike, and his wife Penny. In less than two years, OHSU raised more than $500 million, including $200 million in bonds from the legislature for two new buildings, triggering the match. The institute will raise an additional $200 million and use the $1 billion to recruit researchers and focus on finding ways to detect cancer in its earliest and most treatable stage, along with other cures like Gleevec.

BUILD AND THEY WILL COME

Druker is one of the most dramatic examples of how Kohler's vision, and that of Laster before him, came to fruition. Kohler essentially adopted his own version of farmer Ray Kinsella's dictum in the 1989 film *Field of Dreams:* "Build it, and they will come." Instead of a baseball diamond in an Iowa cornfield, though, OHSU was building research laboratory space on Pill Hill. And instead of trying to draw legendary baseball players from the past, Kohler was going after rising star researchers with promising futures.

He described his rationale for this approach in August of 1993 in remarks he prepared for the Congressional Committee on Science, Space and Technology chaired by Representative George E. Brown Jr. (Democrat from California). He was defending OHSU's choice to build its $63-million Ambulatory Research and Education project, which would become the Hatfield Research Center, in a partnership of federal and private money. Brown saw the project as an example of what he called academic earmarking by Hatfield and other powerful senators and congressmen. Kohler wrote:

> An article by Clark Kerr in the May/June 1991 issue of *Change* supports the belief that the attraction of research stars is a key variable in research reputation. It is likewise clear that research facilities are a key ingredient in the attraction of research stars, which then allow you to grow your own outstanding scientists as we are now doing. In this context, I am pleased to report that Congress' decision to direct funding to support facilities at Oregon Health Sciences University has been a pump-priming technique for Oregon's economy that has enhanced the university's competitiveness for peer-reviewed awards.[12]

Kohler was echoing OHSU's Thomas G. Fox, vice president for development and public affairs, who a year earlier had given Kohler a memorandum that argued the efforts of Kohler and his predecessor, Laster, to build more space at OHSU with help from Hatfield between 1987 and 1992 had been a "pump-priming technique for Oregon's economy by enhancing the university's competitiveness for peer-reviewed awards. Furthermore, it has also provided the best means to assure the university's survival."[13]

During that five-year period, OHSU added 735,000 square feet of new space for everything from the Vollum and Casey Eye institutes to hospital renovations and the sky bridge connecting the university and VA hospitals. Between 1986 and 1991, the university's research volume roughly doubled from $26 million a year to $50 million.

"Likewise, these data suggest the availability of up-to-date facilities has enabled the institution to recruit individuals that previously would not have been attracted to the university," wrote Fox.[14]

As OHSU expanded and drew more researchers and research money, Fox noted, its "ability to attract private gifts has likewise increased dramatically." Between 1987 and 1992, the OHSU Foundation saw a 300 percent increase in gifts, and the funds under its management climbed from $52 million to $100 million.[15]

Kohler also knew that by attracting top faculty and researchers, OHSU Hospital and clinics could offer the most highly-skilled and trained physicians in Oregon. And they were necessary to generate more revenue to support the research, about 15 percent of which typically must be subsidized by the university. Top doctors would attract paying, insured patients, improving the university's revenue flow. Kohler set out to "help somebody who hadn't showed up yet," said former Governor Goldschmidt.

"He set out to help get people we couldn't have hired otherwise," he said. "He set out to help patients who were never going to show up there unless we did the job right, and I suppose above all things, he set out to make live and real this connection between medical research, high quality medical care and medical education."[16]

While they shared aspirations to expand OHSU's research capacity, Kohler and Laster had different visions for how to do so, noted Bagby. Laster understood the importance of building OHSU's research capacity, but he concluded the university should focus on building one area of excellence, a vision he successfully fulfilled in the Vollum Institute and its focus on neuroscience.

"Peter had a grander view," Bagby said. "He wanted surgery to be better. He wanted internal medicine to be better. He wanted pediatrics to be better. He wanted Doernbecher [Children's Hospital] to be better. He had a very big idea. His goal was to get the university itself lifted up, and he knew it would take more than one foundation to do that. You can't just build up the corner of a building. He did things the right way and gave us the kind of space that we needed to accomplish our plans."[17]

Even without much space, Kohler started going after talent soon after he arrived at OHSU, though it was rough going without more to offer.

"The first recruitments in the early nineties were hard work," said Hallick, who as provost oversaw the university's research enterprise, including new hires. "I mean really hard. You sold the mountain over and over."[18]

She is talking about Mount Hood, symbol of Oregon's vast natural beauty. John Kendall, former dean of the medical school, said in the early 1980s, when Lewis William Bluemle was president, the mountain was worth about $10,000 in annual salary. Later in Kendall's tenure, he said, it was worth $20,000.

"It was true," he said. "It was worth money. You could sell it on the Mount Hood Factor. You could sell it on the basis of livability."[19]

Kohler put the value of the mountain at $40,000.[20] But he knew he needed to offer more than the mountain to get good researchers and faculty.

"You wanted to be a major biomedical research institution, and to do that, we had to have capacity," he said. "We were constrained, particularly in the area of research space, but also investigators. We need to be able to do some key recruitment and build-out our research activities. . . . Making sure we had the faculty, the space and the right people who could interact with each other in a coordinated way."[21]

Kohler also sought out strong department chairs who would appeal to good research professors, said Hallick. Federal research grants included money for indirect costs such as maintenance, administration, and other overhead. But for a time Kohler funneled those federal indirect cost allocations into more competitive salaries and what administrators called "dowries" for department chairs, allowing them to recruit new people to their programs. That meant that departments didn't necessarily collect as much of their indirect costs on research grants, but they drew some key people. Using indirect costs in this way is a kind of financial finesse that can work for a while when an organization is in a growth mode, Hallick said.

The indirect money "isn't gravy," she said. "It's just at the moment you get it, it's not embedded, and if the state or some other resources help you cover those infrastructure costs, then you're basically liberating that to invest."[22]

So Kohler and Hallick worked with the medical school to recruit research-oriented chairs with successful track records. They also gave them money to recruit good colleagues, Hallick said. The aim was to use the department chairs as the catalyst for boosting the entire research enterprise.

"It wasn't about recruiting a single person," she said. "It was about recruiting a team that was chosen by the new chair."[23]

Among the promising new department chairs recruited by the university was Magdalene "Maggie" So, hired in 1991 from the private Scripps health system in San Diego to become chair of the molecular microbiology and immunology department. With So came a package of other people. So wanted to bring Jay Nelson, a mid-career virologist and rising star in understanding virology and herpes simplex, who would later take charge of a new OHSU Vaccine and Gene Therapy Institute. In addition, So brought another promising researcher named Fred Hebner, who was her ex-husband. Hebner, in turn, wanted to bring his new wife, a medical student.

"We had to convince the medical school to accept transfer students, which they didn't really do," Hallick said, "but they finally made an exception in this case."[24]

In the early 1990s, the university also recruited Robb E. Moses, a promising young geneticist to head the department of molecular and medical genetics. Moses had a special interest in researching Fanconi anemia, a rare bone marrow disease that increases risks for leukemia. Bagby and Dr. Markus Grompe, a researcher and pediatrician who joined the genetics department in 1991, also had a special interest in the disease, which afflicted three of the daughters of David Frohnmayer, former Oregon Attorney General and University of Oregon president. Frohnmayer and his wife, Lynn, lost three of their daughters to the disease: Katie died in 1991 at age twelve, Kirsten in 1997 at age twenty-four, and Amy in 2016 at age twenty-nine, nineteen months after Frohnmayer himself passed away.

In 1994, Kohler hired M. Susan Smith, a professor in the physiology department at the University of Pittsburgh with a special interest in neuro endocrinology, to be director of the Oregon primate center. He was planning to fully integrate the center into the university after OHSU became a public corporation. Smith wanted to bring some other researchers with her, and she wanted a job for her husband, Bill Smith, an English professor at the University of Pennsylvania.

"It wasn't exactly our wheelhouse," Hallick said.[25]

But she learned that the English professor was computer savvy, so she made him head of educational communications, in charge of helping other professors learn to handle technology. He also proved to be an excellent grant writer. Hallick was fond of saying he was OHSU's first English professor.

EARLY EXPANSION

Shortly after Kohler arrived, many of the projects launched by Laster and others came to fruition, giving Kohler a lot more to sell in his recruiting than the mountain. The Casey Eye Institute opened in 1991 as an independent project led by Dr. Fraunfelder, head of OHSU's Department of Ophthalmology, and sponsored by an organization called Research to Prevent Blindness. Casey was the seventh and last regional eye research institute supported by the organization, which led the capital campaign to build it. The institute was named after James Casey, founder of United Parcel Service, and his brother, George Casey. There were other donors to the privately funded project, too. Shortly after Kohler arrived at OHSU in 1988, he and Fraunfelder invited donors for a bid opening to celebrate the project in the OHSU Auditorium. But upon opening the bids, the two administrators discovered the lowest was $5 million over the university's budget.

"We drew all of these people out there expecting to hear who was going to be the successful bidder," Kohler said, "and we had to tell them we needed more money."[26]

GBD architects, a Portland firm, designed the white, five-story building with clean lateral lines and ever-changing light, as though to say that the place where some of the top ophthalmologists in the world teach, do research, and treat eye disease should be pleasing to the eye. The 82,000-square-foot building, with an adjoining 320-car garage, includes the nation's largest glass floor designed by New York artist James Carpenter.[27]

The $23-million building crouches on the east brow of Marquam Hill as a striking, elegant gateway to the OHSU campus.[28] When the Department of Ophthalmology moved into its new quarters, it already had a good national reputation because of its many accomplished researchers. Fraunfelder, for example, was a world expert on surface eye cancer and on clinical ocular toxicology, the adverse side effects of drugs on the visual system. The additional research laboratories, offices, surgery suites, and outpatient clinics gave the institute space to flourish. The institute later expanded in 2006 into an 11,000-squre foot ambulatory care center in the Center for Health & Healing on the South Waterfront at the bottom of the tram and into 20,000 square feet of laboratories in the university's new Biomedical Research Building. Over the two decades following OHSU's conversion to a public corporation, the number of surgery patients at the institute quadrupled, research tripled, and patient visits and staffing doubled. In 2011, the institute ranked second in the nation in drawing NIH money for eye research.[29]

Several projects initially planned by Laster (with help from Hatfield) were also completed before OHSU became a public corporation. The $13.4 million library, or Biomedical Information Communication Center, was completed in 1991. In the following year, the $13.8 million School of Nursing building and the Center for Research on Occupational and Environmental Toxicology building were completed.[30]

The center, now called the Oregon Institute of Occupational Health Sciences, gets its own stream of state funding from Oregon's Worker Compensation Division. It houses one of the first research centers in the world to combine the use of molecular and cell biology in the study of adverse effects of chemicals on the nervous system and body[31]. Oregon is a fitting place for such a center as its residents place a premium on the environment. Oregon was, for example, the first state to pass a law requiring bottles and cans to be sold with refundable deposits.[32] The state also has some of the strictest land-use laws in the nation, and its entire coast belongs and is open to the public.[33]

In 1993, more space opened on the OHSU campus with the completion of the modern outpatient building called Physicians Pavilion. The development became key in providing the university not only with more parking, but also more revenue. And as noted earlier, the privately funded building gave OHSU administrators a glimpse of what was possible when they had control over raising capital for construction and could enter into business-like partnerships.[34]

FREE TO GROW

OHSU's expansion in the early 1990s gave the university momentum and a base to build on, but as Kohler argued before lawmakers, the growth and momentum would have ended without the university's conversion to a public corporation. As a more independent institution, OHSU could more readily raise revenue and donors were more inclined to give, assured their contributions would go for what they intended and not be absorbed or supplanted by the state.

That's become apparent to Druker in recent years since he started spending more time out of the lab working with donors. Contributors are accustomed to state university systems with big bureaucracies, Druker said, but as a public corporation, OHSU had the independence to raise money, erect buildings, and determine its fate much as a private university could do.

"Donors get that, and it resonates with them," he said. "When we talk about putting up a building or doing new things, we actually can execute on those projects very quickly. They are all on board."[35]

OHSU could now go to Wall Street on its own to get money without long delays. It was free to keep growing. So instead of losing momentum with the completion of all the projects launched during the Laster era, OHSU embarked on its biggest growth spurt in history.

With the initial $215 million bond package it received in January of 1996, it upgraded its hospitals, clinics, and labs and started a project to replace Doernbecher Children's Hospital. Kohler also was working with Hatfield to build a new federally-funded research center adjacent to the hospital, the name of which was changed from University Hospital to OHSU Hospital in 1996.

In February of 1998, the $60 million, 14-story, 266,000-square-foot research building, constructed in three phases, rose to completion between the hospital and library. The Mark O. Hatfield Research Center provided space for a variety of research enterprises scattered across the campus, including the OHSU Clinical Research Center, Doernbecher Pediatric Research Laboratories, Neurosurgery Research Laboratories, the Oregon Cancer Center, the Oregon Hearing Research Center, and a new emergency room.[36]

Three months after the Hatfield building was completed in 1998, the new, $73 million state-of-the-art Doernbecher Children's Hospital opened. The four-story tower spanned a canyon on the Pill Hill campus. *Oregonian* reporter Steve Woodward called the hospital, built with university bonds and $35 million in donations, "the most visible triumph for OHSU since it freed itself from state control in 1995."[37]

Randy Gragg, *The Oregonian*'s architecture and design critic, weighed in on the hospital and many of the other near forty new and old buildings on the 116-acre campus. The campus was beginning to look like "a mini-Hong Kong in the woods," he said.

> From the high idealism of its beginnings to the pragmatic urban mutation it's become, the OHSU campus is an 89-year lineage of architectural highs and lows. . . . Offering a promise of success as a medical facility, the Doernbecher nevertheless remains strained as a work of architecture. In much the same way it forces its way into

the landscape, it uncomfortably exhibits the clash between technology and nature.[38]

RESEARCHERS COME

Part of that conflict stemmed from the absence of flat land, forcing the university to put its buildings on slopes and across canyons and to connect them with bridges. Still, gleaming new laboratories rose on Pill Hill, and the researchers arrived—hundreds of them—and some became leaders. The university, for example, hired Dr. Mark A. Richardson, from Johns Hopkins University, where he was a professor, to become chair of OHSU's Department of Otolaryngology—head and neck surgery. In five years, he tripled the department's NIH funding, lifting it to among the top five otolaryngology departments in the nation. In 2007, he became OHSU's dean in the School of Medicine, a position he held until his death on September 2, 2016, after a steep fall while completing a home repair.[39] Dr. John G. Hunter left his post as a gastrointestinal surgeon and professor of surgery at Emory University School of Medicine in Atlanta to be professor and chairman of the Department of Surgery at OHSU. Hunter is among the pioneers of laparoscopic gastrointestinal surgery. OHSU lured Dr. Ron Rosenfeld, an internationally renowned endocrinologist and authority on the biology of growth, to be its chairman of pediatrics. He left in 2002 to become a senior vice president at the Lucile Packard Foundation for Children's Health in Palo Alto, but he is still on the OHSU faculty, still operates a research laboratory on Pill Hill, and has drawn continuous NIH research support for three decades.[40]

Along with researchers came new research initiatives. One, for example, was the Vaccine and Gene Therapy Institute at the Oregon Regional Primate Research Center in Hillsboro. Even before it was operating, Kohler used it as something to attract good researchers in much the same way he used the promise of a new cancer center to retain Bagby. In 1999, Kohler and Jay Nelson, head of the gene therapy institute, invited another rising star to join OHSU as a senior scientist at the institute and in the Pathobiology and Immunology Division at the primate center. He was Dr. Louis Picker, an associate professor of pathology at the University of Texas Southwestern Medical Center at Dallas. The institute and primate center were on the West Campus in Hillsboro, and Kohler had plans to erect a new building there by 2000 that would house both the Vaccine and Gene Therapy Institute and the Neurological Sciences Institute. The offer to Picker reflected the complexity of the university's funding. In the offer letter signed by Kohler and other administrators, Picker was told he would be tenured in the School of Medicine with a salary of $180,000 plus benefits. The primate center and the gene therapy institute would contribute $150,000 and another $30,000 would come from the pathology department. The letter goes on to explain that half his salary would be considered an X component funded by the university and the other half a Y component that will "be obtained from external sources and is to compensate you for special assignments, conditions or services."[41]

But Picker wasn't being offered just a job and salary. He also was given authority to establish a research program in vaccine development using monkeys at the primate center. He would "recruit three additional immunologists, each with a package of $650,000, thus bringing the total faculty recruitment package to $1.95 million." The money would cover salary, start-up costs such as equipment and supplies, technical help and relocation expenses. The new recruits would be expected to establish research programs within three years that would pay for half their salaries from NIH research grants and other sources. And Kohler told Picker he expected him and his team to shoot high.

"The faculty should make this unit one of the premier vaccine institutes in the world," he said.[42]

The offer included more. Picker would be expected to create a "vaccine testing facility." The offer stated "we will provide $182,000 to equip this laboratory and a total of $90,000 over three years for supplies. A total of $5,000 for personnel travel during the set-up of the laboratory will also be provided." The Vaccine and Gene Therapy Institute would occupy one wing of a $35 million, 100,000-square-foot building, which would be built near the primate center with funds from the NIH. Picker's laboratory would have 1,200 square feet of space for biochemistry, another 200 square feet for a biosafety Level 2 space, an office with a secretary, and additional office space for postdoctoral fellows.

The offer stated that in order to help Picker outfit his laboratory for primate research, the university would provide $750,000 in salary support for technical help, $360,000 for supplies, $260,000 for equipment for the vaccine testing facility, $260,000 for two cytometers, $40,000 for service contracts, $240,000 to support two additional core technicians, $200,000 for supplies for the cores, $400,000 for the molecular biology core laboratory, and $39,539 to pay rent for nine months at the VA Hospital while awaiting the completion of the Vaccine and Gene Therapy Institute's new building.[43]

The institute also would provide centralized or shared core services that Picker and his research team could tap. They would have access to an immunology cell flow core with two cell sorters, two cell analyzers, computers, and service contracts for instruments; a monoclonal core devoted to producing monoclonal antibodies to use in primate studies; an imaging core, which includes a state-of-the-art confocal microscope and a technician; and a molecular biology core with sequencing, oligonucleotide generation, microarray analysis, and chip preparation.[44]

The letter made it clear that Picker was being offered a chance to help lead in the creation of an ambitious new research institute.

"We were trying to create something special here," Kohler said.[45]

Four months later, Picker and Jay Nelson, the institute's director, outlined an $18.5 million, five-year plan for the institute that envisioned five investigators and a support staff of another dozen or so research professors and technicians.

"The time has come to 'breathe life' into the Vaccine and Gene Therapy Institute and set the institute on a course to become a world class research center," they wrote Kohler.

During his work in Dallas, Picker had studied the immune system and had ideas about how disease-causing microorganisms in blood and tissues trigger memory T cells that stay in the body for years and will remind the immune system to attack again should the invaders return. The T cells could be the basis for a vaccine against diseases such as HIV/AIDS and tuberculosis, but Picker could not test his ideas on humans. So the OHSU offer appealed to him because it would put him next door to primates—in particular, the only pathogen-free colony of macaque monkeys in the nation.[46]

But he also was drawn by the chance to be part of something bigger than himself, to join a team that shared his drive to make a difference. He had an additional attractive offer from Emory University. "But at Emory, I wouldn't have had the opportunity to start from scratch to build this new institution," he said.[47]

FREEDOM

Picker may have also sensed another quality at OHSU that often comes up often in interviews with researchers there—freedom. It both draws and keeps researchers at the university. Freedom reflects a core value of the institution that drew its founders to break away from the Willamette Medical School late in the nineteenth century, that drew the academic medical center to break away from the University of Oregon in 1976, and, finally, to break away from the state and the state higher education system in 1995 when it became a public corporation. Freedom helped draw and hold Druker.

"One of the things I've said I like about being here, besides the collaborative collegiate environment, is that you can pretty much do whatever you want," he said. "There aren't any people that tell you to 'do this," and there aren't people that tell you 'you can't do that.' There are lot of other institutions where you'll bump up against either competition for space, for resources, for ideas, whereas around here, people let you explore and actually help you explore."[48]

Giving researchers that kind of freedom became the centerpiece of Bagby's management style. He admired a professor at Harvard's medical school named David Nathan, who had trained at least ten of the heads of pediatrics departments across the country. Nathan told Bagby that he was so successful because he hired people who were smarter than him and then he got out of the way.

"So I worked that way," Bagby said.

OHSU would not be a place where researchers would be told what they couldn't do, he said.

> My feeling is you should do precisely what makes you the happiest and what is the biggest challenge you can face. For me, it became at that period of time personally how leukemia starts. So you have a normal person and the next day they have something wrong that leads to leukemia. That's what I want to understand. Part of that had to do with personal stories. When I was a resident, I took care of a woman with acute leukemia who died within 10 days after coming to the hospital, and that really had an impact on me. I said, "This is something I really need to figure out."[49]

Bagby also became friends with Frohnmayer, who lost his daughters to Fanconi anemia.

"To understand how they get leukemia I think is leading us to understand how other people without Fanconi get leukemia as well," he said. "I am driven now to finish that story, figure it out, and to more importantly get other people interested in that story."[50]

OHSU's culture of freedom spurs researchers to pursue their own interests and collaborate, Bagby said.

"Those are the two parts of freedom," he said, "the freedom of somebody saying, 'I'm going to get out of your way and be supportive,' and that's a very personal person-to-person thing, and that has to do with leadership. And the other thing is sort of a culture. The culture at OHSU is, 'Oh, you're interested in that? Go get a grant and then we'll talk to you, and we won't get in your way.'"[51]

BUSINESS OF GROWTH

OHSU also aggressively exercised its new freedom as a young, autonomous, entrepreneurial public corporation. Kohler and his team looked everywhere for opportunities to find profitable partners and enterprises, to grow not only through construction and new hires, but also through partnerships and mergers. The university was operating like a corporation, looking for ways to stay lean, to compete and to grow.

Because the university was so physically constrained on Pill Hill, Kohler's team looked west for opportunities. Once freed from the state, OHSU fully merged with the Oregon Regional Primate Research Center so that it was not just an affiliate but an integrated part of the university, adding 160 acres to the university's assets and a major source of new research money. For example, the center in 1998 pulled in $17.6 million in federal research grants, more than the $9.8 million in research money flowing to the Vollum Institute and second only to the university's School of Medicine, which drew $68 million in federal money.[52] Adopting the primate center immediately lifted OHSU's research ranking among the nation's academic health centers. In addition, Jean Bates, a nurse and alumna, along with her husband, a dentist, had donated to OHSU property adjacent to the primate center property. So in all, OHSU had 247 acres on its West Campus by 2000.

In anticipation of OHSU integrating the primate center, another merger was orchestrated earlier by Paul Bragdon, former longtime president of the private, prestigious Reed College in Portland. He had been hired in the early 1990s to head the Oregon Medical Research Foundation, which owned the primate center, managed its research grants and also provided start-up grants for other Oregon scientists. The foundation board did little fund-raising, operated independent of OHSU and saw its primary duty as overseeing the primate center, which had a director "who did pretty much what he wanted to," Bragdon said.[53]

"I really thought it was dangerous that they were in charge of the primate center," Bragdon said. "They really had no control of what was happening there."[54]

Because the foundation did little for OHSU and was at times at odds with the university, Laster, during his presidency, had created a second foundation for the university called the OHSU Foundation. With Kohler's expectation that the primate center would become part of the university, Bragdon concluded the two foundations should merge. The merger appealed to Kohler, Bragdon said, with the medical foundation's endowment of about $20 million, its acres of land and its handling of primate center research grants. It made no sense for OHSU to have two foundations, which created confusion for donors. Merging them into one provided a useful clarity and efficiency, said Davis, the communication director.[55]

Bragdon and Kohler worked out the merger over three years, eventually sealing a deal in 1994 that left Bragdon without a job. The day after he left the foundation, however, he stepped in as president of the Oregon Graduate Institute of Science and Technology, which had financial problems that would eventually drive it to propose also merging with OHSU.

The graduate institute was a privately funded computer engineering school established by Howard Vollum, then-Governor Hatfield, and other business leaders and chartered by the 1963 Oregon Legislature to provide research and graduate-level training in support of the state's rapidly expanding high-technology industries such as Intel and Vollum's Tektronix. So many companies were expanding nearby in Hillsboro and Washington County that the region was nicknamed the Silicon Forest. The graduate institute spread over twenty acres that adjoined OHSU's West Campus. By the late 1990s, with a small enrollment of about 350 graduate students, the institute was struggling financially. It was heavily invested in research, which falls about 15 percent short of paying for itself, and it was not getting the philanthropic support it needed to make up the deficit. In 2000, Kohler visited Ed Cooley, chair of the institute's board, in OHSU Hospital, where he was on his death bed. Cooley urged Kohler to save the institute by merging it with OHSU.[56]

In August of 2000, Kohler and Edward Thompson, president and CEO of the institute, signed a memorandum of understanding pledging to merge. The engineers could collaborate with OHSU medical researchers on biomedical engineering, biomedical computer science and environmental and biomolecular systems. The merger plan called for a $20 million budget that would include the hiring of eight new faculty and for a five-year, $37 million fund-raising campaign to eventually hire twenty more faculty. The memorandum described the merger as a win-win plan.

"Activities at the two institutions are largely complementary," it said, "and combining the two will produce critical mass that will attract major new funding and research distinction while enhancing services to their current constituencies."[57]

After the merger was completed in 2001, the university changed its name from Oregon Health Sciences University to Oregon Health & Science University, acknowledging that it was expanding its scope beyond the health sciences into computer engineering. Again, as with the primate center, OHSU also was adopting another batch of research money, about $20 million a year, by merging with the Oregon Graduate Institute. The additional research awards would help OHSU boost its NIH ranking.[58]

Yet another research group joined the university during this period, too. The Neurological Sciences Institute at Legacy Good Samaritan Medical Center in Portland asked OHSU to adopt it. The institute had been harassed by animal rights activists for its use of cats in research, and its leaders felt their research would find a better fit at OHSU. The Vollum Institute, with its focus on the microbiology of the brain, seemed like the logical place to put it. But the neurological institute was more involved in clinical research with humans as opposed to the pure basic science at Vollum, so OHSU found a home for it in 1998 on the West Campus as its fifth institute. The research group got space along with the Vaccine and Gene Therapy Institute in the new West Campus building when it opened in 2001.[59]

OHSU brought together the City of Hillsboro and neighboring educational and research enterprises to craft a twenty-year plan for its West Campus. The organizations involved included the Capital Center, a nearby building offering career education through a consortium of public and private schools and businesses; AmberGlen, a biotech development park; and the Oregon Graduate Institute. The plan protected the campus from being bisected by major roads, as Hillsboro at one time envisioned, and put it right next to the Portland metro area's light-rail network, known as MAX.[60] Hallick described the expansion:

> So by taking advantage of the primate center resources and the interest in AIDS vaccine testing in primates, you can use those resources to bring in the talent that you eventually want to have in immunology and genetics to do gene therapy. The time was ripe. I mean, we had to do it then.[61]

OHSU's aggressive and entrepreneurial moves to establish a substantial presence west of Portland in Washington County, home to a major branch of Intel and world headquarters for Nike Inc., caught the attention of Portland leaders. OHSU was among the city's top three employers. In the five years following its conversion to a public corporation, it added 3,500 jobs, most of them high-paying, and grew to 10,000 employees. The university had become a powerful economic engine for the city, one that Portland leaders did not want to see drift elsewhere. But containing OHSU growth in Portland offered big challenges because Pill Hill was so crowded and ill-suited to more development with its slopes and canyons. The university had added thousands of employees without any more parking spaces, a problem it handled by persuading its workers to take buses, reducing the share driving single cars to 50 percent, a record unmatched just about anywhere. After seeing OHSU break ground for its new West Campus building in Hillsboro, Portland leaders realized they could lose one of their most valuable businesses, Hallick said. City officials were ready to start looking for new space on Pill Hill for OHSU's expansion, even though the hill already seemed saturated with buildings.

"Literally, almost the first shovelful [on the West Campus] suddenly induced Portland to be more accommodating to us," Hallick said, "because it became obvious that what we'd been saying for years—that if we couldn't grow in Portland, we were going to grow out there—suddenly became a reality."[62]

ENTERPRISE

OHSU's new entrepreneurial energy also gave rise to another enterprise launched by its physicians: one that would have been much more difficult if the university had not become a public corporation. The doctors created a 501(c)(3) nonprofit for a physicians' billing group. The OHSU Medical Group unified more than thirty-three independent practice groups into one unit that included the clinical practice plans of OHSU faculty. The group contracted with the university as a separate entity to provide patient care. For a time, the participating faculty members would get one check for their research and teaching duties and another through the medical group for their clinical work.

"It gave us bargaining power, and the ability to contract with insurance entities like Blue Cross and others without having to go through state contracting [rules] that would slow that process, if not kill it," said Dr. Swanson, the skin cancer expert who worked with Kohler and others in creating the medical group, and who saw Kohler as a patient.

Physicians in the group paid an expense, a sort of tax, to help support the medical school. The group "basically was funding and running the school because of the lack of state support," said Swanson. He went on to work in OHSU's Center for Health & Healing on Portland's Southwest Waterfront, a building constructed with more than $105 million in bonds financed in large part by the physicians group.[63]

In another enterprise promoted by an Oregon contingent of the national Campaign for Women's Health and a group of prominent Portland women, OHSU in May of 1998 began raising money to build space, possibly on the South Waterfront, for the Center for Women's Health, an enterprise already taking shape with a director and staff. The center embraced a holistic, team-based approach to integrate health care services focused on women, including outpatient clinical care, clinical research, mental health care, and consumer education services. The university eventually found space for the center in the Physician's Pavilion. More recently, it moved into OHSU's newest patient care facility next to the hospital.

Also in 2000, OHSU entered a joint venture with Management of Medical Innovation (MMI), a company in Cambridge, England, to help turn its research into spin-off businesses. Profits would be divided among MMI, OHSU, and the spin-off companies. The venture never got off the ground, but it revealed OHSU's rising stature in the medical research world. British newspapers noted OHSU's Brian Druker had helped develop the genomic "cancer pill" to cure leukemia. They also mentioned OHSU researchers recently had cloned a healthy female rhesus monkey named Tetra, the first cloning of a primate in the world. Researchers at the primate center had drawn global headlines when they revealed that they had, on September 7, 1999, delivered a healthy cloned female monkey.[64] One British newspaper called OHSU "one of the world's leading research centers."[65]

As if Kohler did not have enough going on as the university approached the new century, he sent Hallick to talk with Michael Mooney, president of the private Lewis & Clark College in Portland; and Edward Thompson, president of the Oregon Graduate Institute of Science and Technology; about establishing a private research university in Portland that could attract at least $1 billion in donor support. That venture, too, died, but talks among the three schools went on secretly for months without ever leaking into the public or the press. The leaders saw the creation of a research university as a way of boosting Portland's economy just as major research universities were doing in Seattle, San Francisco and San Diego. But Kohler believed that OHSU could become the institution to fulfill that role.[66]

THE PAYOFF

OHSU's investments into research generally, though not always, reaped the kind of benefits Kohler and his team envisioned. As the Vollum Institute made plans to add ten more laboratories, many of the university's other research ventures also blossomed. A good example is the Vaccine and Gene Therapy Institute. Less than a year after Picker was hired in the summer of 1999, Nelson, the institute's director, hired many more prominent researchers. The institute hired Klaus Frueh, principal scientist and virology group leader at the R.W. Johnson Pharmaceutical Research Institute in San Diego. Dr. Janko Nikolic-Zugic, a rising star in immunology at the Memorial Sloan-Kettering Cancer Center, also joined the institute. So did Mark Slifka, a scientist in the Department of Neuropharmacology at the Scripps Research Institute in La Jolla, California.

In late September 2001, the institute opened with a staff of sixty in a 44,000-square-foot wing of the new building. The wing housed seven research laboratories and four highly secure biosafety rooms for the study of infectious diseases. The dedication was postponed a year because the September 11 terrorist attacks barred transportation for some scientists from around the world who would want to attend.[67]

By the end of 2014, the institute had brought in more than $240 million in research grants, nearly twenty times what it spent on its initial five-year plan. Picker's team alone, which includes Nelson and Frueh, has brought in millions of dollars in research support for its efforts to develop a vaccine for the HIV virus that causes AIDS. The Bill & Melinda Gates Foundation gave the team $8 million for its research in 2012 and another $25 million in 2014.

Picker's team began recruiting volunteers in June of 2016 for human trials for a potential HIV vaccine and cure for those who already have AIDS. Picker said it is "quite likely" the vaccine he used to eradicate Simian Immunodeficiency Virus in half of infected primates would work in humans. The vaccine also posed a promising technique for fighting other infectious diseases, such as malaria and hepatitis C. Picker's work is being closely watched around the world for its promise in combating AIDS, which kills 1.5 million people each year.[68]

The institute's initial five-year plan worked out just as designed, Picker said, although he noted that it could have benefited from making subsequent long-range plans.

"But from the 10,000-foot level, it is all good," he said. "We have done what we said we were going to, and the university is proud of that. . . . We developed a great team here. The team they allowed us to assemble, it is still here, and we have the freedom to do what we think is right and it has worked."[69]

In its first five years as a public corporation, OHSU expanded its research space alone by 42 percent, from 243,000 square feet to 345,000 square feet. It spent $77 million on new research buildings, $16.8 million on renovations of research laboratories, with nearly half the financing coming from bonds, 27 percent from federal grants and only 3 percent from the state.

Research income climbed during that period by 95 percent to $168 million in 2000. Kohler created an Office of Technology Management to help the public corporation push patent applications, which increased from an average six per year to sixteen per year.[70] OHSU's national ranking among academic health centers as measured by its research money had climbed from eighty-seventh in 1986 to sixtieth in 1995, and to thirty-third by 2000, which put it within striking distance of Kohler's goal of twentieth.[71]

The university made gains on other fronts in its first five years. It was now operating the hospital of first choice rather than last resort. In a survey of 1,031 households, residents ranked OHSU Hospital the best of five in the Portland metropolitan area for reputation, having the best doctors and being best at caring for those who could not pay.[72]

The OHSU endowment doubled to about $225 million, its hospital and university revenue climbed 46 percent to $714 million a year, and it increased its professional teaching and research staff by 24 percent, or 461 people, to a total of 2,363.[73] Kohler created new administrative positions to oversee the university's growth: a vice president for research, vice president for development, and vice president for clinical programs.

An accrediting organization, the Commission on Colleges of the Northwest Association of Schools and Colleges, in a 2000 interim report concluded: "Oregon Health Sciences University is a dynamic institution led by a group of very capable leaders. In many respects it is remarkable that the institution has not only survived, but has increased its stature in a time of dwindling state resources."[74]

The state gave the university between $53 and $56 million for each of its first five years. Despite nearly flat state funding, the university was able through its increased efficiencies and business practices to preserve programs that would have been cut were it still a state agency. The university raised tuition, pushed physicians and basic researchers to pay more of their own salaries, and saved costs it was no longer paying to the state for services. Through more revenue and less costs, OHSU was able to cover its inflationary increases for its first five years as a public corporation despite no significant increases from the state, Hallick said.

"In fact," she said, "we gave significant salary increases to bring people to market, and we didn't eliminate any education programs."[75]

Many other academic health centers, however, were not faring so well. The forces of rising drug costs, reduced Medicare payments, and low-paying managed care insurance plans were forcing teaching hospitals, particularly large ones in inner big cities, to make dramatic cost cuts that usually meant reducing staff. The Detroit Medical Center lost $160 million in 1998 and $93 million in the first half of 1999. Five academic medical centers in New York City collectively saw their operating income drop by $100 million in 1999. The University of Pennsylvania Health System in Philadelphia saw its operating revenues drop $288 million over 1997 and 1998.[76] In a 1999 survey, 40 to 50 percent of forty-nine academic health center hospitals were operating with negative margins. Nearly half of sixty-one hospitals reported reducing staff.[77]

In an attempt to cope with rising costs and declining revenue, the University of California at San Francisco Medical Center and Stanford University Health Services merged their teaching hospitals in 1997, hoping to gain economies of scale. But the merged health center produced a new layer of bureaucracy that only drove up costs more. By 1999, when it called in the Hunter Group, a seventy-member management consulting firm that specialized in helping medical schools balance their budgets, the two hospital systems were hemorrhaging $2 million a month in operating losses. The consultants told the troubled UCSF-Stanford merger it would have to lay off 2,000 employees to be financially viable. The schools made cuts and dissolved the merger. The Hunter Group became viewed as the slash-and-burn cost-cutter for ailing academic health centers across the country. Under Hunter's guidance, the University of Pennsylvania Medical Center in Philadelphia cut 2,800 out of 14,000 health service jobs in 1999 and 2000. The George Washington University Medical Center in Washington, DC, sold 80 percent of its hospital to the for-profit Universal Health Services in 1997.[78]

Many of these academic medical centers had prestige and big endowments, price tags, and profits. They were not accustomed to operating with lean administrations and belt-tightening efficiencies as OHSU was and were caught off guard by the forces of managed care and lower

Medicare payments, said Jim Walker, OHSU vice president for finance and administration.

"The whole world changed in a pretty short period," he said. "It was harder for them to come to grips with it. . . . They weren't used to having to cut costs."[79]

OHSU, by contrast, had trimmed down to a lean operation in its first years as a public corporation and had entered a growth surge, where it added rather than cut workers. Its challenge was to avoid hiring too many workers, Walker said.[80]

David Hunter, chief executive officer for the Hunter Group, told the University Health System Consortium, a national organization serving academic health centers, "One of the most significant factors leading to deteriorating performances is the attitudes of Academic Medical Center Leadership." He said the health center leaders displayed denial, complacency, inflexibility, lack of urgency, slow consensus decision-making, and the inability to make tough decisions. These are all debilitating qualities in a competitive health care market, and they were all scarce at OHSU.[81]

MORE MONEY, MORE PROBLEMS

Though OHSU grew and asserted its dominance in the Oregon health care market, Kohler and his team still had their share of headaches during the university's early years as a public corporation. These ranged from problems integrating its new partners, such as the primate center or the Oregon Graduate Institute of Science and Technology, to disgruntled workers, an unfounded Medicare fraud investigation, and animal rights activists.

In the fall of 1999, Smith, director of the primate center, told Kohler that the merger was forcing her scientists to slow down; ironically, because of OHSU bureaucratic obstacles.

"We are losing efficiency and some of the service provided by OHSU has been of very little added value," she wrote. "It can take a very long time to get anything done at OHSU."

The OHSU human resources department was "adversarial" and taking nine months to approve a new hire, a process that previously took a month, she said. Payroll information was slow, contracts were sloppy, and the OHSU travel services were "terrible" and "costing more money." She said her employees regretted the merger and would prefer to go "back to the way things were" when the primate center was more independent.

"We need some independence to manage our affairs if we are going to maintain our current level of services and effectiveness," she wrote.[82]

An independent group of researchers who came to review the merger the following spring reached similar conclusions:

"During our visit, however, it became apparent that interactions with the Central Campus are far from ideal," wrote John H. Nilson, chair of pharmacology at Case Western Reserve University near Cleveland, Ohio."[83]

Kohler winced at what he was seeing.

"I realized that after escaping the bureaucracy of the state, we had created one of our own," he said.[84]

The merger, he concluded, had created a clash of cultures between the primate center, where a small group of people were focused on a narrow research operation, and the larger university with its complexity and multiple missions. In addition to working to improve communications and operations between the two organizations, the merger also required that Kohler learn to live with occasional confrontations with animal rights protesters. Groups opposed to using live monkeys in research, such as the Coalition to End Primate Experimentation, staged protests outside the primate center. Sometimes they would try to break in. In June of 1999, about thirty protesters gathered outside Kohler's home.[85] And on one late October day, Kohler recalled, a bus of about thirty animal rights activists with a national group parked outside his house. He happened to be in his basement when several of them came up to his basement windows and rattled the bars over them as though looking for a way inside.[86] Groups also distributed tracts attacking OHSU, such as one by the Coalition to Abolish Animal Testing of Portland that questioned the benefits of primate research. At the primate center, the tract said, "research alone cost the public about $25 million, yet the center has not produced a single cure from its animal research in 40-plus years."[87] Activists at times went to the homes of researchers, put graffiti on their homes or put their addresses and photos of their children on the Internet, Hallick said.

"Some of those groups were scary," she said. "It was a very difficult time for our faculty who used animal research models."[88]

One day about eight-to-ten protesters made it to the president's suite in Baird Hall and chained themselves to the desks, said Carol Reinmiller, Kohler's secretary. The president was gone at the time. The protesters chanted against the primate center until security workers and Portland police forced them out.

"They had all that chain stuff all over them and tattoos," Reinmiller recalled. "Half of them had leather boots, belts."[89]

Kohler and his leadership team also contended with some unhappy employees who in some cases defected, sued the university, or threatened to strike. While many if not most employees noticed few changes after the university converted to a public corporation, the shift put more pressure on some, particularly middle managers, as well as doctors and scientists who were expected to generate more of their own pay through clinical practices and research.

In the spring of 1997, a group of twenty doctors, nurse practitioners, and support staff left the university, pooled their money, leased a building in southwest Portland, bought some furniture, and opened the Fanno Creek Clinic. The group objected to the aggressive belt-tightening OHSU was going through to stay solvent while the university continued to provide more charity care than any other hospital and to treat some of the state's sickest, costliest patients. The university had brought together its primary care specialties—internal medicine, family medicine, pediatrics, and women's health—to share resources. OHSU Hospital also discharged patients more quickly and used hospitalists, doctors specializing in hospital care who freed primary care doctors from time-consuming rounds. The Fanno Creek group did not like these changes.[90]

Two years later, representatives of the Oregon Nurses Association at OHSU threatened to strike in the fall of 1999 because the university nurses' pay, an average $22.97 per hour, was not as high as that for nurses in other Portland hospitals. The low pay contributed to a nursing shortage at OHSU that the union also wanted the university to correct. OHSU argued the generous 12 percent of pay it was sinking into each nurse's retirement fund put their compensation on a par with other nurses.[91] More than six months after the negotiations began, the university and union settled in November of 1999 on a compromise that gave the nurses a 3 percent increase for the current year and a 2.5 percent raise the year after. They also got some small bonuses to help offset the rising costs of their health benefits.[92]

In the summer of 2000, two researchers sued the university after administrators concluded they were engaged in a conflict of interest with their private company, Clinical Research Group of Oregon, which conducted clinical trials for drug and food companies. The researchers, kidney specialists Dr. David McCarron and Dr. William Bennett, together ran the university's division of nephrology, building it from four faculty members in 1977 to a division with twenty-two faculty members and a clinical, research, and support staff of sixty people. Kohler's administrators accused the doctors of improperly using employees and funds to operate their private business. Other researchers also charged their research was biased because of their sponsors. Based on his findings, for example, McCarron promoted the health features of milk and Campbell's Soup as a food that reduced high blood pressure, cholesterol, and blood sugars. His research was supported by the dairy industry and Campbell's Soup.[93] While Kohler wanted his staff to be entrepreneurial and foster spin-off companies, he didn't want them engaging in research for profit that marred their scientific integrity. He also didn't like seeing news about the lawsuits appearing on the front page of *The Oregonian* among other places.

"I may be overly sensitive," he wrote to Davis and other staff members, "but I think the stories are doing some harm."[94]

There were other potentially harmful stories about OHSU in *The Oregonian* during the summer of 2000, including three front-page accounts of federal investigations into Medicare billing fraud allegations at the university involving 768 procedures performed by scores of doctors. In addition, auditors for the state Office of Medical Assistance Programs concluded doctors in the University Medical Group improperly charged Medicaid $338,000 in 1995 and 1996, including payments for services physicians couldn't prove they delivered.[95] The medical group repaid the overcharges to the state while the federal investigation, which involved the FBI, fizzled without charges or sanctions. Kohler said the charges were bogus claims from an employee who had been fired.[96]

And not everything the public corporation did during those early years worked. Two institutes adopted by OHSU—the Oregon Graduate Institute of Science and Technology and the Neurological Sciences Institute—would ultimately fail to survive. It became clear that the dream of using the graduate institute as a vehicle to create a sizable bioengineering program was too expensive and ambitious. The Oregon Graduate Institute's merger with OHSU would also prove to be another "clash of cultures," Davis said. While OHSU researchers raised money for their salaries through research grants, she said, the Graduate Institute researchers were accustomed to a guaranteed salary and to working in small, independent units rather than as part of a large institution.

"They were all part of the Oregon Graduate Institute, but they basically were a bunch of completely different businesses that did their own thing," Davis said.[97]

Portland State University and OHSU negotiated a transfer of at least ten of the institute's computer science faculty to PSU in 2004, and within a few years, other Oregon Graduate Institute faculty were absorbed into other OHSU departments, but the institute was closed and its West Campus buildings were sold or leased.[98]

During the same period, the Neurological Sciences Institute also closed, and its scientists were spread elsewhere in the university, most in faculty appointments, said Hallick. The institute's twenty or so investigators came from Legacy Good Samaritan Medical Center "like orphans," placed on the West Campus and never really integrated into the university, she said.[99] After the neurological institute closed, the thriving and expanding Vaccine and Gene Therapy Institute took over its space in the West Campus building.

THE BIG ASK

As a result of its aggressive expansion, OHSU had within four years spent its initial $215 million in bonds and some additional borrowing through a few smaller bond issues and was just about tapped out for capital. And one member of the OHSU board, still one of the most influential political leaders in the state, expressed his concerns about the institution's health in a memo to Kohler and board Chair Fred Buckman. Former Governor Goldschmidt wrote that "after two or more years of conversation," the university still was failing to attract many more "clients from the private insurance marketplace."[100] He acknowledged the university showed promise in that it had increased hospital occupancy levels, reduced costs, won more federal research money, expanded its foundation staff and private fund-raising efforts, and pursued partnerships to offer specialty care for outlying hospitals across Oregon. But he was concerned that the university depended so heavily on its hospital and clinical revenues, yet was not making progress in competing for paying, privately insured patients.

The university was opening some primary care clinics in Portland, but it was not aggressively marketing health plans to potentially lucrative customers such as Nike Inc. or the City of Portland.[101]

Kohler wanted to add more laboratories and researchers, but he and Walker also were sensitive to Goldschmidt's concerns about university finances and were cautious about taking on too much debt.

"If things are going well, people are going to lend you more money than you should have," Walker said.[102]

Borrowing to expand research is also risky because research doesn't fully pay for itself and actually requires a subsidy from somewhere—hospital and clinical revenue, an endowment, or state support. But Kohler needed to keep expanding the research enterprise if he was to reach his top twenty goal. So he and his team looked elsewhere for money and a way to strike a proper balance between debt and growth. They soon had their eyes fixed on the massive settlement that forty-six states made in November, 1998, with the tobacco industry. The industry would give the states annual payments totaling $206 billion over the next quarter century, $2.2 billion of which would flow to Oregon, to help cover their Medicaid costs for damage to smokers' health. The payments would start in 2000,[103] and Kohler and his team thought they could make a good case for using some of that money to pay for research that could lead to health improvements. In a move both audacious and ironic, Kohler proposed to his board that the university ask for money of the state from which it just five years earlier had declared independence. At the OHSU board's annual retreat, the major topic would be how to approach the legislature for $20 million in tobacco settlement money.

The retreat was organized for October 15 and 16, 1999, at Skamania Lodge, a secluded resort near Stevenson, Washington, about a forty-five-minute drive northeast of Portland. The lodge spreads over a hillside overlooking the scenic Columbia River Gorge. The retreat agenda focused first on guiding the board to reflect on OHSU's goals, mission, and values and how best to meet its challenges. Kohler's team raised questions for the board to ponder: Is our goal research growth or financial strength? How do we address the financial gaps in the strategic plan? What should we stop doing? Can our entire strategy be premised on the hospital making money?[104]

The team reminded the board of OHSU's vision: "to improve the lives of Oregonians and others by being a national and international leader through excellence and innovation in health care delivery, education and research."[105]

It also reminded them of OHSU's core values: Creation of new knowledge, education of high-quality health professionals, a commitment to excellence in all we do, integrity and collegiality that makes OHSU a good place to work, and compassionate care for our patients.

And finally, the team listed the institution's goals, which included the following:

- Meet the state's need for health care professionals.
- Become the regional leader in the care of adult and pediatric patients with neurological diseases, cancer, cardiovascular, and related ailments.
- Achieve financial stability, including 175 days of cash on hand and an endowment worth at least $500 million.[106]

Walker showed the board financial documents and graphs and charts that projected the university's revenue would plunge into the red in a year or two if nothing changed. But, he said, if the university invested $140 million to expand and upgrade the hospital, $162 million for two new buildings and an additional 400,000 square feet of research space, and $112 million to hire 212 renowned researchers, it could put itself on a trajectory to net $10 million or more in annual income by 2006. Walker's scenarios, however, included an assumption that the state would increase its annual support by $20 million, which would normally seem unlikely.[107] Board members were skeptical.

"I remember having conversations with board members who said, 'You guys are out of your mind,'" said Davis. "They're not giving you

$20 million. Because at that point the state had not invested in research. They did not see that as their job. They invested in education."[108]

But maybe it was not such a stretch if OHSU aimed for the tobacco money. As the meeting unfolded, board members began to suggest that OHSU not only ask for tobacco money, but ask for more than the $20 million Kohler had proposed. Kohler had reminded board members that OHSU was aspiring to be among the top twenty medical schools in NIH research revenue and already had climbed from a rank of sixtieth in 1995 to thirty-ninth in 1998.[109]

The board then focused on what Fred Buckman, the chair, would call the Big Ask. They discussed how to make a case for tobacco money. Not only would health research directly address the harm caused by smoking, but it also would bring in researchers whose discoveries would lead to spin-off biotechnology businesses and more jobs. The investment would be good for the state's health and economic development. By the second day, the Big Ask had climbed to $100 million. OHSU could match that with a fund-raising campaign, giving it $200 million to expand its research operations. Then, as the retreat was about to wrap up, Goldschmidt dramatically raised the stakes, recalled Buckman.

"He said, 'I think it should be $200 million.' It went from $100 million to $200 million at the 11th hour and 45th minute, and it was one of the really good things we did."[110]

Hallick, who was sitting across the table from Goldschmidt, remembers the moment.

"It was completely arbitrary," she said. "It was not based on what we thought we could get. It was, 'Why not? We go through all this trouble, we might as well ask for what we need.'"[111]

Over the next year, Kohler's team and the board agreed that if the legislature would give it $200 million, the university would raise an additional $300 million from donors. As with its drive to convert OHSU into a public corporation, Kohler and his team again were raising their sights. What had begun as a weekend retreat to consider asking lawmakers for

$20 million had grown into a half-billion dollar proposal for what would be called the Oregon Opportunity Initiative, all devoted to expanding the university's research power, economic health, and national stature.

Notes

1 Brian Druker, MD, interview by Edward Keenan, Nov. 30, 2011, Biomedical Information and Communications Center, OHSU, interview no. 114 11/30, 2011, transcript, OHSU Oral History Project, p. 9. Druker said, "I decided at that point I was going to make a difference, and I was going to do whatever it took. And it was for me the difference between giving 90 percent effort and giving 110 percent effort. And I realized that's what I needed to do. And I needed to leave. I needed to find my own, set up my own laboratory. And it was going to be outside of Dana-Farber. And I needed that kick."

2 Brian Druker, MD, interview, Feb. 11, 2015, in his OHSU office.

3 Druker, interview, Nov. 30, 2011, p. 10.

4 Druker, interview, Feb. 11, 2015.

5 Druker, interview, Nov. 30, 2011, p. 10.

6 Grover Bagby, MD, interview, April 14, 2014 at the Heathman Hotel in Portland.

7 Druker, interview, Feb. 11, 2015.

8 Druker, interview, Nov. 30, 2011, pp. 10-16.

9 Lois Davis, interview, March 9, 2015, in her Portland State University office.

10 Peter O. Kohler, MD, interview, Dec. 5, 2014, Baird Hall, OHSU.

11 Kristina Breeneman, "Mr. OHSU: Pill Hill Enters 2000 in Good Fiscal Health," *The Business Journal*, Oct. 8, 1999, p. 19.

12 Peter O. Kohler, "Remarks to the U.S. House of Representatives Committee on Science, Space and Technology." Kohler was prepared to deliver these remarks on Aug. 3, 1993, but that meeting was canceled. His speech was put into the committee hearing record. In the speech, Kohler goes on to say, "The latest National Science Foundation data, based on 1991 fiscal year, show that Oregon Health Sciences University now ranks 73rd in the amount of federal research and development dollars that have been awarded. This is up from a rank of 105th in 1986, just five years earlier. One can easily infer that the university's recruitment of outstanding scientist-clinicians is directly related to the availability of new facilities that have permitted the institution to alter its economic circumstances. . . . The presence of these research stars has functioned as a magnet, attracting to OHSU the best and brightest of Oregon's own young research community, so that the recruitment of these stars has enhanced local potential, providing career opportunities that previously had not existed for young Oregonians."

Kohler drew on a Dec. 11, 1992, memorandum from Thomas G. Fox, vice president for development & public affairs, titled "Using Space to Enhance University Reputation." Fox noted that Clark Kerr, in an article for the May/June 1991 issue of *Change* argued that "the attraction of research stars is the key variable in university reputation." Kerr added, it is "reasonable to suggest that facilities are a key ingredient to the attraction of research stars."

13 Thomas G. Fox, vice president for development and public affairs, to Peter O. Kohler, memorandum titled "Using Space to Enhance University Reputation," Dec. 11, 1992, pp. 1–2. Peter Kohler collection, OHSU Archives.

14 Ibid., p. 4.

15 Ibid., p. 7.

16 Neil Goldschmidt, interview, Jan. 15, 2015, in his Portland home.

17 Bagby, interview.

18 Lesley Hallick, interview by Charles Morrissey, Sept. 10, 2001, History of Medicine Room, OHSU, interview no. 87 9/10, 2001, transcript, OHSU Oral History Project, p. 17.

19 John W. Kendall, MD, interview by Joan Ash, June 23, 1999, Biomedical Information and Communications Center, OHSU campus, interview no. 75 6/23, 1999, transcript, OHSU Oral History Project, p. 18.

20 Randy Gragg, "Sight Lines News and Views on Architecture: What's the Prognosis," *The Oregonian,* Sept. 22, 2002, p. D01. Gragg quotes Kohler saying the campus's Mount Hood views are worth "$40,000 in salary."

21 Kohler, interview.

22 Lesley Hallick, interview, Feb. 18, 2015, Portland, Oregon.

23 Ibid.

24 Ibid.

25 Ibid.

26 Kohler, interview. Kohler said he and Dr. Frederick Fraunfelder, head of OHSU's Department of Ophthalmology, presented to the disappointed crowd for about a half hour. Kohler said, "Fraunfelder is a natural entertainer anyway, so it went okay. People were disappointed to know they had to keep working. I remember telling a joke there, one of the old light bulb jokes popular in those days."

27 "OHSU Casey Eye Institute," GBD Architects, http://www.gbdarchitects.com/portfolio-item/casey-eye-institutue/.

28 Randy Gragg, "Casey Eye Institute: Meier, Money and Myopia," *The Oregonian,* Oct. 6, 1991, p. D1.

29 Frederick Fraunfelder, MD, interview, July 14, 2014, his office at the Casey Eye Institute.

30 "OHSU: 125 Years of Connection," OHSU website, http://www.ohsu.edu/xd/about/facts/history.cfm.

31 "Institute History," Oregon Institute of Occupational Health Sciences, http://www.ohsu.edu/xd/research/centers-institutes/oregon-institute-

occupational-health-sciences/about/history.cfm.

32 Sophia Bennett, "Oregon's Bottle Bill a Leader Yesterday and Today," *Recycle Nation*, July 29, 2013, http://recyclenation.com/2013/07/oregon-bottle-bill-leader.

33 "Land Use—Overview," *Oregon Blue Book*, http://bluebook.state.or.us/topic/landuse/land05.htm.

34 John Woodward (San Francisco health finance specialist who helped OHSU during its transition to a public corporation), interview, Oct. 8, 2014.

35 Druker, interview, Feb. 11, 2015.

36 Oz Hopkins Koglin, "OHSU will Renew Spirit of Research," *The Oregonian*, Feb. 15, 1998.

37 Steve Woodward, "Millions in Donations Realize Vision; New Doernbecher Ready to Let Healing Begin," *The Oregonian*, May 3, 1998, p. A01.

38 Randy Gragg, "Hong Kong on the Hill," *The Sunday Oregonian*, June 7, 1998, p. F01.

39 "OHSU mourns loss of School of Medicine Dean Mark Richardson," OHSU press release, Sept. 6, 2016, https://www.ohsu.edu/xd/education/schools/school-of-medicine/news-and-events/OHSU-mourns.cfm.

40 Lesley Hallick, and Peter O. Kohler, MD, interview, Pacific University campus, March 5, 2016.

41 Peter O. Kohler, MD, Joseph Bloom, MD (dean of School of Medicine), Susan Smith (director of the Regional Oregon Primate Center), Jay Nelson (director of the Vaccine & Gene Therapy Institute), to Louis Picker, MD (professor in the pathology department at Southwestern Medical Center, University of Texas, Dallas), letter of offer of employment, Aug. 13, 1999.

42 Ibid.

43 Ibid.

44 Ibid.

45 Peter O. Kohler, MD, interview, April 9, 2015, his office in the Medical Research Building, OHSU campus.

46 Peter O. Kohler, letter to Chares S. Rooks (executive director of Meyer Memorial Trust), Oct. 28, 1999.

47 Louis J. Picker, interview, Jan. 26, 2015.

48 Druker, interview, Feb. 11, 2015.

49 Bagby, interview.

50 Ibid.

51 Ibid.

52 OHSU, "*The Value of Healing, Teaching & Discovery: A Report to the Oregon Legislative Assembly*, 1999, pp. 14, 15. OHSU provides a report to the Legislature each biennium. OHSU Strategic Communications.

53 Paul Bragdon, interview, Sept. 16, 2014, University Club, Portland.

54 Ibid.

55 Davis, interview. Davis said merging the two foundations "was more efficient. It helped bring more people maybe to contributing to the foundation that might oth-

erwise have contributed elsewhere."

56 Peter O. Kohler, MD, interview, Sept. 17, 2014, OHSU campus.

57 Memorandum of Understanding between OHSU and OGI [Oregon Graduate Institute], Aug. 15, 2000. The memorandum went on to say, "Both institutions have an entrepreneurial culture and a strong proclivity to help existing industries and foster new ones . . . . This merger not only buttresses our ability to support the area high-tech industry's research and education needs, but it also stakes out ground for Oregon in the emerging field of biotechnology, where it is becoming clear that states that hesitate to establish their position will be left behind."

58 Ryan Frank, "OGI: An Educational Gem Hidden in Suburban Washington County," *The Oregonian*, April 29, 2003, p. B1.

59 Aaron Fentress, "OHSU Looks West to Hillsboro for Research Site," *The Oregonian*, July 20, 1998, p. B1. Also, David R. Anderson, "OHSU's Westside Campus Adds Research Facilities to OHSU: Campus Planning Includes Low Area Impact," *The Oregonian*, June 15, 2000, West Zone, p. 1.

60 Ibid.

61 Hallick, interview, Sept. 10, 2001, p. 35. Hallick said, "We had long had that hold in the primate center science, the money was there in NIH to do it, and we were building a building. So we made this decision to build two wings in this building, totally unrelated, really, the Neurological Sciences Institute and this Vaccine and Gene Therapy Institute."

62 Ibid., p. 36. Hallick said, "We were building a 100,000-square-foot building because we didn't think we could ever be allowed to grow here (on Pill Hill). So it had a pivotal effect on both campuses."

63 Neil Swanson, MD, interview, July 9, 2014, is office in OHSU's Center for Health and Healing.

64 Oz Hopkins Koglin, "OHSU Researchers Clone Monkey," *The Oregonian*, Jan. 14, 2000, p. A01.

65 Tony Quested, "US Seizes the Chance to Tap Bioscience Pipeline," *Business Weekly*, July 13, 2000.

66 The private university plans are outlined in two memoranda: Norm Eder and Gary Conkling to Dr. Michael Mooney, "Murdock Discussion of a New Private University," Sept. 2, 1999; and Norm Eder, Gary Conkling to Dr. Michael Mooney, Dr. Peter Kohler, and Dr. Ed Thompson, "A Plan to Pursue a New Private University in Portland, Nov. 5, 1999, both Box 9/72, Peter Kohler collection, OHSU Archives.

67 Oz Hopkins Koglin, "Medical Research Institute takes up fight against diseases," *The Oregonian*, Sept. 26, 2001, p. B01.

68 Nick Budnick, "Oregon Health & Science University HIV Vaccine Researcher, Louis Picker, Wins $25 Million," *Oregonian/OregonLive*, Sept. 3, 2014.

69 Picker, interview.

70 Joe Rojas-Burke, "A whole new research race," *The Oregonian*, Feb. 4, 2001, p. B01.

71 Breeneman, "Mr. OHSU"; Peter O. Kohler, MD, "Look Again," speech by Kohler to

the Greater Portland Chamber of Commerce, Feb. 16, 2000; "Building Bioscience in Portland," a research assessment by Batelle Memorial Institute for the City of Portland; Jim Pasero, "OHSU President Peter Kohler's Prescription for Oregon: Opportunity or Gambler," *Brainstorm Magazine,* February 2003, http://brainstormnw.com/Business/BankingOnBiotech.html.

72 "Portland Residents Rank OHSU as #1 Hospital," OHSU press release, Nov. 23, 2000, http://www.ohsu.edu/xd/about/news_events/news/2000/11-23-portland-residents-rank.cfm.

73 Brenneman, "Mr. OHSU".

74 Richard J. Sperry, MD (associate vice president, University of Utah), *Regular Interim Report, Oregon Health Sciences University,* Commission on Colleges, Northwest Association of Schools and Colleges, April 24–25, 2000, p. 3.

75 Lesley Hallick, interview, Oct. 1, 2014, Beaverton.

76 Milt Freudenheim, "Bitter Pills for Ailing Hospitals," *The New York Times,* Oct. 31, 1999, Money and Business section.

77 Association of American Medical Colleges, National Association of Public Hospitals, University HealthSystem Consortium, *Short Survey of Quarterly Data,* 1999.

78 Freudenheim, "Bitter Pills for Ailing Hospitals".

79 Jim Walker, interview, Feb. 25, 2015.

80 Ibid.

81 David Hunter, CEO of the Hunter Group (presentation to the University HealthSystem Consortium board, Sept. 16, 1999).

82 M. Susan Smith to Dr. Peter Kohler, interoffice memorandum, "Issues Related to Merger," Nov. 8, 1999, Peter Kohler collection, OHSU Archives.

83 John H. Nilson (professor and chair of pharmacology, Case Western Reserve University near Cleveland, Ohio) to Susan Smith (director of the Oregon Regional Primate Research Center), letter, July 27, 2000, Peter Kohler collection, OHSU Archives.

84 Peter O. Kohler, MD, interview, May 15, 2015, his office in the Medical Research Building at OHSU.

85 Richard Colby, "Police Arrest 12 Fighting Research," *The Oregonian,* June 10, 1999, p. C02.

86 Kohler, interview, May 15, 2015.

87 The Coalition to Abolish Animal Testing, "What do these two have in common? OHSU is hurting them both," says the tract, which features a photo of a monkey and a young man. Portland, Peter Kohler collection, OHSU Archives, ca. 2004.

88 Hallick, interview, Feb. 18, 2015.

89 Carol Reinmiller, interview, Oct. 21, 2014, Baird Hall, OHSU.

90 Steve Woodward, "Rebel group defects from OHSU," *The Oregonian,* May 22, 1997, p. Co1.

91 Joe Rojas-Burke, "OHSU nurses reject contract offer by resounding margin," *The Oregonian,* Sept. 10, 1999, p. C06.

92 Joe Rojas-Burke, "OHSU nurses accept two-year pact," *The Oregonian*, Nov. 16, 1999, p. B14.

93 Joe Rojas-Burke and Oz Hopkins Koglin, "OHSU, physician tangle over research," *The Oregonian*, June 12, 2000, p. A01.

94 Peter O. Kohler, MD, to Lois Davis and to others identified only as Marlys, Bob, and Jon, email, June 25, 2000.

95 Kim Christensen and Brent Walth, "Doctors Overbilled Medicaid, State Says," *The Oregonian*, July 10, 2000, p. A01.

96 Kohler, interview, May 15, 2015.

97 Davis, interview.

98 Aliza Earnshaw, "Portland State snaps up OGI faculty," *Portland Business Journal*, Sept. 20, 2004.

99 Hallick interview, Feb. 18, 2015. Hallick explained, "It was sort of like a stranded family. They felt like they had to stick together. It was sort of one for all and all for one . . . . They certainly did not all justify the same sized programs, but when they came there was a sense that everybody had a lab and everybody had some guarantee that when their grants ran out they would continue to be funded. . . . I would say the Neurological Sciences Institute didn't make a lot of sense in the end, but we didn't invest very heavily into it either, frankly. Fortunately, some of these faculty joined OHSU departments where they had logical colleagues, and a few are still active researchers."

100 Neil Goldschmidt to Peter Kohler and Fred Buckman (chairman of the OHSU board), memorandum, "Directions and Concerns," Nov. 30, 1998.

101 Ibid. Goldschmidt wrote, "My limited perspective alerts and alarms me to our 'national security' issue—the fragile inverted pyramid of a vulnerable hospital at the bottom, on top of which we are heaping re-modeling, and new investment on the hill, plus the primate center, and which is being kept upright by a revenue structure funded 50 percent from sources other than the private insurance market."

102 Walker, interview.

103 Joe Rojas-Burke, "Tobacco Money Proposals Offer Separate Paths," *The Oregonian*, Nov. 3, 2000, p. A18. Also see, *Turning Intellectual Property into Jobs: The Oregon Medical Research Initiative*, paper by OHSU staff, Peter Kohler collection, OHSU Archives.

104 OHSU Board of Directors 1999 Retreat, detailed agenda and presentation materials, OHSU Archives.

105 Ibid.

106 Ibid.

107 Ibid.

108 Davis, interview.

109 OHSU Board of Directors 1999 Retreat.

110 Fred Buckman, interview, Dec. 10, 2014, Beaverton, Oregon.

111 Hallick, interview, Feb. 18, 2015.

Chapter Seven

Reaching for the Top

Kohler opened his campaign for the Big Ask from the legislature in much the same way he did with his push for the public corporation bill—by floating it in public with a major speech to the Portland Regional Chamber of Commerce on February 16, 2000. He didn't mention that the university planned to ask the legislature for $200 million, but he did describe why OHSU must continue to expand and how doing so would benefit Oregon. In an argument he would use across the state, he reminded the audience of how far OHSU had come since becoming a public corporation and that it was now well-positioned to take advantage of a new revolution in biotechnology emerging with the US Human Genome Project, an international effort to for the first time identify and map all of a human's genes. Kohler said the university now was Portland's largest employer with ten thousand workers, and had added $380 million to its annual budget over the previous five years and nearly two million square feet of space over the last decade.[1] OHSU, he said, had climbed from about sixtieth among the nation's 125 academic health centers in NIH research dollars to thirty-third. Kohler noted that Dr. Druker and his cure for leukemia had been featured the previous Friday on the national ABC program, *20/20*.

"It was a struggle," he said, "But now in our fifth year as a public corporation, we are hitting our stride."[2]

Kohler argued that if OHSU grew to his goal of reaching the top twenty medical centers in research funding, it would be a powerful economic engine for Oregon. It could create jobs and bring $250 million or more a year in research money to the state. It could also foster spin-off biotechnology businesses and be the catalyst for Oregon's biotechnology industry. OHSU scientists already had spun off 15 businesses and introduced 340 inventions, he said. To reach its full potential, Kohler said, OHSU needed space.

"Our academic reputation is already good enough right now to recruit world-class researchers who can bring most of their own money, but we simply lack the space to house them," he said. "We want to add 150 more research scientists over the next seven years. To do that, we will need to double our laboratory space and space for health care delivery research."

So without saying how OHSU proposed to get money for more space, Kohler made the case for why it needed to do so. Soon after, he and others on his team would talk about their hope to win $200 million in tobacco settlement money from the legislature.

In the following months, they sharpened their arguments. In May of 2000, the OHSU government relations office put out a three-page paper titled "The Oregon Medical Research Initiative." The paper said the university wanted to invest $155 million in upgrading its clinical programs and another $400 million in expanding research space and recruiting scientists over an eight-to-ten-year period. The university could self-finance the clinical upgrades and raise $200 million more through private fundraising. In addition, OHSU would "propose to ask the state to invest the additional $200 million as a one-time investment."[3]

Kohler and his administrators knew they couldn't win that much money from the state without putting up a private match, Davis said. Initially, they looked at a one-to-one match, but soon realized they'd need more. "What we were really trying to accomplish was bigger than $400 million," she said. "It was $500 million."[4]

A brief description of the plan surfaced in a short story in May tucked deep inside *The Oregonian.* "During the next six years, the university hopes to raise $500 million, its most ambitious fund-raising goal ever," the newspaper said.[5]

Over the summer, Kohler's team refined its campaign, arguments, and numbers. The team changed the name of the initiative to Oregon Opportunity. It persuaded some of the state's business and political leaders to serve on a steering committee "to advise our executive team as we discuss this investment opportunity with the governor and Legislature."[6] The committee was chaired by former Senator Hatfield and included Tom Imeson, Portland lawyer and former chief of staff to Governor Goldschmidt, and other Portland leaders. But most members on the committee were leaders from other parts of the state such as Steve Forrester, publisher of *The Daily Astorian*; Dr. Charles Hofmann, a Baker City physician; William Thorndyke Jr., president of Medford Fabrications; and Elizabeth McCool, chair of Western Communications, which published newspapers in Central Oregon including *The Bulletin* in Bend. Again, Kohler was employing the strategy that worked so well in selling the public corporation plan by bringing rural leaders into his camp.

He traveled to small towns across the state such as Lincoln City on the coast to sell Oregon Opportunity before civic groups, business leaders, and newspaper editorial boards. His core argument was that OHSU was poised to capture the benefits of the genetic revolution, marked by the coming map of the human genome, for the entire state. With the Oregon Opportunity investment, OHSU could seize the moment, claim a stake in the biotechnology boom, and create jobs through its own expansion and spin-off businesses.

What's more, he argued, the university had proved itself worthy of the investment. In fifteen years, its research awards had climbed sixfold to $168 million a year,[7] putting it among the top 2 percent of the more than 2,000 grant-receiving institutions nationwide. In the next year, 2001, it would merge with the Oregon Graduate Institute and open its new building for the Vaccine and Gene Therapy Institute. OHSU already employed a critical mass of some of the world's most accomplished researchers,[8] and the Oregon Opportunity investment could double OHSU's research funding over the next decade.

By fall of 2000, the university was describing Oregon Opportunity in detail. Of the $300 million private investment it was raising, it planned to spend $66 million on endowments and scholarships for the schools of medicine, dentistry, and nursing; $132 million on faculty endowments and facilities for cancer, heart disease, women's health, and children's health; $25 million to expand the Casey Eye Institute; $20 million for the Oregon Graduate Institute; $16 million for neurosciences programs; $10 million for the Center for Healthy Aging; and $5 million for hearing research programs and facilities. It would also spend $80 million of the $200 million state investment on building a patient care building and a biomedical research building, $75 million to recruit scientists, $25 million on the Oregon Graduate Institute, $10 million for an advanced imaging center, and $5 million for a statewide education network.

Oregon Opportunity would also reserve $5 million for the creation of the Oregon Rural Practice-based Research Network. The network would allow rural doctors and their patients to participate in clinical trials and other OHSU research, an unusual practice that would "realize the dream of sharing the benefits of medical research across the entire state," said an OHSU discussion paper on the proposal.[9] The university had shown its commitment to a statewide, 98,000-square-mile campus, the paper said, with its development of Area Health Education Centers, rural rotations for its medical students, and a nursing education program that was offered on three regional university campuses: Southern Oregon and Eastern Oregon universities and the Oregon Institute of Technology in south-central Oregon's Klamath Falls. The research network would work with health centers in Oregon's hinterlands to get research grants and contracts for research projects that involve rural Oregonians and their issues. It could create jobs that grow out of new technologies and biotech spin-off companies and bring some of OHSU's claim on the biotech boom to the countryside.[10] The network would prove successful in making OHSU a national leader in tapping rural practitioners for relevant, needed clinical studies on their medical practices.[11]

"It was fundamentally how we went about getting the public corporation," Davis said. "We figured out that, yes, the single biggest block of legislators are in the Portland metro area, . . . but if you can't get the support of the other [rural] folks, then you have problems."[12]

THE BIOTECH DEBATE

Kohler promoted the potential benefits of investments in bioscience as the centerpiece of his campaign for Oregon Opportunity. The biotechnology industry emerged as a force across the nation during the 1990s, mostly as small companies, many born in the research labs of the nation's academic health centers, including OHSU.

For example, two scientists and an officer at OHSU's Vollum Institute in 1993 founded Northwest NeuroLogic Inc., which developed melanocortin receptor and neurotransmitter transporter technologies that could be used in developing drugs for stroke, head trauma, diabetes, and many other diseases. The company had grown to six employees five years later when it was sold to a San Diego company for $4.2 million in common stock.[13] Dr. Richard I. Lowensohn, a nationally prominent OHSU obstetrician-gynecologist, developed OBLink, an electronic medical records system, for Health Outcome Technologies Inc. The company was founded in 1991 and merged with MedicalLogic Inc., a larger Hillsboro, Oregon, company in 1998.[14] OHSU had shares in both of these companies and more.

Even so, OHSU's nascent biotechnology enterprises were small and brought in little revenue. But the industry was thriving elsewhere in the country, and Kohler saw it as a potential new source of support for OHSU in the years ahead. He was not alone. The Oregon Economic Development Department focused its efforts on twelve key industries, one of which was biotechnology. The Portland Development Commission in 1998 had identified bioscience as a key industry for the city, and Portland's then-Mayor Vera Katz had created a biotechnology committee to work on recruiting bioscience and pharmaceutical companies to the city.[15]

The biotech industry already was exploding near major universities elsewhere in the country, including the Massachusetts Institute of Technology in Cambridge, the University of Washington in Seattle, and the University of California at San Diego. A 1995 study showed that UC San Diego had spun out more than 7,000 jobs in the region, largely in biotechnology, and a 1997 report said MIT had created 14,000 jobs in Cambridge alone. An analysis by the Milken Institute in Santa Monica, California, concluded the high-tech sector could account for 65 percent of economic growth in metropolitan areas, largely determining which cities succeeded, and the presence of major research centers and institutions was the most important factor in creating high-tech companies.[16] A *New York Times* article explained:

> The university is an increasingly powerful force in the knowledge economy, both because its brains are greater assets than ever before and because of a growing trend in which institutions of higher education see themselves as generators of business, whether professors' start-ups or technology licensing deals. "There's a great awakening that we're sitting on top of a gunpowder keg" of growth, said David Lampe, author of two books on high-tech locales.[17]

Kohler took these findings to the leaders and people of Oregon, arguing that OHSU not only should be part of that gunpowder keg, but that it could be with the Oregon Opportunity investment. He and Edward Thompson, president of the Oregon Graduate Institute of Science and Technology, wrote an op-ed column for *The Oregonian* and were interviewed by *Oregon Business* magazine, and in both they pressed the case for how the merger of their two institutions would give the state a competitive edge in the emerging biotech industry.[18] As Kohler made that argument in talks across the state, the university did the same in its marketing publications.

"The benefits far outweigh the costs," said a flier, one of many brochures, papers, Q-&-As, and other publications OHSU churned out in support of the campaign. "The biotech boom created more than 437,000 new jobs in 1999 alone, on U.S. revenues approaching $47 billion. And that's just the tip of the iceberg. Financial analysts project the biotech industry to grow at a 35 percent annual rate for the foreseeable future. The genetic revolution is underway."[19]

OHSU already was a "national and international leader in biomedical research" with its potential barely tapped, wrote Davis, now OHSU vice president for communications, in a memo to Felicia Trader, executive director of Portland's development commission.

"Just as the University of North Carolina, North Carolina State University and Duke University spawned the Research Triangle Park and the University of California at San Francisco gave birth to Genentech and other biomedical companies, OHSU is poised to serve as the catalyst for development of the biomedical industry in Oregon," she wrote.[20]

Another OHSU paper underscored the urgency of the investment in OHSU by describing how Oregon lost a major opportunity when Druker's cancer drug ended up as Gleevec, a major moneymaker for Novartis Pharmaceuticals Corporation in New Jersey and Switzerland.

Druker "sought to identify companies that were furthest along in developing cancer or leukemia inhibitors," said the flier. "There was no such company in Oregon, no culture of biotechnology to foster his work and share in the financial rewards. This opportunity has been lost forever."[21]

However, claims by Kohler and other OHSU leaders about the university's potential to still become a biotech powerhouse met some skepticism. Oregon had yet to lure or spawn a major biotech company on the scale of Glaxo-Wellcome or Genentech, and it was not putting pressure on its universities to churn out product ideas and companies. Brock Metcalf, cofounder of Oregon Life Sciences LLC, one of a handful of Oregon venture capital firms investing in biotech, said the biotech industry in Oregon was still struggling. "There has to be a critical mass," he said.[22]

Successful small biotech firms created in Oregon found it hard to stay because of their isolation from larger industry centers. A successful six-year-old biotechnology venture called Bioject Medical Technologies, which made devices to shoot medicine under the skin without a needle, moved from Oregon to New Jersey in 2001 because it wanted to be near three of the world's biggest pharmaceutical makers.

"When you are a small company like ours," said Jim O'Shea, the company's president, "there just isn't anything like New Jersey or the Boston area for access to pharmaceutical and biotechnology companies."[23]

OHSU was getting into the biotech game too late, said Joe Cortright, an economist with Impressa Consulting in Portland and lead author of a 2002 economic report on the biotech industry by the Brookings Institution, a nonprofit research foundation in Washington, DC. More than forty states were engaged in drives to get into the biotechnology game.

Research centers already well established in Boston, Baltimore, and seven other cities had the critical mass to draw top scientists and federal research funding, but Portland wasn't one of them, Cortright argued. OHSU could not expect to compete. His study showed that the nine top-tier biotech communities in the United States—including Seattle, San Francisco, and San Diego—claimed 88 percent of all venture capital for biotechnology drug development and 96 percent of the estimated value of research alliances with drug companies.[24]

Portland, the study showed, ranked among twenty-eight third-tier cities. Four second-tier cities competed with those at the top for research dollars.

"Our studies show not just that the industry is concentrated, but that it is becoming more concentrated over time," Cortright said. "The fact that everybody wants to be the next biotech Mecca says more about the herd instinct of the economic development fraternity than it does about the technology of biotech."[25]

Four months before Cortright's report was published, Portland's Bureau of Planning and the Battelle Memorial Institute produced an assessment of OHSU's research prospects and Portland's bioscience economic potential titled *Building Bioscience in Portland.* The report noted OHSU had developed a thirty-year plan for growth that would require adding 1.2 to 1.5 million square feet of facility space elsewhere than on Pill Hill. The report concluded Kohler's aspiration to see OHSU become one of the top twenty NIH-funded bioscience centers in the nation was achievable, provided it "could move forward quickly" in adding research and support buildings—more space. The Oregon Opportunity fund was "crucial," the report said, in making that happen.[26]

Kohler argued that even if OHSU captured just a sliver of the burgeoning biotech industry, just 1 percent, it could mean another billion dollars flowing into Oregon. "Presently, Oregon's biotech industry pales compared to those in San Diego, San Francisco, or Seattle," he told a US Senate subcommittee. "But we need not—nor can we afford to—think of biotech as the exclusive province of our larger neighbors to the north and south."[27]

In retrospect, the argument by Kohler and other advocates for creating a biotech hub in Portland were probably overblown, said Daniel Dorsa, a neuroscientist and OHSU's senior vice president for research.

"The press got the idea that what was going to happen was that in September of 2001 this [Oregon Opportunity] money would hit the ground, and in 2004 Pfizer would announce it's placing a 10,000 person facility on the waterfront," he said. "The point being, it wasn't driven by biotech, per se; it was driven by OHSU's need to expand."[28]

The university did need space. But the bioscience industry has also boomed in Oregon. In 2010, the behemoth drug maker Genentech opened a $400 million factory and distribution center in Hillsboro, and in May of 2016, Pinnacle Economics, Inc., reported that biotech research at Oregon universities and hospitals, which occurs primarily at OHSU, produced $587 million in economic activity, including $356 million in wages and

4,085 jobs. Pinnacle, which the Oregon Bioscience Association commissioned to do the study, also reported that 793 private bioscience establishments in Oregon generated $5.6 billion in economic activity in 2014. So private and university biotech research produced a total $6.2 billion of economic activity in the state, six times the goal Kohler had set in his campaign for Oregon Opportunity.[29]

SELLING OREGON OPPORTUNITY

None of this growth was certain when Kohler first focused on the promise of biotech while pressing his case for Oregon Opportunity to the legislature. Nevertheless, as the result of OHSU's statewide advocacy, its Big Ask emerged in 2001 as Senate Bill 832, also called the Oregon Opportunity Act, and like the public corporation bill, it was sponsored by rural Republicans from north central Oregon: Senators David Nelson of Pendleton and Mark Simmons of Elgin. The bill would allow the state to use its tobacco money to finance $200 million in bonds for OHSU's research expansion.

Kohler made some trips to the legislature, but not near as many as when he pushed for the public corporation bill. Even so, the legislation won broad support, and Governor Kitzhaber signed it on August 8, 2001, with an audience of about one hundred legislators, business leaders, and university officials. Kitzhaber said the investment would help Oregon take "advantage of the incredible opportunity for medical advances offered by the fast-growing world of genetic research." Kohler said the money would put OHSU on a platform to help the state "catch the coming biotechnology wave."[30]

This marked the final victory for the administrative team that had helped Kohler transform OHSU into a rising star among the nation's academic health centers. The team had slowly been losing its cohesion as each member took on bigger and bigger responsibilities in the rapidly expanding medical center. The demands of their individual duties left them little time to meet together on university-wide initiatives such as those for a public corporation and Oregon Opportunity bonds. Hallick had become provost and vice president for academic affairs, which included overseeing the university's rapid research expansion until Dorsa arrived in 2001 to become vice president for research. Billups had assembled a growing legal team, including medical malpractice, contract, and employment lawyers. In 1999, after she adopted her daughter, she had reduced her own hours, and Stadum, the real estate lawyer, was hired to serve as General Counsel for her office. As vice president for finance and administration, Walker was putting in sixty-hour weeks overseeing not only the university's finances, but its administrative operations, including finance, risk management and purchasing. Davis, vice president for public affairs and marketing, oversaw the university's promotion and lobbying duties while serving as its chief spokesperson for news events. Goldfarb orchestrated the university's expanding clinics and hospital operations as director of hospitals and the health care system. Kohler, too, was pulled in other directions. While overseeing the rapidly expanding medical center, he was gaining more jobs on boards and professional groups. For example, he served on and chaired the board of the Association of Academic Health Centers; chaired the Committee on Quality in Long-Term Care for the Institute of Medicine; and was on the boards of the Alzheimer's Disease Center of Oregon and the Portland Chamber of Commerce.

Goldfarb became the first member of Kohler's leadership team to leave OHSU. He departed in 2001 as the university sealed its Oregon Opportunity plan with the legislature. He moved on to more hospitals—this time in Gainesville, Florida, where he became chief executive officer of Shands HealthCare. The health care system is affiliated with the University of Florida Health Science Center. That put Goldfarb in charge of a primary teaching hospital, two children's hospitals, a cancer hospital, two specialty hospitals, two home care agencies, and other outpatient services. The Florida job was one of three offers that came to Goldfarb in a period of about sixty days. The two others were from public universities still affiliated with their state higher education systems—the University of Washington and the University of Wisconsin. He turned those down because they were still state agencies, which was what he and Kohler's team fought so hard to get away from in making OHSU a public corporation. He said he had decided to move on because he was no longer happy.[31]

OHSU was not making enough money, he said. "Peter was unhappy about that. I was unhappy."[32]

Kohler was happy, however, to get his hands on $200 million in bonds to spend on research expansion. Yet if the state could give, it also could take away. The legislature allocated OHSU about $96 million for its 2001–03 budget, down more than $10 million from the previous biennium.[33] That meant OHSU would have $10 million less for its academic and indigent care missions. Kohler broke that news in his *Message from President Kohler* newsletter, which came out on campus in late September, 2001, just weeks after the September 11 terrorist attacks. The $10 million "can only come out of services and programs," he wrote.[34]

Among other adjustments, Kohler downsized the OHSU satellite nursing program at the Oregon Institute of Technology in Klamath Falls, raised tuition for incoming medical and dentistry students, and trimmed services at its statewide programs for children with disabilities and special needs in the Child Development and Rehabilitation Center. By this time, state funding accounted for only 6 percent of the university's operating budget.

"Cuts in state support meant that, more than ever, OHSU's survival depends on its ability to function efficiently as a business, competing in the marketplace," Kohler wrote in the newsletter.[35]

NURSES STRIKE

Another strain on OHSU's resources emerged in late fall of 2001 when its nurses went on strike. Unlike the earlier strike by the American Federation of State, County and Municipal Employees, which Kohler characterized as almost "friendly," the nurses dug in for a tough, two-month battle that drew regular newspaper coverage. About 71 percent of OHSU's 1,500 registered nurses, members of the statewide Oregon Nurses Association, voted to go on strike on Monday, December 17, 2001, the first time nurses in any Oregon hospital had gone on strike since 1990. As organizers stacked picket signs, OHSU management began hiring replacement nurses.

Citing the same concerns as when they had threatened to strike two years earlier, the nurses complained they were underpaid, earning about $2 to $3 less per hour than nurses at other Oregon hospitals, and worked in hospitals and clinics that were understaffed. OHSU argued again that their lower pay was offset by 12 percent of their pay that OHSU put into their retirement plans. OHSU management offered to raise wages 14 percent over twenty-seven months; the nurses demanded a 20 percent raise over twenty-four months.[36]

The strike began Monday with hundreds of nurses and supporters picketing in front of OHSU and Doernbecher Children's hospitals as OHSU security guards, whose ranks had been increased by fifty temporary hires, stood sentry at the hospital entrances. OHSU was forced to divert some emergency cases to other hospitals and to postpone non-urgent heart procedures.[37] One day, as the strike unfolded, Mark Dodson crossed the nurses' picket line to meet with Walker. The strikers were shouting, "Jim Walker is ugly. Jim Walker is ugly," Dodson recalled. And then Walker appeared to greet Dodson, and the strikers muffled their voices, even as they continued to repeat, "Jim Walker is ugly."[38]

The strike was in part rooted in OHSU's remarkable growth. The university had added 200 registered nurses over the previous two years, a 17 percent increase. But even that rate of new hires, nurses said, failed to keep up with the growth in patients. Emergency room traffic had jumped by 8,500 patients over the previous year to 38,392. The hospital inpatient count had soared from a daily average of 288 in 1998 to 339, which kept the hospital humming at 90 percent to 95 percent occupancy.[39] Hospital administrators say the optimum occupancy is about 85 percent; anything higher strains the staff.

"It's gotten to the point where you always seem to be one nurse short," said Kristin Kidd, a nurse on the picket line.[40]

Four days into the strike, *The Oregonian*'s editorial board weighed in, faulting both sides for failing to settle. The nurses were loud and unruly on the picket lines, disturbing patients, and OHSU management was not taking the nurses seriously, the board said.

"Stirring a deep anger in your workforce is not a sign of effective management," the editorial said. "OHSU has had less and less state oversight, making it less publicly accountable than even other higher education institutions."[41]

Pat Southard, a nurse and the interim hospital director replacing Goldfarb, challenged the editorial in an op-ed article. She said OHSU was offering the nurses the best deal in the local market.[42]

The nurses continued to walk the picket line through cold and windy winter days, including Christmas, into January, then February. Finally, at 6:30 a.m. on February 13, 2002, about 200 nurses walked into the lobby of OHSU Hospital to report for work. OHSU had agreed to give the nurses a 20 percent pay increase over three years, rather than two, to improve working conditions and to seek national hospital accreditation for nursing excellence. The two-month strike, one of Oregon's longest labor disputes in a generation, had cost OHSU at least $6 million, a rift between management and nurses, and lingering enmity between nurses who crossed the picket lines and those who didn't.[43]

The strike, slashed state funding, and more patients incapable of paying for care had suddenly "clouded the future of Oregon Health & Science University," said *The Oregonian*. It explained:

> In dollar terms, the recently ended strike by registered nurses almost fades in comparison to such looming problems as the proposed $9.4 million reduction in state funding for serving the poor,

> a projected 35 percent increase in uninsured patients seeking charity care and a likely $26 million net loss for the schools of medicine, dentistry and nursing. Dr. Peter Kohler, president of OHSU, remains optimistic about carrying out the institution's ambitious strategic plans, which include expanding the hospital by as many as 100 beds, building thousands of square feet of laboratory space and recruiting dozens of leading scientists to make Portland a hotbed of biotechnology.[44]

But before Kohler could begin building new lab space, the university needed to turn to Oregon voters to settle another issue with its finances. The state and OHSU wanted the university to use its Oregon Opportunity money to finance general obligation bonds, which were funded with the tobacco settlement money, and have lower interest rates than revenue bonds. The latter are riskier because they depend on revenue from what they are used to build. If the university, for example, were to use revenue bonds to build a hospital, it would figure on paying back the bonds with revenue generated by the new hospital. The state gave OHSU $16 million a year in tobacco settlement money to finance bonds. That was enough for OHSU to finance $200 million in general obligation bonds, but only $165 million in revenue bonds because of their higher interest rate. State law, however, limited what general obligation bond money could be used for, and it did not include all of OHSU's plans to hire new researchers and build research laboratories and clinics. The state would have to amend the constitution to allow OHSU's broader use of general obligation bonds, which meant putting the proposal up for a vote of the people.

So Kohler's team persuaded legislators to propose House Joint Resolution 46-A, which would go on the ballot the following spring. The resolution passed and showed up on the May 21, 2002, election ballot as Measure 11. As with previous OHSU initiatives, Measure 11 won broad support. *The Oregonian* editorial board called support of it "a no-brainer."[45] Former Senator Hatfield, a member of the OHSU board, and Governor

Kitzhaber co-chaired a committee in support of Measure 11. In a guest opinion column for *The Oregonian*, Hatfield wrote the measure would reduce bonding costs, create jobs, save lives, and improve health care for all by allowing Oregon Opportunity to go forward with a full $200 million in bond money. "It's simply too good to miss," he wrote.[46]

Voters solidly approved Measure 11 in May, with 76 percent voting in favor, 24 percent against. After weathering the election, budget cuts, and a nurses' strike, Kohler could finally proceed on a project that he expected would lift OHSU's stature. On September 17, 2002, the OHSU board approved a $321 million contract with Hoffman Construction and Anderson Construction, both of Portland, to build the Biomedical Research Building and a fourteen-level patient care center. The financing would come from a combination of revenue bonds and Oregon Opportunity money.[47]

On October 10, 2002, a cool, but dry and pleasant day in Portland, Kohler gathered with university officials; three state legislators, including Senator David Nelson, who sponsored the Oregon Opportunity bill; OHSU board members, and other leaders, including Randall Edwards, state treasurer; and Oregon's Democratic US Congressman David Wu to break ground on the Biomedical Research Building on the west side of campus.

"Today is the first step in fulfilling the promise of the Oregon Opportunity," Kohler said. "The new research building cannot come too soon. It will allow us badly needed space to recruit new scientists and expand existing research projects. . . . Architecturally, the building will promote functionality by connecting the existing research quadrangle with the outpatient clinics."[48]

Additional Oregon Opportunity money would be used to renovate two research buildings on the West Campus in Hillsboro, to establish the rural health research network, and to recruit scores of researchers. By early 2003, work also was underway on the new patient care facility, a twelve-story building that would rise like a 100-yard-long, curved glass cliff facing east and stretching north off OHSU Hospital.

This was all part of a thirty-year plan that in early 2000 Kohler had enlisted his staff to work on with City of Portland planners. The two-year project, called the Marquam Hill Plan, created a blueprint that was to guide development on Pill Hill through 2032. The plan recognizes the intersection between "OHSU's vision and Portland's economic development priorities," said Stadum, OHSU's general counsel at the time the plan was adopted.[49] Marquam Hill had been zoned residential from the time the University of Oregon Medical School moved onto it in 1919. So every time the university wanted to build anything—a hospital, research building, a library, a parking lot—it had to apply to the city for permits and re-zoning. The process was slow and cumbersome and sometimes ended in denials.

In 2002, the city council adopted the Marquam Hill Plan, which re-zoned one hundred acres as a "central employment" zone and designated it a plan district. This allowed OHSU to move forward on construction projects as needed provided that they conform to the thirty-year plan. The blueprint organized development into three zones that reflect the university's three missions—research, patient care, and education. The plan included measures for constructing buildings, new parking structures, road improvements, parks, and walking paths. It envisioned the need for an additional 2.2 million square feet of building space by 2032, some of which would be developed on OHSU's West Campus in Hillsboro. Some also would be developed on the South Waterfront along the Willamette River at the base of Pill Hill.

SOUTH WATERFRONT PROJECT

It was not long after OHSU became a public corporation that Kohler and his administrative team and board were looking at the possibility of taking a giant leap off Pill Hill to the vacant industrial land below. OHSU and city planners had been working for years on development plans for the area long before Kohler created his thirty-year plan. In fact, Kohler and his leadership team were looking to the waterfront even before they retreated to Skamania Lodge to devise the Big Ask. The 130-acre swath of land stretches south from Portland's Marquam Bridge about a mile along the Willamette River. It had served industry from the 1880s, when the Portland Lumber Company was established there, through most of the twentieth century. The land appealed to industries that relied on access to the river, roads, and railways. The Portland Lumber Mill operated on the South Waterfront as did a metal fabrication plan, chemical manufacturers, an aluminum smelter, a barge-building operation, and various salvaging operations. Industrial waste from some of these industries was dumped on the site and into the river. By the 1960s, though, the South Waterfront's industrial development was on the decline. The construction of two freeways—Harbor Drive in the 1940s and Interstate 5 in the 1960s—limited access and isolated the waterfront, contributing to the demise of industry. By the 1970s, the South Waterfront had become dead space in the city, a barren brownfield. The Portland Development Commission acquired seventy-three acres of the South Waterfront District in 1978, removed Harbor Drive and made plans to redevelop it as part of the Portland Downtown Urban Renewal Plan. This led to a series of revitalization plans—the South Waterfront Redevelopment Program of 1979, the Central City Plan of 1988, and the North Macadam Renewal Plan of 1999, named for Macadam Avenue, which parallels part of the South Waterfront.[50]

In late 1997, Mayor Katz created a twenty-five-member steering committee to study the development possibilities of the land, including use for OHSU expansion. She urged the panel to come up with a more creative name than the North Macadam District. By its second meeting, the committee was discussing whether a big gondola or tram might be the best way to move people between the waterfront and Pill Hill. Former governor and OHSU board member Neil Goldschmidt had come up with the tram idea as he and OHSU administrators discussed possibilities for expansion on the South Waterfront.[51]

"He was the first to mention the tram," said Davis, who served on

Katz's South Waterfront steering committee for years. "He mentioned it to me early on. We began to look at it, and it started to make sense."[52]

Goldfarb said he was at the breakfast meeting across from Kohler's office in Baird Hall when Goldschmidt proposed the idea. Also at the meeting was an expert from Bechtel—an international engineering and construction company and one of Goldschmidt's clients—who worked on snow resort trams in Europe. First they talked about a funicular, a tram-like vehicle that would rise from the South Waterfront to Pill Hill on rails.

"I thought that was a pretty good idea because I was stationed in the Navy in Italy in Naples, and they had a lot of them there," Goldfarb said. "Then we talked about a gondola. Then Walker joined us."[53]

Kohler liked the idea of a gondola or tram and appointed Walker to work with the city on exploring the possibilities.[54] They didn't have to worry about regulations because there were none: no US city had ever built an aerial tram, Goldfarb said.[55]

Before long, city and OHSU leaders were considering a tram. "People were juiced by it," Goldfarb said. The Bechtel expert told Goldschmidt a tram connecting Marquam Hill to the waterfront could be easily built. "This is nothing as trams go," he said.[56]

It made sense because no other option for moving people between the waterfront and the hilltop campus seemed feasible. Three two-lane roads led to OHSU from the north, south and west. The one road snaking up the hill from downtown Portland already was clogged with traffic, and any South Waterfront traffic—whether cars, buses, or streetcars—would have to flow through a neighborhood and up the hill, creating unacceptable congestion and delays. Many involved with the project, including Kohler and Davis, would later conclude the South Waterfront project could not have worked without the tram. Yet the tram would be the project's most controversial feature, creating friction with neighbors, a common problem for universities when they expand.

The steering committee brought together the city, developers and OHSU in a plan for the South Waterfront, which would become part of the Marquam Hill Plan. The design, incorporating an earlier vision from the Central City Plan of 1988, proposed an urban mixed-use neighborhood. It modeled the South Waterfront development after English Bay in Vancouver, BC, with restaurants, hotels, thin apartment and condo towers, a river greenway, parks, and a wildlife refuge. OHSU's future patient clinics and biotechnology research and classroom buildings would be mixed with these developments.

"This goes way beyond OHSU," said Homer Williams, a prominent Portland developer. "This is about the city itself over the next 30 years."[57]

The steering committee incorporated city policy objectives that called for affordable housing, job growth, new greenways and parks, new transportation options, sustainability, and the smart growth practice of keeping jobs, restaurants, and living space close. Williams and Dame Development, a real estate development consultant to the committee, said OHSU should serve as an economic development anchor for the waterfront with more buildings for research labs, clinics, and classrooms. Gerding Edling, a real estate investment and development firm, recommended that energy-efficient green practices be part of every building that rose from the brownfields of the South Waterfront.[58]

The city and its consultants produced their first draft for the waterfront development in May of 1999. It proposed a 130-acre district that would support 1,550 to 3,100 housing units and 10,000 jobs in 250,000 square feet of retail space and 1.9 million square feet of space for business offices and university research labs, clinics, and classrooms. The plan also called for a fifty-foot-wide greenway along the Willamette River, eighteen acres of parks and a streetcar connecting its 5,000 residents to the city, a light-rail station, and a tram connecting OHSU workers and patients to Pill Hill. The city would invest $150 million in property taxes in the project. The Portland City Council established the North Macadam Urban Renewal Area.[59]

But planners just kept planning for another two years, as environmentalists pushed for a wider greenway along the river and residents in the neighborhood adjacent to the waterfront district expressed growing concerns about how the development and the tram would affect their quality of life. By the spring of 2001, Kohler and his team were pressing city officials for a clear commitment to the project. If the development was going to become bogged down in controversy, the university needed to consider shifting its focus to its 263-acre West Campus in Hillsboro. That pivot could ultimately lead to OHSU moving its entire center of gravity to Hillsboro, Walker said.

"An academic medical center cannot afford to have two full-service campuses," he said.[60]

By moving west, the university could avoid buying more land as it would have to do on the waterfront, and it would not have to deal with public controversy over the tram or with parking and congestion issues. Portland leaders wanted to keep OHSU's expansion in the city, which meant finding room for it on the South Waterfront. The district had multiple owners, the largest being Zidell Marine Corporation, which was still building barges on some of its thirty acres on the north end of the district. The Schnitzer family, who made its fortune in the steel business, also owned about twenty acres. Planners, consultants, and developers were bogged down in forging intergovernmental agreements for parks, transportation, zoning codes, greenway guidelines, and other details in the complicated plan. But in December of 2001, sensing OHSU's growing restlessness, the North Macadam Urban Renewal Advisory Committee recommended the city concentrate its entire budget, staff, and work on making room for OHSU on the waterfront.

"Do what you need to do for OHSU and let the rest of these fall off the table," said Ann Gardner, member of the committee and development project manager for Schnitzer Investment.

Davis, also a member of the committee, reminded the city that OHSU, now armed with Oregon Opportunity money, had reached a critical point where it needed to start building in the coming summer of 2002.[61]

In the spring of 2002, the Portland Planning Commission organized two public hearings to allow residents to weigh in on the thirty-year Marquam Hill Plan, which was aligned with what was still being called the North Macadam District. Hallick reminded the commission that OHSU was making plans to build with its Oregon Opportunity money and needed to move soon to stay competitive in the rapidly evolving bioscience industry. If city leaders and residents cannot accept an aerial tram, she said, "we would rather build in the West Campus. We think we are in an excellent position to compete, but not if we dawdle."[62]

Three weeks later the Portland Planning Bureau released proposed zoning and design guidelines for what it wanted to rename the South Waterfront development. A group called the North Macadam Investors led by Homer Williams, the veteran urban developer, had bought ten acres in the district with plans to buy eighteen more by July. On the land, they proposed to build a 400,000-square-foot tower of offices, research labs, and classrooms for OHSU. That building would be flanked by four to eight blocks of additional development that would include condominiums and apartments. The greenway along the Willamette River had been extended to 100 feet, and the plan included construction incentives to encourage 150-foot setbacks. The plan allowed buildings to rise to 250 feet and also offered incentives for environmentally friendly building practices.

"This is the most seductive piece of property in the region," Williams said. "Four stories up and you're looking straight into Mount Hood and [Mount] St. Helens."[63]

Randy Gragg, *The Oregonian*'s architecture critic, had earlier been critical of the development plan for lacking ambition and vision. But he changed his tone after seeing the buildings Williams and his partners were proposing to build.

> Sleek, glass "pin" or "blade" towers 240 feet high, surrounded by five- and six-story bases. Following the city's new guidelines . . . the idea is to create a Pearl District-style[64] urbanity of

> active ground floors but topped with Vancouver, B.C.-style skyscrapers—tall, thin and clad entirely in glass, maximizing the light inside and views between them. . . . The first building would be developed by the team who did the award-winning Wieden+Kennedy Building, Gerding/Edlen Development and Allied Works Architecture. Together the concept designs and the developers' approach hold the promise of the kind of new architectural energy the city needs and that OHSU has occasionally aspired to with buildings such as the Biomedical Information Communication Center and Casey Eye Institute. Williams and his Partners clearly are raising the stakes of the North Macadam game, matching, if not exceeding, the city's aspirations.[65]

However, before construction could begin to carry out those aspirations, the city, OHSU and the residents near the waterfront had to come to an agreement on the tram. Without the tram, there would be no waterfront development, said Buckman.[66]

THE TRAM BATTLE

Buckman said he probably spent more time on the tram debate than any other issue during his tenure as chair of the OHSU board from its inception through 2003. He didn't work so much with the neighbors opposed to it, he said, as with members of the city council, Mayor Katz, architects, and engineers who all were feeling the heat of the opposition.[67] The resistance surprised Kohler and other OHSU leaders who thought Portlanders would love the tram because it would be so much better for the environment compared to any alternative.

Residents in Corbett-Terwilliger-Lair Hill, a strip neighborhood eight blocks wide bordering the South Waterfront area, began expressing alarm about the tram in the fall of 2000. About sixty signed a letter by Craig Rowland on behalf of their neighborhood association, notifying

OHSU they were prepared to fight to stop the project. Rowland and many of them lived on SW Gibbs Street, which ran east–west right under the route the tram's cars ride on their climb to Pill Hill. In a letter to Gordon Davis, OHSU's planning consultant, Rowland wrote:

> We cannot conceive how this tram could be built without severely impacting our neighborhood. Our concerns include, but are not limited to, the visual impact of tram and cables and the potential noise from the operation of the tram. Who can honestly say they would welcome a bus-sized conveyance sliding over the street that fronts their house 10, 20, 40 times a day? If there is a positive side for our neighborhood, we fail to see it. . . . We want to hear from OHSU regarding why they might need a tram in the first place and how they intend to address the concerns expressed above.[68]

The battle over the tram would rage for the next twenty-one months in public meetings, newspaper editorials and op-ed columns. The more they studied the idea, the more city and OHSU officials became convinced that the tram was the best, and probably the only, solution for handling transportation in connection with waterfront development. Davis told a Portland planning commission that without the tram, "traffic constraints on both Marquam Hill and in the North Macadam area would make the [the waterfront] site impractical and would ultimately limit growth on Marquam Hill as well."[69]

The tram could ferry sixty or more people up the hill in a matter of two or three minutes whereas buses would take about twenty minutes, said Gordon Davis, the consultant to OHSU, in a public presentation of a preliminary engineering study. The university would have to add ten buses to handle the traffic at the cost of $1.2 million a year compared to about $480,000 a year for a tram system, he said.[70] City officials also argued that the tram was key to keeping OHSU in Portland. Without it, the university would expand at its West Campus in Hillsboro. And without OHSU, the waterfront development would not have the economic engine it needed to support a thriving community of condos, apartments, and small businesses. Without the tram, city officials argued, the Corbett-Terwilliger-Lair Hill neighborhood would continue to live next to an industrial wasteland and nothing more.

"Having a healthy OHSU is a good thing, and far, far better thing than having them go to the suburbs," said City Commissioner Charlie Hales.[71]

The Oregonian's editorial board urged the Portland City Council to use a wider lens in making a decision on the tram, looking beyond one neighborhood's objection to the needs of the whole city to keep OHSU in Portland. Without the tram, the board wrote, OHSU would shift its expansion to its West Campus and "Hillsboro would reap much of the biotechnology benefits that could have been Portland's—a huge economic blow for Portland."[72]

Neighbors were livid.

"What occurs to me is, 'How dare you?'" said lawyer Mark Eves, whose office was on Gibbs Street. "How dare you step into our neighborhood so you can save a bunch of money and damage the value of our properties?"[73]

Opponents argued the tram would block views, mar a historical district, intrude on their privacy, lower their property values, and offer them no benefits.

"Design cannot remove the fact that it's intrusive," said Sean Brennan, a technical writer and Gibbs Street resident. "They keep talking engineering; they can't see that it can't be mitigated. It doesn't matter whether you make the towers look like trees."[74]

Stephen Leflar, a neighborhood activist and designer, objected to the way the proposal flouted community guidelines and scenic protections.

"I'm against bankrupting 100 years of planning," he said. "Also, it bankrupts my heart to know all the work I've done for the city" may be for nothing. If the tram is built, he added, "I won't do it anymore."[75]

In the spring of 2001 and again in the fall, Gragg, *The Oregonian*'s architect critic, argued the tram could integrate OHSU, "a castaway on an island," with the city. He urged the city to see it as more than a transportation solution, but as "part of a comprehensive effort to link two important places—public places—in the city. It means designing the cars, towers and surrounding plazas as objects and places of beauty."[76]

Gragg urged city leaders to seek one of ten $50,000 grants the National Endowment of the Arts was offering to cities to fund architectural design competitions for projects such as the tram.

> The tram could be the most important project this city builds in the next 25 years. It will link Portland's landlocked largest employer to 130 acres of prime, largely empty waterfront acreage where it will seed thousands of jobs and housing units. It will become a major landmark in one of the city's verdant vistas, an instant tourist draw and another chapter in Portland's 25-year history of transportation alternatives. If designed, not just well, but beautifully, the tram's towers and cars could become an international icon for the city. Its landings at OHSU campus and North Macadam could grow into dynamic civic gathering spaces.[77]

In the spring, tram supporters created a private nonprofit called Portland Aerial Transportation Inc. to design and build the tram. The nonprofit would also oversee other improvements, including a pedestrian bridge, to reconnect neighborhoods west of Interstate 5 and under the tram to the Willamette River and restore some cohesion to a community that had been fragmented by decades of freeway and arterial construction. The group's board included representatives from OHSU, South Waterfront property owners, residents of the Corbett-Terwilliger-Lair Hill neighborhood and a member of the city council. The organization also created a citizens advisory committee to recommend priorities for the tram and related projects.

But the battle continued. A consultant on the project, Battelle Memorial Institute, told the Portland Planning Bureau that the tram could serve as a catalyst for civic development and an aerial icon for "an emerging bioscience center." An opposition group called No Tram countered the tram would only connect two parts of OHSU.

"A single-purpose transit system with such a limited scope brings no more benefit to the city's transit system than would a fleet of carrier pigeons," wrote No Tram.[78]

In late June of 2002, the city council agreed to hear the debate in a series of public hearings and then decide whether to build the tram. Gragg summed up all that was at stake:

> For OHSU, the tram is key to a campus expansion its president, Peter Kohler, hopes will leverage the university into the top 20 medical schools in the country. For a group of developers led by Homer Williams, OHSU's expansion is the backbone of ambitious plans to build a high-density neighborhood on 28 acres of waterfront the developers have acquired south of the Ross Island Bridge. And for the city, the development could begin transforming the 140-acre Macadam District into what city Planning Director Gil Kelley envisions as a "Science and Technology Quarter," supporting 10,000 jobs and 5,000 housing units.[79]

On the eve of the June vote, Mayor Katz said the council would hear all sides and examine all options. But then it must act.

"We need to make a decision," she said. "Period. End of conversation. . . . If Homer [Williams] has a deal and OHSU wants to come down to North Macadam, we need to begin working on it now, plain and simple. And the community needs some resolution."[80]

That resolution came on July 20 when the four-member city council unanimously accepted the recommendation from the city's Office of Transportation for a tram over Southwest Gibbs Street. The decision set the Portland Aerial Transportation Inc. to work setting up a design competition for the project. Mayor Katz said the tram could become the city's postcard image as the Space Needle is for Seattle or the Gateway Arch is for St. Louis.[81]

Now that the tram finally had a green light, so did development plans for OHSU and the South Waterfront—just as construction was getting underway on the Biomedical Research Building and the new patient facility on Pill Hill.

Designers and engineers went to work over the following months on forging a complicated agreement that would outline commitments and plans for the waterfront development over three phases. In the first, developers would build apartment and condo towers, and OHSU would build what would become the OHSU Center for Health & Healing, a sixteen-story building with space for surgery, research, clinics, classrooms, and a fitness center. The OHSU board voted on July 7, 2003, to agree to the building and OHSU's broader role in developing the South Waterfront.

Three days later, the Portland City Council approved a development agreement among the city, OHSU, and developer Homer Williams and his partners. Before anyone could build, though, the developers had to work with state Department of Environmental Quality officials in cleaning the property of contaminants. Work also got underway to extend the Willamette River Greenway from downtown Portland through the South Waterfront District, with an average 125-foot setback. The plan also called for a two-acre Elizabeth Caruthers Park and multiple condominium towers on the waterfront.[82]

The Oregonian's editorial board urged the Portland City Council in August to approve $72 million in development aid for the project, which it did. The board, like most people in Portland, was now looking at the Oregon Opportunity buildings rising on Pill Hill and OHSU's construction on the South Waterfront as all part of one massive expansion.

> If OHSU doesn't expand aggressively, says Dr. Peter Kohler, president, it will shrink in a downward spiral because the costs of training doctors and nurses and serving indigent patients continue to climb. . . . OHSU has wisely decided to tackle its financial ills by slugging it out in the wilderness of biotechnology. . . . Kohler

does not expect Portland to rival Boston, San Francisco or other biotechnology centers. But it is reasonable to expect Oregon to claim at least 1 percent of the more than $100 billion that the industry is expected to produce nationwide over the next decade. Even if OHSU falls short of its new vision, it will be far healthier than if it had never tried to fulfill it. So will Portland.[83]

DEPARTURES

As the university's most ambitious building project in its history unfolded on Pill Hill and the waterfront in the summer of 2003, Kohler was contemplating his retirement. He was sixty-five, old enough to retire, and his wife, Judy, wanted him to. But the president had not yet reached all of his goals. The university ranked thirty-one among US academic health centers in NIH research money, still shy of the top twenty. Kohler's research expansion was not yet complete; his buildings still unfinished. He had had plenty of other opportunities to leave the university for other jobs, too, but he turned all of those down so he could complete his agenda at OHSU.[84] Kohler struck a compromise with his wife. He had hoped to retire in Portland, but Judy wanted to move back to Arkansas where some of their children and grandchildren lived. So Kohler told Judy he would agree to retire in Arkansas if she could give him three more years on Pill Hill. She accepted the deal.

Jim Walker, though, had had enough.

"I had talked with Peter for a number of months about the stress and strain of 60 hour weeks—week after week, month after month, year after year," he said. "It was taking its toll on me. It had become too stressful, and it just wasn't fun."[85]

Kohler kept urging him to stay, but Walker said he had ended up with too much responsibility. He was overseeing almost all operations of the university, including finance, legal, administration, even contract negotiations with the unions. One evening while once again negotiating a contract with the Oregon Nurses Association in a Portland building off campus, Walker collapsed. An ambulance took him to OHSU Hospital where he underwent an emergency appendectomy. The next morning Kohler visited him in his hospital room.

"Pete, this is my wake up call," Walker said. "I know this is caused by stress. This is it. I'm going to have to leave."

So at age fifty-four, early in 2003, Walker retired.

"We were a great team," he said. "I loved working with the rest of the team. But at the end of the day, I retired. I could not face going to work, and I couldn't face going out and getting a job."[86]

But it wasn't long before Lewis & Clark College in Portland called up Walker to help it handle a financial and political disaster. Michael Mooney, president of the small liberal arts college, resigned in June of 2003 after he made an unauthorized loan to an Idaho energy operation and lost $10.5 million of the college's money when the company went bankrupt.[87] Paul Bragdon, the former Reed College president and former head of the OHSU Foundation, stepped in as interim president and brought Walker on board to help him make repairs.

Walker ended up staying two years as chief financial officer.

"That was 40 hours a week," he said. "It was the easiest thing in the world."[88]

So with Goldfarb and Walker gone, and with Billups working reduced hours to care for her daughter, Kohler pressed on with only Hallick and Davis from the old team.

Another big break came his way in the summer of 2004 when the Schnitzer family, represented by Gilbert Schnitzer, donated nearly twenty acres of the South Waterfront property to OHSU.[89] Goldschmidt said he had urged the Schnitzers, whom he represented as a consulting lawyer, to make the donation if they were not going to build on the land themselves.[90] Kohler said the gift, worth about $35 million, was the largest in the university's history and would be used to create a Schnitzer campus for the dental and medical schools.

By the winter of 2004–05, cranes again dominated the university skyline, with construction underway for the Biomedical Research Building, the sweeping patient care building attached to OHSU Hospital, the Center for Health & Healing on the waterfront, and the tram that would connect them. As new buildings rose, so did the precariousness of the university's financing and its danger of getting overextended with debt. A drop in the stock market in 2002–03 discouraged philanthropic donations across the county. The OHSU Foundation was no exception; its gifts declined by a third. Donations rebounded by the fall of 2004, but the foundation still had not raised $67 million of the $90 million it had projected to collect for furnishing the new Biomedical Research Building and the patient care facility, both about a year from completion.[91]

In a memo to the OHSU administration, Lora Cuykendall, the university's new director of media relations and publications, warned that OHSU was vulnerable and open to challenges on numerous fronts.[92] The institution, she wrote, was under unusual financial pressure because of "its expansion and increasingly competitive health care environment in Portland" and more cuts in state funding. It could face public concern over whether it would fulfill its Oregon Opportunity promises, continue to serve the indigent and other people in need and avoid more cost overruns for the tram.

The university hospitals were serving about the same number of Medicaid and indigent inpatients in 2005 as ten years earlier, but their number of commercially insured, that is paying, patients, had climbed by more than 40 percent. Therefore, their low-income patients had become a smaller share of their overall mix, shrinking from 42 percent of all inpatients in 1997 to 34 percent in 2005.[93]

Compared to other Portland hospitals in serving low-income and indigent patients, "OHSU is doing more than its 'fair share,'" wrote Cuykendall. "However, a shift in the payer mix and the hospital's current bottom line may be a flashpoint for media interest."[94]

The tram project also was drawing public fire because of cost overruns. The initial estimate for the project in 2002 was $15.5 million. But in 2003, Portland Aerial Transportation Inc., the nonprofit created to help oversee the project, selected through international competition a bolder design with broader scope and more substantial docking stations at each end, pushing the cost estimate up to $25.9 million. After a building contractor completed building documents, the price climbed to $39.6 million. By January of 2006, as construction got underway, the tram was carrying a $45 million sticker price. Developers, the City of Portland, and OHSU were sharing in the costs of building the tram. The city was in charge of managing the project, but OHSU was on the hook for nearly 70 percent of the costs.[95]

The cost overruns were the result in part of a poorly calculated, grossly low early estimate of only $15 million, officials said. An 85 percent climb in steel prices also contributed to the increase.[96] Stadum, who had moved from general counsel to chief administrative officer at OHSU, noted in an op-ed column for *The Oregonian* that OHSU was on budget and on schedule for the three buildings it had under construction—the Biomedical Research Building, the new patient care wing adjoining OHSU Hospital, and the Center for Health & Healing on the South Waterfront.[97] Two condominium towers were also rising on the waterfront, just the first of numerous high-rises planned by developers. Stadum urged critics to see the big picture.

> But we must not lose sight of the long-term vision. Driven by OHSU's decision to expand within the city, an unkempt segment of Portland's riverfront is being transformed into a vibrant downtown district. The tram is the catalyst for $2 billion in commercial and residential investments and—once it is completed—will take its place as a Portland icon that will add to the city's already great appeal.[98]

By February, five months into construction, the tram's price tag had bumped up another $10 million to $55 million. A small group of angry residents, including some from the Corbett-Terwilliger-Lair Hill neighborhood, showed for a city meeting March 14 on the tram's rising costs. Alan Peterson, who lived in the neighborhood, wore a T-shirt bearing the words: No Tram to OHSU. "It's not necessary," he said. "They could run a shuttle. It's just too expensive."[99]

To continue the project, the city would have to increase its share from $3.5 million to $8.5 million, and OHSU would put up an additional $7.5 million, bringing its total to $40.2 million.[100] South Waterfront property owners also would put up some money. Some city commissioners preferred letting the project die to spending so much more. But Commissioner Dan Saltzman agreed to back the project, giving it a majority vote.[101] The tram now came in at $57.6 million—a price that would hold through its completion in December.

Ted Sickinger, a business reporter at *The Oregonian*, took a hard look at OHSU's expansions and ambitions to grow to financial self-sufficiency.[102] He acknowledged Kohler had "presided over OHSU's transformation from a medical backwater to a behemoth with 11,500 employees, a $1.2 billion annual budget and an array of clinics, hospitals and research centers during the past two decades." [103] He concluded the university's assumptions for growth were "plausible," but also implied they were a long shot. Scott Gibson, a venture capitalist and member of the OHSU board, told him OHSU was making reasonable assumptions.

"As head of finance and audit committees," he said, "I would never let OHSU get out over its skis."[104]

But OHSU's expansion, Sickinger explained, depended on it regularly turning a 6 percent margin, or profit, on its hospitals and clinics, a historically high rate that it rarely achieved. OHSU was counting on the hospital, with its new patient care wing, to increase profits as it made payments on $600 million in debt. At the same time the state was cutting subsidies for charity care and federal deficits were pressuring Medicare to reduce reimbursements.[105]

The university was also assuming it would see significant increases in NIH research grants at a time when the NIH funding was not growing and increasingly difficult to win. One researcher, who left the university to chair neurobiology at the University of Pittsburgh, said OHSU's chronic budget problems and its focus on new buildings rather than existing programs were sapping the institution's vitality and faculty's morale. On the other hand, the university had attracted some high-profile researchers such as a team of anesthesiologists from Johns Hopkins, a new chair of biomedical engineering from Emory University, and a chair of orthopedics from Case Western Reserve University.

Federal money that Senator Hatfield once steered to OHSU at the rate of about $9 million a year had dropped to $1.5 million since he left the Senate in 1997. The university also was relying on its OHSU Foundation to gain momentum and build its endowment so it could support OHSU's new buildings. But much of the money the foundation was raising was targeted for specific projects, programs, and academic support that did not fit the university's expansion goals, leaving it short of the money it needed to equip new buildings.[106]

In short, Sickinger wrote, "the bean counters at OHSU are squeezing the budget in search of savings. That has meant cutting staff, freezing departmental cash reserves, raising tuition and undertaking a host of new measures to profitably manage hospital operations." [107]

OHSU THRIVES

For all the concerns with money, the tram, and politics, the OHSU academic health center bloomed during Kohler's final year and everything seemed to fall into place much as he had envisioned.

The university raised $378 million from more than 78,000 donors to surpass its goal for matching the legislature's $200 million in bonds for Oregon Opportunity projects. And as a public corporation, it also raised

$250 million in its own revenue bonds. So with bonds and a portion of its donations, the university amassed $513 million for its various Oregon Opportunity projects, which included constructing two buildings, luring teams of top researchers, and $44 million to buy land on the South Waterfront.[108] The university had also found fortune in buying steel at a good price for its buildings before prices shot up when the tram construction got underway.

The $145 million, 274,000-square-foot Biomedical Research Building was completed in February of 2006. The eleven-level building included four basement floors, one for a new advanced imaging research center, and seven more floors above ground, six devoted to research laboratories. A crane dropped four huge magnets, each weighing from 15 to 30 tons, onto one basement floor to create one of the most powerful Magnetic Resonance Imaging (MRI) machines in the world. The OHSU Advanced Imaging Research Center would use the MRI system to create images of tissues beneath the skin for experimental studies on both people and mice and rats. The NIH in Maryland was the only other place on Earth with an MRI machine as strong as that at OHSU.[109]

The biomedical building rose on the west side of campus, attached to the Medical Research Building behind the medical school's Mackenzie Hall, blocking Kohler's view of Portland and Mount St. Helens from his office in Baird Hall. The building also connects with the Multnomah Pavilion, the former county hospital. It was renamed in 2015 after Hildegard Lamfrom, an influential molecular biologist who guided Brian Druker early in his career and broke ground in the field of protein synthesis before her death from cancer in 1984. Hallick, the provost, later said the research building added value to the neighboring research and clinical buildings.

"We connected the whole hill into integrated research," Hallick said. "We connected with the old research labs, and we connected with the clinical investigations."[110]

Druker moved in on the fifth floor next to cell biologist John

Scott, and they created a new Center for Cancer Cell Signaling. Both studied kinases—enzymes that change proteins to do work in cells—and sometimes worked together and shared lab space.[111] The new labs also helped OHSU hold onto Dr. Markus Grompe, genetic researcher and professor in the departments of Pediatrics and Molecular and Medical Genetics, who was being recruited by Stanford University, said Dorsa, the vice president for research.

"Stanford was recruiting him because they have a leadership in the stem cell area," Dorsa said. "So one of the things we needed to do with Oregon Opportunity and the space created by it was to give Marcus an opportunity for leadership. So we created the Oregon Stem Cell Center and placed him [in charge of it] in the new building."[112]

On other floors of the research building a scientific staff of more than 350 conducted medical research. Pediatric researchers probed the genetic and molecular causes of childhood diseases, including pediatric cancer and congenital heart disorders, while others scientists studied the viral and environmental causes of asthma, inflammatory eye diseases, and treatments for neurodegenerative diseases such as multiple sclerosis.

The US Green Building Council awarded the research building LEED (Leadership in Energy and Environmental Design) silver certification for a design that is a third more energy efficient than Oregon's code requires. The design features included smart storm water management, erosion control, water efficiency, recycled and local materials, and extensive use of day lighting.

"The design of this building will take this campus to the forefront of biomedical technology," said Dorsa.[113]

Indeed, the building became a magnet for scientific talent. Because the building could offer a custom cardiovascular imaging laboratory, it was able to lure Dr. Sanjiv Kaul and his entire research team from the University of Virginia, even before it was complete. Kaul's team was studying ways to use imaging technology to diagnose causes of chest pain and to deliver medicines to specific body sites with pinpoint accuracy.[114] Charles

Springer came to OHSU from Brookhaven National Laboratory to establish the Advanced Imaging Research Center. The university's Jungers Center for Neurosciences Research established an Advanced Light Microscopy Core Resource in the Biomedical Research Building, which attracted Gary Banker and Fred Robinson, two world-famous neuroscientists, to the OHSU faculty. Stefanie Kaech Petrie, a leader in neuroimaging, also came to direct the new Advanced Light Microscopy Core.[115]

In June of 2006, the university completed the construction of the twelve-story patient care wing sweeping north from the hospital and including a docking station for the tram on its ninth floor. The $216 million patient care facility gave OHSU 335,000 square feet of new hospital and clinical space and a 450-car garage. The gracefully curving, 100-yard-long wing connected to OHSU Hospital at each floor level. It included room for twelve operating rooms and 120 hospital beds, including sixty beds for surgery patients and twenty-four for patients in intensive care. It also included clinics for oncology, cardiac, and neurology services and for the Center for Women's Health.[116]

At its meeting three months earlier, the OHSU board gave the building a name: the Peter O. Kohler Pavilion. The president was caught off guard. The university had not named a building after a living employee since the 1940s, when buildings were dedicated to two nurses, Emma Jones and Katherine Sears. The only other living person to receive that honor from the board was Senator Hatfield, who was on the board when it named the pavilion for Kohler.[117]

"It was a total surprise to me and very humbling," Kohler said. "I was hoping we could find a donor we could name the building for. I showed it to [Nike cofounder] Phil Knight [while it was being built] to try to get him interested in it."[118]

AUDITING OREGON OPPORTUNITY

In January of 2010, Oregon Secretary of State Kate Brown released an audit on how well OHSU had spent its money on its Oregon Opportunity projects. "We found that OHSU met or exceeded its specific goals and measurable targets," wrote state auditor Gary Blackmer.[119]

The report noted OHSU not only had built the Biomedical Research Building, but also expanded research space on its West Campus and created the Oregon Rural Practice-based Research Network, which included 157 physicians in thirty-seven rural communities and a rural high-speed electronic communications network. In addition, the university raised $378 million from private donors, recruited ninety-four scientific investigators, added 175 research staff, and, by 2009, received $217 million in research grants through the investigators it had recruited, more than the money it had spent.[120]

While the glowing report confirmed the Oregon Opportunity investment had produced huge benefits for OHSU and the state, *Oregonian* reporter Ted Sickinger noted that Kohler had failed to deliver on producing a $1 billion biotech industry.

"The biotech industry, the private-sector jobs and the industry activity on South Waterfront have not materialized in a meaningful ways," he said.[121]

But as Kohler prepared to retire in 2006, plenty was happening on the South Waterfront. Both the Biomedical Research Building and the Peter O. Kohler Pavilion were being completed. So also were the tram—designed by the Los Angeles office of Zurich-based Angélil/Graham/Pfenninger/Scholl Architecture—and the Center for Health & Healing on the waterfront. Most residents in Portland saw the overlapping projects as all part of one big surge in growth at OHSU.

The sixteen-story Center for Health & Healing gave the university another 400,000 square feet of space for surgery, research, clinics, classrooms and a fitness center with pools, spas, weight rooms, and lab facilities. The building rose next to the tram docking station so that people descending on the tram cars could look through the center's giant picture windows to see into its fitness area with basketball and volleyball courts. The university paid for 25 percent of the $145 million building, while the OHSU Medical Group, the physicians group, financed the remaining 75 percent. The university started moving 937 staff members into the building on October 23, 2006, but the building was not declared officially open until December 3.

Gragg, the architecture critic, described the building as reaching a "high middle ground between dull and bracing."[122] But he noted some of its exceptional environmental features such as sun shades on the south face with integrated photovoltaic panels, and a solar collector on the roof to heat the building's air and water. Microturbines in the building use its recycled heat and a little natural gas to generate electricity.[123] The building, which won LEED platinum rating, also had toilets that flush with rainwater and staircases ventilated with outdoor air, making it among the most environmentally friendly buildings in the nation.[124]

This new front door for OHSU would become "one of the most important buildings OHSU has ever built," said Stadum. "It will really be a place where all of our missions will come together in one space."[125]

The building also would enable OHSU to hold on to one of its prized researchers, Shoukhrat Mitalipov, a Russian immigrant who developed a new process for creating human stem cells from skin cells. He and other researchers are exploring ways to use stem cells to treat various degenerative diseases. Cincinnati Children's Hospital saw Mitalipov as a rising star and was trying to recruit him, said Dorsa, OHSU's vice president of research, so "I had to retain him." Dorsa made him the director of OHSU's new Center for Embryonic Cell and Gene Therapy in the Center for Health & Healing.[126]

At the new building, the first silver, bullet-shaped pod was attached to the tram cables on November 9, and the tram was unveiled and began carrying passengers on December 9. Almost immediately, all the political and financial turmoil over the tram evaporated as Portlanders marveled over the two pods gliding quietly from one gleaming new building to another.

Two weeks earlier, a streetcar started rolling into a station on the South Waterfront, creating another connection between downtown Portland, the South Waterfront, and the tram station. Mary Pitman Kitch, an editorial writer for *The Oregonian,* took a ride on the tram one rainy day and declared it a success. The tram's cars "dematerialize" against the gray sky exactly as the designers had intended, she wrote. After all the political battles and cost overruns, Portland ended up with an efficient way to move people that "collapses distances," Kitch wrote. "Using the tram will melt misgivings and turn many Portlanders' opinions inside out, like their umbrellas. For all its complications, the tram will soon be known for its functional simplicity and true trademark—speed."[127]

OHSU workers loved the tram. An OHSU shuttle bus trip to the waterfront would take twenty minutes or more each way. The tram took three minutes, almost like an elevator. Like many people who expressed opinions on the project, Ian Schnadig, a fellow of hematology and oncology, said the tram was well worth the cost and expense.[128] In January of 2007, the twin tram pods were named Walt and Jean after Walt Reynolds, then eighty-six and the first African-American to graduate from the OHSU medical school, and Jean Richardson, eighty, the first woman to graduate with a civil engineering degree in Oregon. The pair met for a ride on the tram.

"I must say," said Richardson, as she entered the aerial car and looked at the city below, "I don't care for heights."[129]

Ten years later, residents of the Corbett-Terwilliger-Lair Hill neighborhoods, all part of what has been named the South Portland Neighborhood Association, have come to accept the tram, said Ken Love, president of the association. "It is just part of the landscape now," he said.[130]

Jim Gardner, seventy, who lives near Gibbs Street, which runs directly under the tram, said there are "very few hard feelings about it, and it has benefited us in indirect ways." The pedestrian bridge over the freeway, built in conjunction with the tram project, gives residents living under the tram access to the South Waterfront and its restaurants and parks. Property values did not drop as feared in the neighborhoods, said Gardner, but rather climbed as the housing became prized by people working at OHSU with its close, convenient access to the tram. In an unusual agreement, the City of Portland had offered to buy houses at market rates from residents who did not want to live with the tram, he said, but no one took the city up on the offer. Windows on the tram pods are painted along the bottom so riders can't look directly down into residents' homes as they silently glide over. What residents notice, he said, is not the pod, but the shadow it casts.[131]

KOHLER MOVES ON

By the time the tram was sailing, Kohler had retired. On his final day of work, September 14, 2006, Kohler literally passed the torch, the flickering flames of a backyard tiki torch, to his successor, Dr. Joseph Robertson Jr., an ophthalmologist stepping up from dean of the OHSU School of Medicine. OHSU had adopted the torch flame as its logo, so as Kohler ended his eighteen-year run with a town hall meeting for university staff in the OHSU Auditorium, the torch seemed a fitting symbol for the transfer of leadership.

"Think of this as a great flame," Kohler said. "The flame has become our new symbol, the flame of knowledge, so before this goes out, I'd like to give it to Joe."[132]

Robertson, who had worked at OHSU for twenty-six years, was selected from three finalists to succeed Kohler. The other two were Paul Whelton, senior vice president for health sciences at Tulane University Health Sciences Center in New Orleans, and Jay Gershen, executive vice chancellor of health sciences at the University of Colorado Health Sciences Center.[133]

Robertson, a Yale graduate skilled in performing microsurgery on the retina, grew up in rural Indiana, the only child of a flour miller. Like Kohler, he had an interest in rural health and was committed to reinforcing the rural health network Kohler had built.[134] He said he would set out to develop a ten-year plan that would include a variety of partnerships with other universities and health care organizations to help it train more doctors and continue its role in providing a safety net for the uninsured. Robertson would face a complex set of challenges. It would be up to him to manage the university's physical expansion on the waterfront and hill, absorb scores of new research scientists and clinicians, compete with other local providers for insured patients, and adjust to eroding government support from the state and a decline in federal research funding and Medicaid and Medicare reimbursements. Representative Mitch Greenlick, a Democrat from Portland who previously worked as a professor at OHSU, said Robertson was the kind of leader who could "make sure the culture of growth that Peter built is stabilized."[135]

Three years later, Davis and Hallick would also leave OHSU. Davis left in mid-August of 2009 to become chief of staff and vice president for public affairs for Portland State University. She loved OHSU, she said, but it had arrived, had reached a state of healthy stability, and it was time for a new challenge.

> If you look back over my career, what I always have been most interested in and excited about is working with organizations when they're in the messy phase, at the inflexion point with enormous potential that they have yet to realize. I like being part of helping them build from there. . . . I went to OHSU at a time when they were changing over from [Leonard] Laster to Kohler. Kohler had a very clear vision of where the institution would go, and I was able to play a small part. . . . It was a great team, and we were really able to help move the institution along in realizing its potential. I think Portland State is at the same kind of inflection point. It's messy, there's a ton of work, we've got an enormous amount to do, but it's that time in an organization's life that gives me energy. . . . Now I feel like I'm battling the same battles all over again. . . .
>
> I know we've all said this, but the teamwork at [OHSU] was such an important piece of it, because we came to understand each

> other and what our strengths and weaknesses were, which allowed us to be much more agile. You didn't have to worry about "Does Janet have it? Or does Jim have it?" You knew they had it. Even at a certain point, you could anticipate what they were going to say. Fun ride.[136]

Hallick left OHSU about five months later to become president of Pacific University, a small, private liberal arts university in Forest Grove, twenty-seven miles west of Portland. She wasn't looking to leave, she said, but was intrigued when approached about leading Pacific.[137] When she interviewed for the job, the former president, Phil Creighton, told her the place "just weaves its way into your heart," she said. "I felt that from the moment I stepped on this historic campus."[138]

Of the leadership team that led the battle to make OHSU a public corporation, only Billups remained. She had returned as general counsel, overseeing seven in-house and multiple outside lawyers.

KOHLER'S LEGACY

As Kohler departed OHSU, he received broad recognition for all that he had accomplished, but he also drew some criticism for what the institution had become. *The Oregonian* summed up the "knock" on OHSU: "While the university portrays itself as a sort of Florence Nightingale for the state, outsiders say it has become too big, too insular, even too arrogant for what is still, in effect, a public agency."[139]

The newspaper's editorial board also said Kohler's gains came at some cost to OHSU's goodwill. "The bruising battle over the tram between Marquam hill and the new South Waterfront campus is only the latest and most prominent of the episodes that have damaged OHSU's standing in the community." The paper went on to cite the examples of the university taking a hard line in paying for care of a patient whose brain was damaged during a botched procedure in the hospital, warning it might close the Poison Center for lack of state funding, and threatening to expand on its West Campus.[140]

OHSU had its faults, Kohler said, but his administration made earnest efforts to address them and was never "arrogant." What's more, the problems cited by the *Oregonian* proved to be fleeting issues, eclipsed by OHSU's dramatic transformation. Under Kohler's watch, OHSU doubled its building space to more than 6 million square feet, grew its research awards seven-fold to $294 million, and doubled its employees from 5,800 to 12,000.[141] At the same time, its state funding had dropped to $42 million or about 3.5 percent of its operating budget. An independent rating system ranked its hospital among the fifty best in the nation out of 1,263 hospitals that participated in the 2006 survey.[142] When Kohler departed, the university had become a nationally recognized center of research and teaching with a $1.2 billion annual budget, the largest employer in Portland and fourth largest in Oregon. [143]

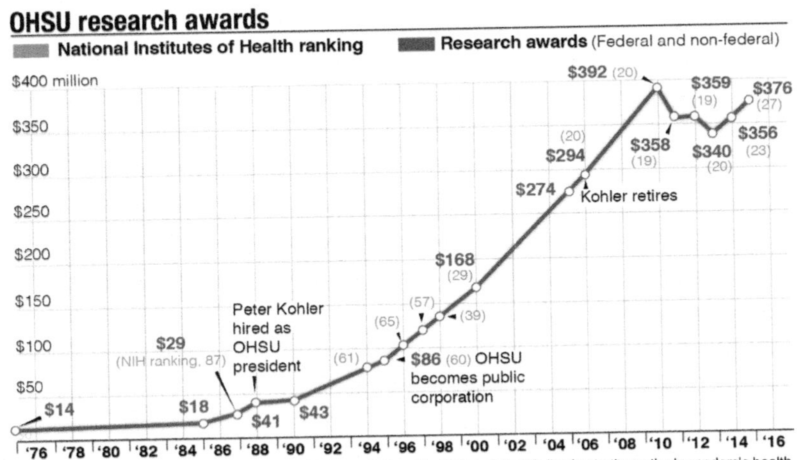

Note: Rankings based on research money solely from National Institutes of Health flowing to the nation's academic health centers, which range in number from about 125 in 1988 to 140 today.

Sources: Oregon Health & Science University and Blue Ridge Institute for Medical Research
Graphic by Mark Graves

The university was a central player in the South Waterfront District redevelopment project, the largest urban renewal initiative in Portland's history. Three years after Kohler left, ECONorthwest, an economic think tank in Portland, conducted an analysis of OHSU's economic impact on Portland and Oregon. The study concluded that in 2007, the absence of Oregon's only academic health center would mean a loss of $2.4 billion a year in net economic output and the loss of 20,748 jobs and $1.1 billion in net personal income. With OHSU and Doernbecher hospitals and with more than eighty primary and specialty care clinics in Portland and throughout the state, the university provided care for patients with the most complex needs in Oregon. OHSU drew more than 40 percent of its patients from outside the metropolitan area and also remained the primary provider of health care for low-income households.[144]

At Kohler's retirement town hall meeting, Keith Thompson, an Intel executive and chair of the OHSU board, named Kohler OHSU's first emeritus president. Kohler, who had just been honored with a beautiful building named after him, was given an honorary degree and a retirement watch: a gentleman's model by Seiko. But perhaps the most valuable gift to the retiring president was a lifetime parking pass on Marquam Hill.[145]

Kohler described to the town hall gathering what he considered his four major accomplishments: making OHSU more of a statewide institution with its rural health network, achieving financial stability, raising OHSU's profile as a nationally recognized academic health center, and converting OHSU to a public corporation, which helped make all those other achievements possible.[146]

Seven months after retiring, Kohler took a new job as vice chancellor at the University of Arkansas for Medical Sciences, where he led efforts to establish satellite medical programs in northwest Arkansas. He worked with local health care providers to establish a campus with rotations for students in medicine, pharmacy, and other health professions from the

University of Arkansas for Medical Sciences in Little Rock. Based in Fayetteville, Arkansas, he leads a major effort to reduce obesity and diabetes among a large migrant population from the Marshall Islands.[147] He moved into semi-retirement in the summer of 2016.

Kohler also continues to keep an office at OHSU. He makes regular visits there, often in connection with meetings as a member of Hallick's board of directors at Pacific University in nearby Forest Grove. He was scheduled to give the commencement address to the medical school graduates in the spring of 2015, but had to cancel because of an eye injury that prevented him from traveling.

"Do the right thing" and "learn to adapt," he was prepared to tell graduates, according to his draft speech. "As long as you are firmly grounded and adhere to your principles, you can survive all sorts of systems change."

Kohler left OHSU having accomplished nearly all twelve of the goals he outlined to the board before he was hired. He had streamlined administration, upgraded OHSU Hospital and replaced Doernbecher Hospital, expanded research, strengthened instruction with a curriculum overhaul, created the Area Health Education Centers, established a focus on gene therapy research, developed new revenue sources, improved parking, and expanded facilities. He was not able to win gains in state support, and though he did increase the university's share of minority faculty and students, he did not make as much headway on that goal as he had hoped.

And what about that driving, overarching quest to lift OHSU's research capacity into the ranks of the top twenty academic health centers in the nation? Hallick, with her penchant for numbers, had predicted that the university would hit that benchmark when it reached $300 million a year in research grants, a little more than half of which come from the NIH. In 2006, as Kohler prepared to depart, OHSU had crept up to the edge of that mark with $294 million in research grants. And that was close enough. The NIH 2006 rankings for medical schools and their departments put OHSU at twentieth.[148]

Notes

1. "Growth and Change at OHSU: 1990–2014," available at OHSU Strategic Communications. The chart shows that the institution's operating budget grew from $499 million in 1995 to $882 million in 2000. It also shows that the OHSU's square feet of building space climbed from 3.1 million in 1990 to 5 million in 2000.
2. Peter O. Kohler, MD, "Genes, Jobs and the Giant on the Hill," speech to the Portland Regional Chamber of Commerce, Feb. 16, 2000.
3. OHSU Government Relations, "The Oregon Medical Research Initiative," May 17, 2000.
4. Lois Davis, interview, March 9, 2015, her Portland State University office.
5. Joe Rojas-Burke, "OHSU Sets Ambitious Goal," *The Oregonian*, May 7, 2000, p. A12.
6. Peter O. Kohler, MD, recruitment letter to candidates invited to serve on the Oregon Opportunity Steering Committee, June 22, 2000.
7. OHSU, *OHSU and Oregon in an Era of Opportunity*, report to the 2001 Oregon Legislative Assembly, p. 15. Available through OHSU Strategic Communications.
8. *The Oregon Opportunity: Medical Research at OHSU benefits all Oregonians*, a flier, Kohler presidential papers, OHSU Archives, 2000.
9. OHSU Rural Health Research Institute, discussion paper, OHSU archives, Sept. 1, 2000.
10. Ibid.
11. OHSU's Oregon Rural Practice-based Research Network (ORPRN) continues to thrive as a statewide network of primary care clinicians, community partners and academicians providing health care to rural residents and reducing rural health disparities. ORPRN uses evidence-based practices to improve preventive health care, identify community health priorities, use information technology, and conduct randomized controlled trials. The network celebrated its 15th year in 2017 with partners in 189 practices involving more than 500 primary care clinicians serving more than a half million patients. Two out of every five rural Oregonians receive their care in a practice affiliated with the ORPRN network. The network includes nine Practice Enhancement Research Coordinators with offices on the campuses of Eastern and Southern Oregon universities and in Hood River, Bend, Eugene and Portland. "We did deliver on the Oregon Opportunity," said Dr. Lyle Fagnan, outgoing ORPRN director, in an email to Dr. Peter Kohler on Feb. 6, 2017.
12. Davis, interview.
13. Steve Woodward, "Microscopic biotech lab makes it big," *The Oregonian*, March 4, 1998, p. C01.
14. Steve Woodward, "Health Firm a New OHSU 'Grad'," *The Oregonian*, April 2, 1998, p. B01.
15. "Dawn of an Industry: Bioscience and Medical Technology in Oregon," *The Business Journal/Bioscience and Medical Technology Directory*, April 10, 1998, pp. 13–17.
16. Carey Goldberg, "Across the U.S., Universities Are Fueling High-Tech Economic

Booms," *The New York Times*, Oct. 8, 1999.

17 Ibid.

18 Edward W. Thompson and Peter O. Kohler, "Let Oregon set pace by joining high-tech, medical resources," *The Oregonian*, Aug. 27, 2000, p. G3; Teri Cettina, "The Best of Both Worlds," *Oregon Business*, Dec. 2000, pp. 22–25. Kohler said in Cettina's article that "the important benefits we'll provide employers through our merger is the growth and development of the biotechnology industry as a result of our research strength; the development of new intellectual property, the new discoveries we're making, and being able to deploy those discoveries [through technology transfer] within the state in such a way that they benefit the state economy."

19 *The Oregon Opportunity: Medical Research at OHSU benefits all Oregonians*, flier, Peter Kohler collection, OHSU Archives, 2000.

20 Lois Davis to Felicia Trader (executive director of the City of Portland's development commission), memo, "Research Growth Potential at OHSU," Nov. 29, 1999.

21 *Brian Druker's Cancer Drug: Oregon's Lost Opportunity*, flyer, Kohler presidential papers, OHSU Archives, 2000.

22 Chris Penttila, "Blip on the Biotech Radar," *Oregon Business*, Dec. 2000, pp. 18-21.

23 Joe Rojas-Burke, "Slow Startup for Biotech," *The Oregonian*, Dec. 16, 2001, p. G01. The company has since moved back to the West Coast with offices in Lake Forest, California, and Tigard, Oregon.

24 Joe Rojas-Burke, "Biotech not Immune from Risk," *The Oregonian*, June 11, 2002 p. C01.

25 Jonathan Brinckman, "City, Biotech Imperfect Match," *The Oregonian*, June 30, 2003, p. D01.

26 Bureau of Planning, City of Portland, Technology Partnership Practice, Battelle Memorial Institute, *Building Bioscience in Portland: An Assessment of Oregon Health & Science University's Research Prospects and Portland's Bioscience Economic Potential*, Executive Summary, Feb. 2002.

27 Peter O. Kohler, MD, testimony before the US Senate Committee on Commerce, Science and Transportation, Subcommittee on Science, Technology and Space, Portland, Ore., April 5, 2002.

28 Daniel Dorsa, interview, Dec. 23, 2014, his office, OHSU.

29 Alec Josephson (president of Pinnacle Economics, Inc.), *Economic Impact Study: Profiling the Growth of Oregon's Bioscience Industry, 2014*, May, 2016.

30 "Governor Signs 'Oregon Opportunity' for OHSU Research," OHSU press release, Aug. 08, 2001, http://www.ohsu.edu/xd/about/news_events/news/2001/08-10-governor-signs-oregon-op.cfm.

31 Timothy Goldfarb, interview, Aug. 7, 2015, his Portland home.

32 Ibid.

33 A table of state contributions to OHSU operations for 1989–91 through 2013–15 shows that OHSU received $96 million from the state in 2001–03, which was down $16 million from the $112 million it received in 1999–01. The table was produced by

OHSU Central Financial Services and the Oregon Department of Administrative Services, Budget and Management, for OHSU 2014 Fact Book, p. 49. Online at: https://www.ohsu.edu/xd/education/library/upload/OHSU-Fact-Book-2014.pdf.

34 Peter O. Kohler, MD. *A Message from President Kohler*, Sept. 2001.

35 Ibid.

36 Joe Rojas-Burke, "OHSU Nurses Vote to Strike," *The Oregonian*, Dec. 16, 2001, p. C01.

37 Joe Rojas-Burke, "OHSU Adjusts as Nurses Picket," *The Oregonian*, Dec. 18, 2001, p. A01.

38 Mark Dodson, interview, Feb. 23, 2006, Multnomah Athletic Club, downtown Portland. Dodson said the nurses "didn't want to say [Jim Walker is ugly] to his face. He thought it was drop dead funny that the nurses were out there saying that about him."

39 Joe Rojas-Burke and Wendy Lawton, "Staffing at the Heart of OHSU Strike," *The Oregonian*, Dec. 19, 2001, p. C01.

40 Don Colburn, "2 Nurses, 2 Views, One who Walked: Kristin Kidd," *The Oregonian*, Jan. 13, 2002, p. B01.

41 *Oregonian* Editorial Board, "Settle this Strike," Dec. 20, 2001, p. C10.

42 Pat Southard (interim hospital director at OHSU), "In Response, Strike isn't about OHSU's Responses to Complaints," *The Oregonian*, p. D07. Southard wrote, "*The Oregonian* draws the erroneous conclusion that the strike is the result of poor labor relations. The majority of nurses and managers at OHSU have wonderful working relationship."

43 Wendy Y. Lawton, "Nurses Return to OHSU, but Strike Tension Chills the Air," *The Oregonian*, Feb. 14, 2002, p. A01.

44 Joe Rojas-Burke, "Q & A, Dr. Peter Kohler, OHSU, State of the University," *The Oregonian*, Feb. 15, 2002, P. B01.

45 *The Oregonian* Editorial Board, "Don't Miss this Opportunity—Measure 11 should be a Slam-Dunk with Voters," April 14, 2002, p. E06.

46 Mark O. Hatfield, "In my opinion supporting Measure 11 will help Oregon's future," *The Oregonian*, May 9, 2002.

47 Joe Rojas-Burke, "Expansion will Begin at OHSU," *The Oregonian* Sept. 18, 2002, p. E06.

48 Peter O. Kohler, MD, prepared remarks for Oct. 10, 2002, ground-breaking of the Biomedical Research Building, OHSU Archives.

49 "Fostering the Future: The Marquam Hill Plan Encourages Intellectual, Economic and Physical Synergy," OHSU summary of the Marquam Hill Plan, OHSU archives, 2002.

50 Christopher De Sousa, School of Urban and Regional Planning, Ryerson University, and Lily-Ann D'Souza, "South Waterfront District, Portland, OR: A Sustainable Brownfield Revitalization Best Practice," a project for the Sustainable Brownfields Consortium, based at the Institute for Environmental Science and Policy, University

of Illinois, Chicago, 2012, p. 1–3.

51 In an interview on Jan. 15, 2015 in Portland, Goldschmidt confirmed the tram idea was his.

52 Davis, interview.

53 Goldfarb, interview.

54 Both Dr. Peter Kohler and former Governor John Kitzhaber remember discussing the tram while dining at a restaurant in Germany (during a trade mission that Kohler had accompanied Kitzhaber on, along with other Oregon leaders) around 2001. Kohler described the tram proposal, but he also asked Kitzhaber whether he would be interested in becoming the next president of OHSU after Kohler retired in 2006. In an interview on Feb. 12, 2016, Kitzhaber said, "I didn't picture being the president of an academic health center. I'm sure it would have been a really good job as it turns out."

55 Ibid.

56 Goldschmidt, interview.

57 Ibid.

58 De Sousa and D'Souza, "South Waterfront District," p. 4.

59 Randy Gragg, "Riverfront Plan Doesn't Hold Water," *The Oregonian*, May 16, 1999, p. F02.

60 Gordon Oliver and Janet Christ, "OHSU Growth a Test for City," *The Oregonian*, April 10, 2001, p. C01.

61 Janet Christ, "City Urged to Focus Effort on OHSU Expansion," *The Oregonian*, Dec. 7, 2001, p. C03.

62 Janet Christ, "Residents Weigh in on OHSU, Marquam Growth," *The Oregonian*, April 2, 2002, C02.

63 Randy Gragg, "North Macadam: Tall, Thin and Glassy," *The Oregonian*, April 28, 2002, p. E01.

64 The Pearl District was a highly successful urban revitalization project that created a vibrant mix of upscale restaurants, shops, condominiums, and apartments in a previously industrial sector of Northwest Portland.

65 Gragg, "North Macadam".

66 Fred Buckman (former president and CEO of PacifiCorp), interview, Dec. 10, 2014, in Beaverton, Oregon.

67 Ibid.

68 Craig Rowland, representative of the Corbett-Terwilliger-Lair Hill neighborhood to Gordon Davis, planning consultant to OHSU, letter, titled, "North Macadam District: Transportation Components of Plan Proposed Tram Alignment from North Macadam to OHSU," Sept. 17, 2000.

69 Janet Christ, "OHSU Tram's Ride Turns Bumpy," *The Oregonian*, Dec. 8, 2000, p. B03.

70 Janet Christ, "OHSU, Neighborhoods Square Off over Tram Proposal," *The Oregonian*, March 1, 2001, p. B01.

71 Janet Christ, "OHSU's Aerial Tram Idea Stirs Fuss," *The Oregonian*, Nov. 3, 2000,

p. B03.

72 "The Escalator up the Hill," Editorial, *The Oregonian*, March 11, 2001, p. G04.

73 Christ, "OHSU Tram's Ride Turns Bumpy," p. B03.

74 Christ, "OHSU, Neighborhoods Square Off," p. B01.

75 Ibid.

76 Randy Gragg, "Planning, Commentary: A New Tram Line," *The Oregonian*, April 1, 2001, p. F01.

77 Randy Gragg, "OHSU Tram is a Project for Portland to put its Heart Into," *The Oregonian*, Oct. 28, 2001, p. B01.

78 Spencer Heinz, "Desires in Conflict over Idea of Tramway," *The Oregonian*, May 26, 2002, p. B01.

79 Randy Gragg, "Tram Plan Creates Heat on the Hill," *The Oregonian*, June 23, 2002, p. A01.

80 Randy Gragg, "Tram Debate Muffles Voices of Moderation," *The Oregonian*, June 26, 2002, p. E01.

81 Janet Christ, "Aerial Tram Envisioned as Portland 'Postcard,'" *The Oregonian*, July 15, 2002, p. B01.

82 De Sousa and D'Souza, "South Waterfront District," http://citeseerx.ist.psu.edu/viewdoc/download?doi=10.1.1.593.1545&rep=rep1&type=pdf.

83 "OHSU must grow to survive," Editorial, *The Oregonian*, Aug. 10, 2003, p. F04.

84 Buckman, the board chairman (interview, Dec. 10, 2014), said at one point the board was concerned about losing Kohler. "We talked about things we could do to retain him," said Buckman, who left the board himself in 2003. "Had we lost him about that time, it would have been a big loss."

85 Jim Walker, interview, Feb. 25, 2015.

86 Ibid.

87 Steven Carter and Jeffrey Kosseff, "Mooney Resigns as College President," *The Oregonian*, June 17, 2003, p. A01.

88 Walker, interview.

89 Patrick O'Neill and Fred Leeson, "Schnitzers Donate Land to OHSU for Campus," *The Oregonian*, June 16, 2004, p. A02.

90 Goldschmidt, interview.

91 Patrick O'Neill, "OHSU Names New Leader for Fund Raising," *The Oregonian*, Feb. 23, 2005, p. D01.

92 Lora Cuykendall (director of media relations and publications), memo titled "Upcoming Communication Challenges," Dec. 14, 2005, Peter Kohler collection, OHSU Archives.

93 Ibid.

94 Ibid.

95 Steve Stadum, "Portland's Tram Troubles: Stop the Overruns, but Keep Sight of the Vision," *The Oregonian*, Jan. 17, 2006, p. B07.

96 Ryan Frank, "Tram Anxiety: How Flimsy Math, Shaky Design and Scorching Steel Prices

Nearly Tripled its Cost," *The Oregonian*, Jan. 12, 2006, Metro Portland Neighbors, p. 10.

97 Stadum, "Portland's Tram Troubles," p. B07.

98 Ibid.

99 Ryan Frank, "City's Tram Meeting Brings out More Foes than Friends," *The Oregonian*, March 15, 2006, p. C02.

100 Ryan Frank and Jeff Manning, "Tram Deal a Dud at City Hall," *The Oregonian*, March 17, 2006, p. A01.

101 Ryan Frank, "Saltzman Vote Gives OHSU Tram Plan a Lift," *The Oregonian*, April 7, 2006, p. A01.

102 Ted Sickinger, "OHSU Bets on Profits in Lofty Expansion," *The Oregonian*, Feb. 5, 2005, p. A01.

103 Ibid.

104 Ibid.

105 Ibid.

106 Ibid.

107 Ibid.

108 OHSU, "Overview of 2002 OHSU Revenue Bonds and Oregon Opportunity GO Bond Financing Program," Dec. 3, 2002, Peter Kohler collection, OHSU Archives.

109 Andy Dworkin, "OHSU Boasts a Magnetic Advance," *The Oregonian*, Jan. 2, 2006, p. A01. (Andy Dworkin, a health and science reporter for *The Oregonian*, later enrolled at OHSU and studied to become a physician.)

110 Lesley Hallick, interview, Feb. 18, 2015, Portland.

111 Andy Dworkin, "A Building Fitted for Discovery," *The Oregonian*, Feb. 22, 2006, p. A12.

112 Dorsa, interview.

113 "OHSU Breaks Ground on New Research Building," OHSU press release, Oct. 10, 2002.

114 Patrick O'Neill, "A Hearty Ambition Pulses at OHSU," *The Oregonian*, July 5, 2005, p. A01.

115 "ROI: Biomedical Research Building", OHSU Foundation, https://www.ohsu.edu/xd/about/foundation/about/ohsu-extra/roi-brb.cfm.

116 "Media Sneak Peek of OHSU's New Peter O. Kohler Pavilion," About OHSU, May 25, 2006, http://www.ohsu.edu/xd/about/news_events/news/2006/05-25-media-sneak-peek-of-ohsu.cfm.

117 Joe Rojas-Burke, "New OHSU Building to Honor Peter Kohler," *The Oregonian*, March 20, 2006, p. E02.

118 "Plan Ahead," *The Oregonian*, May 25, 2006, p. C09.

119 Kate Brown, Secretary of State, "State Funds Resulted in Expanded Research at OHSU," *Secretary of State Audit Report*, Jan. 2010, p. 1.

120 Ibid., pp. 1–3.

121 Ted Sickinger, "OHSU State Funding Audit Positive, but Others Disagree," *OregonLive*, Jan. 21, 2010.

122 Randy Gragg, "Waterfront Lift-Off Building 1, OHSU's Glass-Fronted Temple of Wellness, Will Anchor Plans to Redevelop the South Riverfront," *The Oregonian*, April 19, 2004, p. D01.
123 Ibid.
124 Dylan Rivera, "OHSU Takes Green Building Higher," *The Oregonian*, Dec. 2, 2005, p. B01.
125 Gragg, "Waterfront Lift-Off Building 1," p. D01.
126 Dorsa, interview.
127 Mary Pitman Kitch, "Editorial Sketchbook: Tram does its Job of Collapsing Distances," *The Oregonian*, Dec. 15, 2006, p. D08.
128 Joseph Rose, "Fast-Acting Analgesic: The Tram," *The Oregonian*, Dec. 16, 2006, p. B01.
129 Joseph Rose, "Tram Gives Walt, Jean their Due," *The Oregonian*, Jan. 19, 2007, p. A01.
130 Ken Love (president of South Portland Neighborhood Association), interview, March 25, 2016.
131 Jim Gardner (resident near the tram's path in South Portland), interview on March 25, 2016.
132 Ted Sickinger, "Kohler Farewell Toasts the 'Health' in OHSU," *The Oregonian*, Sept. 15, 2006, p. D01.
133 Joe Rojas-Burke, "Three Make Shortlist to Succeed OHSU President Kohler," *The Oregonian*, June 16, 2006, p. D01.
134 Ted Sickinger, "Prescription for Change," *The Oregonian*, Nov. 12, 2006, p. B01.
135 Ted Sickinger, "OHSU Picks President from its own Ranks," *The Oregonian*, July 12, 2006, p. A01.
136 Davis, interview.
137 Ted Sickinger, "OHSU Copes with Leadership Exodus," *The Oregonian*, Sept. 18, 2009, business section.
138 Wendy Owen, "OHSU Provost Hallick Picked to Lead Pacific," *The Oregonian*, May 20, 2009, local news section.
139 Sickinger, "Prescription for Change."
140 "A Pledge to Look Outward from the Hill," editorial, *The Oregonian*, July 13, 2006, p. B06.
141 Sickinger, "Kohler Farewell."
142 Joe Rojas-Burke, "Survey Puts OHSU among Nation's 50 Best Hospitals," *The Oregonian*, Oct. 18, 2006, p. E1. The Leapfrog Hospital Quality and Safety Survey scored hospitals in nine areas, including their progress in using computer order-entry to prevent medication errors, staffing intensive-care units with trained specialists and implementing a set of twenty-seven practices know to reduce errors. OHSU reached full compliance in five of the nine areas.
143 "OHSU and Oregon: Looking to Tomorrow," report to the 2007 Oregon Legislative Assembly, pp. 4, 6, 28.

144 "The Economic Impacts of Oregon Health & Science University," *ECONorthewst*, Dec. 2009, pp. i–iii.

145 Sickinger, "Kohler Farewell."

146 Ibid.

147 Ted Sickinger, "Ex-OHSU Chief Returns to Work in Arkansas," *The Oregonian*, April 26, 2007, p. C01.

148 Blue Ridge Institute for Medical Research 2006 rankings for medical schools and their departments, http://www.brimr.org/NIH_Awards/2006/NIH_Awards_2006.htm.

Chapter Eight

OHSU Inc.

In the months following Kohler's departure, OHSU continued to expand with the momentum of a freight train. The medical center had successfully built a positive cycle of growth so that as it added space, it attracted more donors, researchers, and patients, who in turn gave it revenue to expand more and draw even more donors, researchers, and patients. The vision Kohler and his team had worked for continued to unfold like a flowering rose on the South Waterfront, beginning with the opening of the Center for Health & Healing and the tram that gracefully ferried people up to the Pill Hill campus through docks in the new Peter O. Kohler Pavilion. An anonymous donor gave the university $40 million, its largest gift ever, to help it expand its innovative medical school in a new building on the nineteen acres of the South Waterfront donated to the university earlier by the Schnitzer family. The 2007 Legislature gave OHSU one of its first increases for operations in years, a 3.1 percent raise. The hospital was generating net income of $19 million on revenues of $756 million. OHSU scientists delivered a breakthrough when they took DNA from Semos, an adult rhesus monkey at the primate center, inserted it into an egg, and used it to make a line of embryonic stem cells. *Time* magazine put that achievement on its list of the top ten scientific discoveries for 2007.[1]

The new president, Dr. Joseph Robertson, was keeping OHSU on the course Kohler had charted, and the university seemed to be thriving.[2] But Robertson also saw developments piling up on the road ahead that threatened to slow the medical center's momentum. Congress was proposing to reduce federal payments to medical schools, a pending lawsuit could mean an increase in malpractice insurance premiums, and the medical school was seeing its annual financial losses climb. After a long string of annual increases in grant funding, the NIH budget was flat.[3] And with all of its construction, OHSU saw its debt up more than 300 percent since 1995 to about $750 million, which was draining cash reserves and jeopardizing its credit rating. Robertson knew that while the university was thriving for the moment, its prosperity was precarious. The university had to be financially vigilant.

"It's no longer sufficient to say a program is exciting," Robertson said. "It has to have a sound business plan from the start that doesn't create a liability that has to be borne by other programs. . . . There's no room for anything but a lean and mean operation."[4]

ECONOMIC SETBACKS

By fall of 2007, the university was seeing losses in laboratory research and the medical school projected to reach $50 million. Another blow came in December. Though a public corporation, the medical center was still affiliated with the state and, as other state agencies, was protected by a liability cap of $200,000. But the Oregon Supreme Court ruled the cap violated the constitutional rights of Jordaan Michael Clarke, a nine-year-old who suffered permanent brain damage in 1998 while in intensive care at OHSU Hospital.[5] In addition to driving up the potential payouts on malpractice and other damage claims, the ruling also drove up OHSU's cost of malpractice insurance by millions.

Robertson began cutting costs. The university sold a parcel of land on the South Waterfront to a retirement home developer, and it sold the campus of the former Oregon Graduate Institute to an investment group. It also sold another parcel on its West Campus. Those sales gave it a one-time windfall of about $30 million.[6] OHSU also closed some community primary care clinics, raised tuition by 20 percent, and laid off 300 employees, containing losses for the 2007–08 fiscal year to about $10 million. Plans for a $350 million expansion of the Kohler pavilion were put on hold. Despite the losses, Robertson paid performance bonuses totaling about $1.4 million to about fifty administrators, drawing critical attention from the press.

Then banks began to fail, the stock market plunged, and the country fell into the Great Recession. OHSU saw investments drop by $23 million, its endowment by $100 million. Hospital profits plunged.[7] Robertson scrapped bonuses, ordered more layoffs, froze hiring, restricted overtime, canceled holiday parties, cut the medical school class size by five students to 115, reorganized to reduce administrative costs, cut rural clinics, cut custodial contracts by 40 percent, and vacated space it leased in the VA Hospital. In all, he had cut about 500 jobs as the economy tanked in late 2008 and early 2009, mostly from central services such as information technology, human resources, and public safety.[8]

OHSU, of course, wasn't alone. Faced with more indigent patients, fewer paying patients, losses on investments, and tight credit, hospitals across the country, including those connected to academic health centers, cut staff and other costs. In 2008, hospitals recorded the highest level of mass layoffs—defined as cuts of fifty or more people under a single employer—in a decade, with about half of hospitals reporting layoffs.[9]

During the first two years of the Great Recession, Robertson, the ophthalmologist, had become a fiscal surgeon, wrote *Oregonian* reporter Ted Sickinger.[10] In February of 2009, he brought back Jim Walker as interim chief financial officer after Walker's successor resigned. The administrators were able to refinance $238 million in debt, reducing interest costs. A variety of other developments helped them shore up OHSU's wobbly financial status. The legislature approved a new tort cap of $2 million, reducing the university's annual malpractice insurance premium by $12.5 million. Lawmakers also approved $50 million in bonds to help OHSU build a life sciences center, where it could expand its medical school on its South Waterfront property in collaboration with other institutions in the Oregon University System. About $12 million of the federal stimulus issued in the recession to curb the nation's economic crisis flowed to OHSU.[11] And it didn't hurt that the Phil and Penny Knight Foundation created by the Nike founder pledged in the fall of 2008 to give the university $100 million over seven years for the cancer institute, which would help offset the leveling of NIH funding.

By July of 2010, Robertson was still taking measures to cut costs—such as reducing visits by the Office of Rural Health to rural clinics and cutting nursing support to the Child Development and Rehabilitation Center. But there were signs OHSU had survived the Great Recession and was on the upswing. OHSU Hospital and its clinics were earning more money and raising OHSU's net income.

"We have weathered the economic downturn and global recession remarkably well—better than we might have expected 18 months ago—but that has not been without incredible sacrifice and hard work," Robertson said in the summer of 2010.[12]

In retrospect, this rough patch would prove to be little more than a "hiccup" in the history of OHSU's financial health, said Robertson. Soon, the health center fell back into that virtuous cycle. It built space for more hospital beds and added clinics and research laboratories, enabling it to earn more money and attract more top researchers, who in turn brought more research money, giving the university resources for further expansion. The layoffs, handled mostly through attrition, lasted little more than a year. It was a "painful" time of "great strain," said Robertson, but it was brief.

"If you compare the activity level, growth, any financial parameter of OHSU compared to any other major business enterprise in Oregon during that time," he said, "we sailed through the recession in comparison. It was just a very, very mild inflection point in the growth curve. It wasn't the Great Recession for us. It was a blip."[13]

But the recession brought new discipline to OHSU, pushing it to look for ways to be even more entrepreneurial. Rather than buying more land and constructing new businesses alone, Robertson adopted a strategy used often by Kohler and looked for partners who could help share the cost and increase the value of OHSU investments. He and Portland State University President

Wim Wiewel in October of 2010 announced they had struck a strategic alliance. They pledged to conduct joint research, share faculty, and create a collaborative School of Public Health. Some legislators, including Representative Mitch Greenlick (Democrat from Portland), former OHSU professor, had long advocated merging the two institutions. Greenlick argued that was the only way the state could create a major, top-ranked research university in Portland like the University of Washington in Seattle. But Robertson and Wiewel said a merger would be expensive and counterproductive. A close partnership, Robertson said, achieves many of the same benefits "at a fraction of the costs in a fraction of the time."[14]

OHSU BLOOMS

As the health center forged partnerships, it also saw steady growth in philanthropic support that in some cases enabled it to draw more support from the state. In September of 2011, Bob and Charlee Moore, who had amassed a fortune milling stone-ground grains near Oregon City for Bob's Red Mill Natural Foods, donated $25 million to OHSU.

"These people are helping so many others," said Bob Moore, whose donation established the Bob and Charlee Moore Institute for Nutrition and Wellness at OHSU.[15]

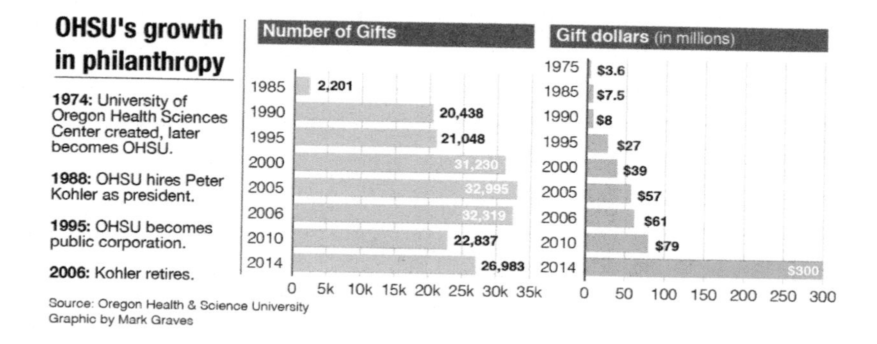

A year later, Nike cofounder Phil Knight and his wife, Penny, stepped up again with another record donation to OHSU—$125 million to establish the OHSU Cardiovascular Institute. Two years later, Knight stunned OHSU leaders and guests gathered in a downtown Portland ballroom of the Nines Hotel to celebrate and raise money for the university's Knight Cancer Institute. Knight promised to give $500 million to the institute if the university could come up with a match within two years. Dr. Druker, the institute's director, had already been recruiting some top cancer researchers to OHSU. Another billion would enable him to expand that brain trust dramatically.

"There's no reason that we can't, and won't, become the premier cancer institute in this country," he said.[16]

OHSU not only raised the $500 million, which included $200 million in bonds from the legislature, it did so in less than two years, drawing from 10,000 donors. Remarkably, 75 percent of the money came from donors in Oregon, which is not a wealthy state. The state bond money will be used to construct two buildings on the South Waterfront with one million square feet of research and clinical trial space for the cancer institute. The institute also plans to raise another $200 million. Phil Knight and Druker appeared on ABC's *Good Morning America* in late June of 2015 to announce they had met the $1 billion goal. Druker said the institute would be focusing first on detecting cancer at its earliest stages.

"We want to go after cancer as aggressively as it comes after us," he said.[17]

Druker set out to recruit 300 more research scientists, including twenty-five considered to be among the world's top. "I can take a congratulatory lap, but then I have to go back and start a marathon," he said.

Phil Knight said he had confidence Druker's team would put a stop to a disease that touches all people.

"These last 22 months have shown what is possible when people of vision focus on a single goal," he said. "We are more convinced than ever that cancer will meet its match at OHSU, and we are proud to play a role in this history in the making."[18]

Some OHSU faculty had misgivings about concentrating this infusion of $1.2 billion on one institute, just as they did with the Vollum Institute, arguing it would cause OHSU to stray from basic science and education. Two anonymous faculty members wrote a letter to legislators, urging them not to give OHSU $200 million in state-backed bonds because money was being misused to support executive bonuses.

"There has been a lot of angst around the Knight challenge," said Bonnie Nagel, a neuropsychologist and president of the OHSU Faculty Senate.[19]

Dr. Lynn Loriaux—an endocrinologist, veteran chair of the Department of Medicine, and longtime friend of Kohler's—expressed concern about big donations flowing into OHSU specialty centers, such as the heart and cancer institutes, rather than the medical, dentistry, and nursing schools. He and others feared, he said, that "what we have lost is a sense of academic excellence."[20]

But Lawrence Furnstahl, OHSU's executive vice president and chief financial officer, noted that a big gift like Knight's has a synergistic effect on the university that helps everybody by raising the medical center's stature and attracting more researchers and donors. "These tremendous gifts allow us to have core facilities" like advanced imaging and gene sequencing equipment, he said.[21]

SOUTH WATERFRONT TAKES SHAPE

As part of its growth, OHSU's footprint expanded, and its campus began to spread over the once barren brownfield that the Schnitzers had donated to the university. In the fall of 2014, OHSU opened its $160 million Collaborative Life Sciences Building, a joint venture with Portland State University and Oregon State University and a symbol of the kind of partnerships Robertson would continue seeking to leverage OHSU's resources and talent. The building provides space for biomedical research, for medical, nursing, and pharmacy school classrooms, and for the new OSHU/ PSU School of Public Health. Adjoining it is the $135 million Skourtes Tower for the School of Dentistry, and together, with parking, the building gives the university partners 650,000 square feet of space.[22]

They rise next to the new Tilikum Crossing, a gracefully arching, cable-stayed bridge which opened in September 2015, as the only one of its kind in the nation. It is designed to carry Portland's newest light-rail line across the Willamette River to neighboring Milwaukie along with buses, streetcars, bicyclists, and pedestrians—but no cars. The Life Sciences Building stands at the hub of nearly every form of transportation Portland offers except the tram, which glides 800 yards to the south from OHSU's Center for Health & Healing.[23]

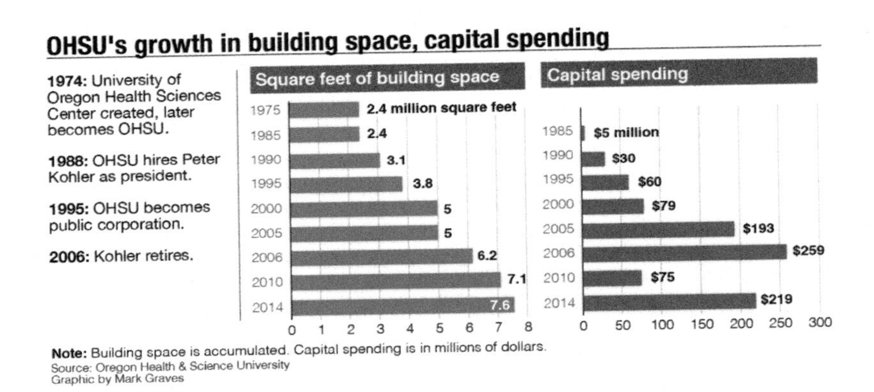

A small city of sleek, thin, glass-and-steel apartment and condominium skyscrapers tower on the south flank of the OHSU health center along with other apartment buildings, shops, and restaurants, all served by the Portland Streetcar. The thin towers allow Portlanders to see Mount Hood and the Cascade Mountains between slices of buildings on the South Waterfront.[24] The development includes The Ardea, a thirty-story apartment building; the twin Meriwether Condominiums, double towers reaching twenty-one and twenty-four stories high; the John Ross Condominiums, a 325-foot-tall tower with a community garden on its roof; Atwater Place, a twenty-two-story tower for 212 condos; and the Mirabella Retirement Community, a thirty-story building for a continuing care retirement community that features apartments for independent living, assisted care, and rooms for skilled nursing and memory care support. The South Waterfront development also includes Caruthers Park, urban gardens, and open lawns amid the skyscrapers and an 800-foot greenway on the banks of the Willamette River that eventually will stretch along the entire border of the development district into downtown Portland.[25]

Other projects are still in the works. The Zidell family, which still owns its barge-building business on the South Waterfront, struck a deal with the City of Portland in June of 2015 to redevelop another thirty acres nearby into 1.4 million square feet of new office, residential, and commercial space. The development will include at least two office buildings and an apartment building. The city agreed to contribute $24 million of public money for parks, roads, and other improvements, and the Zidell family committed to including affordable housing in the ten-year project. And, of course, OHSU also has plans to put two new buildings for the OHSU Knight Cancer Institute on the South Waterfront.[26]

Since it became a public corporation in 1995, OHSU has added 3.8 million square feet of building space, doubling its total to 7.6 million square feet. That has allowed it to hire more people and increase enrollments in its medical, dental, and nursing schools and graduate programs. Since becoming a public corporation, its number of employees more than doubled from 6,600 to 15,100, and its student enrollment climbed from 1,795 to 2,895. It employs about 1,100 principal investigators, each leading a team of scientists. The university operated on an annual budget of $2.5 billion in 2016, five times what it was when it became a public corporation. While the US Gross Domestic Product grew since 1995 at an average 4 percent a year and health care spending climbed at 6 percent a year, OHSU grew at the rate of 9.5 percent per year.[27] It pulled in $376 million in research awards in 2015, more than four times what it was drawing in 1995, and it currently ranks twenty-seventh among academic health centers in NIH research funds. President Robertson described the university's financial health:

> If you look at any of our programs, you will see tremendous growth by any of the conventional numbers. Our financial heft, status and performance has continued to improve. Our balance sheet has expanded at double-digit rates, and over the last four or five years, we've gone from a triple B-plus bond rating to double-A minus. We have launched major new initiatives with partners in each of the mission areas. . . . Last year [2014–15], we trained the most students ever, we had the most house staff ever, we did the most research ever, we had another big increase in clinical activity, we had had our best financial performance ever, and I think we have greater presence out in the community than ever.[28]

A NATIONAL PLAYER

OHSU has found its place on the national stage in neuroscience, infectious disease, immunology, cancer, and stem cell research, and it is gaining strength in cardiovascular disease and stroke, diabetes, metabolism research, imaging, and aging. Its medical school is nationally recognized for its patient-centered curriculum and emphasis on rural rotations. The *Annals of Internal Medicine* in 2010 ranked OHSU eleventh in the country among the nation's medical and osteopathic schools for meeting its social mission to the state as measured by the percent of graduates who practice primary care, work in underserved areas, and who are minorities. The university medical school's primary care and family and rural medicine consistently rank high as do OHSU's biological sciences, clinical medicine, nurse midwifery, and physician assistant programs. For example, *US News and World Report* magazine in 2016 rated OHSU's medical school fifth in the nation in primary care among the nation's 130 accredited medical schools and twenty-six accredited osteopathic schools.[29] *Times Higher Education* in 2016 ranked OHSU the seventh best small university in the world.[30] OHSU Hospital also has distinguished itself in focusing on patients with the most complex and severe medical needs. The OHSU case mix index, a measure of the degree and complexity of illness among its patients, ranks among the nation's highest.

"We are in the top ten of the group of the 130 some hospitals that receive the sickest patients," said Robertson. "So with regard to complexity of care, we are elite in the elite."[31]

OHSU is among the top 10 percent of academic health centers in research funding as a percent of overall funding and in the bottom 10 percent for state funding. In the 2015–16 academic year, OHSU received about $36 million from the state, which covered less than 2 percent of its operating budget and is far less than the $53 million it received in 1995. Because of its small endowment and low state funding, OHSU has had to be disciplined, entrepreneurial, and innovative, said Robertson.

"We are larger but leaner," he said. "We are more nimble and responsive to the marketplace trends and community needs. Being in charge of your own destiny creates a sense of urgency that has been a big part of our success."[32]

MORE PARTNERS

One factor in OHSU's new responsiveness is its interest in fostering partnerships with other organizations. In the fall of 2015, it joined Salem Health, which includes Salem hospital, to form a $2.5 billion-a-year integrated health system throughout the northern part of the Willamette Valley, where most of Oregon's residents are concentrated. It also signed a similar agreement to bring Tuality Health Alliance in suburban Portland into the network. Robertson outlined the health center's statewide ambitions:

> We are in the process of forming what I believe will ultimately be a statewide health care system that will be integrally linked with

> key payers as well. A flow of patients, particularly complex patients, is essential to maintain an academic health center. We can't assume in today's era that patients will automatically arrive on our doorstep. We have to set up a system that ensures those patients will continue to have access to OHSU. . . . We see patients currently being hospitalized at OHSU that could be treated at their local hospitals, particularly with OHSU backup. . . . We are at capacity. Most community hospitals are not. It's really about sharing responsibility.[33]

OHSU has also formed partnerships with Intel to help it with computer-based cancer research, and even has Intel workers and staff from FEI, an electron microscope company, working part-time at the university. Having become a public corporation with little operating support from the state has both forced and allowed OHSU to be more entrepreneurial, Robertson said. The university also would have had difficulty striking agreements with other private organizations if it were still part of the state system. Being a public corporation has enabled OHSU to go to the bond market, chart its own course with its own board, and create its own infrastructure for contracts, purchasing, payroll, and legal and human services. That has made it more sophisticated than other academic health centers in the ways it allocates costs and rewards its staff on the basis of productivity, said Robertson. OHSU also has been able to draw more philanthropic support as a public corporation. The university would not have the stature to draw Knight's $500 million gift or to raise the money to match it if it had not grown as a public corporation.

"We needed the public corporation to get to the point that we would be credible having a $500 million campaign for cancer," Robertson said.[34]

The university's success as a public corporation, ironically, also has enabled it to draw more money from the state than it ever received as a state agency, but for projects rather than operations, such as the $200 million in bonds for Oregon Opportunity, $200 million for the Knight Challenge and more than $100 million for the Life Sciences Building on the waterfront.

"We have a very deep, rich, and strategic relationship with the state," Robertson said. "It is also a mutually opportunistic relationship. When there is something we can do together, where OHSU can leverage that action, the state has demonstrated it is willing to step forth and work with us."[35]

Though the university still doesn't draw much state money for daily operations, with the notable exception being stable Medicaid funding, lawmakers are more willing to give it one-time boosts for projects that help it build capacity, sustain its missions, and lift the local economy—a seismic shift from the days when legislators were proposing to close the university's hospital.

TRUE TRANSFORMATION

The shift in lawmakers' views of OHSU is indicative of the transformative nature of the change that took place during its rebirth as a public corporation. Unlike the incremental change experienced at some institutions, OHSU's conversion was truly a transformation, "a clear break with the organizational structure and functioning of the past," observes Barbara Archer.[36]

OHSU went through a culture shift after becoming a public corporation, Robertson said, that firmly took root over seven years, making it more nimble and entrepreneurial, which in turn has enabled it to sustain enormous growth with more comprehensive services. Certainly, it changed. But was it transformed?

Archer began exploring that question one sunny morning on May 24, 1995, when she was headed for work in Hood River, cruising in her car down Interstate 84 through the scenic Columbia River Gorge. As she drove, news came on her car radio that Governor Kitzhaber had just signed a bill allowing OHSU to leave the Oregon University System to become a public corporation. She was stunned.

"I nearly drove off the road," she said. "How did they do that without a huge public uproar? It just blew my mind."[37]

At the time, Archer was working as chief executive officer for a federally-qualified health clinic in Hood River and working on her doctorate degree in public administration from the University of Southern California.

"I have to figure out how this happened," she told herself.[38]

It wasn't long before she was studying OHSU's conversion to a public corporation as the topic of her doctoral dissertation. Archer made the case that OHSU's conversion to a public corporation was not just an incremental change, but a true transformation. Every one of her professors challenged her thesis.

"They said, 'Public organizations don't transform. They can change. They can change rapidly. But they don't transform.'"[39]

Archer postulated that four forces are necessary for transformational change in an organization: the organization must have supportive policies, face economic pressures pushing it to change, be steered by an entrepreneurial leader, and establish a clean break from its principal overseer, which in OHSU's case was the state and system of higher education. Based on interviews with OHSU administrators and staff, Archer determined all of these forces aligned in sufficient force at OHSU to foment transformational change.

> There was a general belief that the combination of a good policy idea at the right time, tightening economic times at the state level and in the health care marketplace, and the ability of OHSU to gracefully leave the Oregon State System of Higher Education were critical to the success of the conversion process. These elements, combined with the internal and external entrepreneurial activities that created the vision and negotiated the agreements associated with the conversion process, resulted in the success of the initiative. It must be also said that respondents believed that luck also played a part in the process.[40]

Archer believes that "need, opportunity and action" converged in sufficient strength at OHSU to "foster organizational transformation."

OHSU's structure and functions, such as personnel, finance, and procurement changed dramatically in a short time, she writes. State funding dropped. The university's culture shifted in the face of immediate marketplace competition and the need for capital financing. OHSU's mission to serve the indigent remained intact, but the way it carried out that mission changed. President Kohler and his administrative team were able to promote the change within and without the university. And all of this occurred in a political climate receptive to innovative change.

"It was a time," she concludes, "when a series of decision and action streams converged at the right moment with sufficient strength to create a climate that fostered and propelled a transformational change in OHSU."[41]

TRANSFORMING STRUCTURE, PRESERVING MISSION

Kohler and his team and all of the people interviewed for this book agree that this radical, relatively sudden transformation was key in making OHSU a superior institution, lifting it from mediocre status to the upper tier of the nation's academic health centers. But not everyone agrees that this change was all for the best. Michael Warren Redding's doctoral research compared OHSU's transformation to changes at the University of Virginia and the College of William & Mary in Virginia, which each got more autonomy from the state in exchange for agreeing to meet certain performance outcomes. Neither, though, made a clean break from the university system as OHSU did. Redding concluded that after their changes, the Virginia public universities have been better able to remain true to their public missions than has OHSU. The Virginia schools were given more autonomy, he said, but they also were required to comply with ongoing requirements to meet state public higher education goals.[42]

OHSU's more transformative shift away from state oversight, on the other hand, resulted in greater freedom to "operate unencumbered in the health care marketplace" with far fewer state accountability requirements and performance goals. Further, because of declining state support, it was under pressure to earn money. As a consequence of their differing circumstances, OHSU was more focused on market pressures and private funding, and more distracted from its public missions, than were the Virginian universities, concludes Redding.

"Due to the increased flexibility granted through the public corporation legislation, there has been a gradual transition regarding the investment decisions for capital facilities that have changed the focus and the client base for OHSU in order to improve the institution's bottom line," he writes.[43]

Redding said OHSU's shift to a heavier dependence on the marketplace "has strained" the medical university's capacity to fulfill its historic public missions—teaching, research, and health care for the indigent.[44] He recommends states follow the path of Virginia and balance autonomy for their universities with accountability measures to keep them attentive to their public missions and with sufficient funding so they are not forced to turn to the market for money. "Findings from the Oregon case," he notes, "illustrate the challenge of a market-based autonomy policy framework, while the Virginia case offers contrasting evidence of the benefits of policies that balance the demands of the contemporary environment with the important societal mission of public higher education."[45]

Former Governor John Kitzhaber told Redding that OHSU's focus on "high profile construction" had "overshadowed" its community mission.[46] In a later interview, Kitzhaber said he supports Knight's "amazing gift" of $500 million to the cancer institute, but OHSU is "spending money on things that to me to some extent is about getting recognition." Eighty percent of the forces affecting health are socioeconomic factors such as lifestyle, diet, housing, and income, said Kitzhaber, so OHSU should be showing some commitment to "population health," especially since a large share of its income is from public dollars through Medicare and Medicaid. He said OHSU should, for example, put up $50 million for public housing and challenge developers to do the same.[47]

"A little would make a huge difference, and it would say so much," he said. "I think they [OHSU leaders] have become more obsessed with becoming recognized as a world class research center, which I'm all supportive of, but they have sort of lost that community connection. I worry about that."[48]

Contrary to Redding and Kitzhaber's concerns, Kohler and his team argue that by winning more autonomy as a public corporation, OHSU was able to not only sustain its public missions, but enhance them. And like Virginia's universities, it also maintains some state performance benchmarks it is expected to reach. OHSU has increased its number of students and overhauled its medical school curriculum twice. It has continued to serve more indigent patients than any other Oregon hospital, though OHSU, like all hospitals, has seen its share of indigent patients drop precipitously as a result of the Affordable Care Act, pushed through Congress by President Obama in 2010. The act expands Medicaid and subsidizes the costs of health insurance premiums for even middle-class families, extending insurance to about 400,000 more Oregonians and seventeen million more people nationwide. As a result, OHSU's share of indigent patients dropped to about 1 percent of the roughly quarter million patients it serves each year.[49]

"We did not abandon the public mission, and we carried over the educational mission, and we didn't change the mission at all," Hallick told Redding. "Unfortunately, I think there is a perception on the part of one or two people [that its mission has shifted to the bottom line] and that became a kind of clarion calling card kind of thing."[50]

Furnstahl, OHSU's current chief financial officer, worked for more than two decades with other academic health centers, including those at the private University of Chicago and Stanford University and the public University of California at San Francisco. He found a different culture at OHSU when he arrived in 2011. What he found most striking, he said, was how committed everyone was to OHSU's goal to "improve the health and well-being of Oregonians." Whether cleaning rooms in the hospital or doing research in the labs, people working at the university would verbally state that goal, he said. In contrast to Kitzhaber's view that the university needed to show more concern for population health, Furnstahl found the health center put improving the health and well-being of Oregonians at the center of its work.[51] In July of 2016, OHSU issued $100 million in new bond debt, twice what Kitzhaber suggested, for population health initiatives, such as Propel Health—collaboration among OHSU, health systems, and insurers to share data and promote improved health care use across Oregon.[52]

In addition, OHSU joined four other major Portland hospitals and a nonprofit health care plan in taking the kind of action Kitzhaber recommended—they pledged in September, 2016 to donate a combined $21.5 million toward the construction of 400 housing units for the city's homeless and low-income population.

OHSU President Joe Robertson said he was excited about the example the group was setting.

"Most of the story is already written by the time these people show up in our health system," he said. "So we have to do something and do it in a manner that is different than what we've done before."[53]

EFFECTS ON WORKERS

While there has been considerable attention devoted to the public and external impacts of OHSU's transformation, the internal impact on staff and faculty is also important to consider. Dana Director, a third-generation Oregonian who is now vice president of research operations and student affairs at OHSU, explored the effect of OHSU's transformation on staff and faculty for her 2013 doctorate in public affairs and policy.[54] She interviewed Kohler and his leadership team, about twenty faculty members, and about twenty OHSU employees who were members of the American Federation of State, County and Municipal Employees (AFSCME), most of whom were there during the university's transformation to a public corporation.

A large majority of the AFSCME staff solidly favored the transformation, saying it made them feel more valued, added worth to their work, and increased their pay and overall job satisfaction. About half said they felt more pressure. All said the overall impact of the transformation was for the better.

Faculty members, though, were more divided over whether the overall impact made OHSU better, whether their pay increased, and whether promotion or tenure improved. Most said shared governance had declined, and more than 70 percent, including all former faculty, said they felt expectations for their productivity had climbed. Ninety percent said they felt more pressure.[55]

Director described her findings:

> So what I found with AFSCME employees was that really quite significantly the people I talked to felt [the transformation to a public corporation] sort of pushed everyone out of their comfort zones, like they didn't know definitely what they were supposed to do, and there wasn't a lot of job clarity. But overall people felt it was a really positive move—that the processes got more efficient, they had more freedom to get things done the way they wanted to get them done rather than the way the state said you had to do them. So it was pretty clear that the AFSCME population felt pretty good about the public corporation, that it really improved their quality of life. . . .Faculty were more mixed about things. . . . In general, the feeling is, particularly with the basic science faculty [as opposed to the clinical faculty] that when OHSU became a public corporation, they lost a large part of what is traditionally known as the academic culture. It became much more business oriented. . . . They were very close to unanimous on the fact that, thankfully, they don't feel their academic freedom was impinged upon at all, so that is a good thing.[56]

Director quotes anonymous staff and faculty members who say they experienced a significant entrepreneurial shift in operations when OHSU became a public corporation. "Everything definitely became streamlined and more efficient," said an administrative worker in the school of dentistry. "Systems all got a lot better and processes all got a lot better," said a classified employee. Another staff member said, "We could have our own systems; I know we could not have done that as part of the state."

Many faculty members experienced that change too. "When they decided to get serious about research funding, they decided to pursue a more professional operation," said one basic science faculty member. Another basic scientist said, "Initially, yes, there were some old dusty processes that were eliminated. And people really thought about what they were doing." And yet another faculty member said, "at the outset there seemed to be a feeling of empowerment—everybody go find ways to be more efficient and think of better ways to do things."

But not everyone saw big changes. "It seems that the red tape is about the same length as it always was," said one staff member. "There are a lot of people and a lot of steps. And that's when I want to ask, 'Are you sure we're not [still] a state institution?'" Unknowingly echoing Kohler's earlier observations about the primate center, one faculty member said OHSU replaced one bureaucracy with another by "recreating a new bureaucracy. It has become as big as what we walked away from at the state, and then some."[57]

However, all of the staff and more than half the faculty said OHSU's conversion to a public corporation made the university a better place.

"It was a great idea," said one faculty member. "And it was in fact probably brilliant, and the best thing that happened since they laid the first brick up here. In fact, I think it was transformational for the institution, and I doubt we would be in the position we are today without this step."[58]

Just three years after OHSU became a public corporation, J. Peter Bentley, a researcher in the division of experimental biology, describes himself as an "entrepreneur" and attributes the rise of OHSU's national stature to it becoming a public corporation.

"You don't have to say Oregon Health Sciences University anymore," he said. "Everybody knows OHSU or what it is. . . . If you go to national conferences, this place is really recognized as a place where very good research is going on."

The university is "streamlined," he said, but its growth has also put more emphasis on bringing in money and high-powered researchers over good teaching.

"We're a big, money-making corporation," he said, "and people can get lost in it."[59]

Other faculty who lived through OHSU's transformation agree that it opened new avenues for the university to expand and prosper. Dr. Joseph Bloom, dean of the medical school from 1994 to 2001, says that OHSU was unique in that the entire academic health center, not just the hospital, broke ties with the state, allowing it to keep its research, teaching, and health care missions integrated. By doing so, it avoided the money conflicts that often emerge between researchers and medical schools on one hand and privatized hospitals on the other.

"As far as I know, there are no other national models like this [public corporation]," he said. "What happened nationally is most of these places, facing the same pressures we were facing and wanting to change, spun the hospital out. . . . Once a hospital starts thinking how important they are, and they are free, they start acting like it."[60]

Grover Bagby, the researcher who helped Kohler build the Oregon Cancer Center, said the university prospered after it became a public corporation and probably, at least in part, because it did.

"We developed our campus, we developed our visibility, we increased our levels of National Institutes of Health support," he said. "I attribute that all to the public corporation status."[61]

PILL HILL TODAY

When he became OHSU's second president, Leonard Laster said he found the academic health center a "dispirited institution" mired in mediocrity, without self-confidence, and facing an uncertain future. Today, he would find a different place, where research thrives and the quality of health care and education routinely earns high marks. The institution brims with confidence and busy purpose and has become a place where researchers, medical students, and patients want to be, and in many ways the place he hoped it would become.

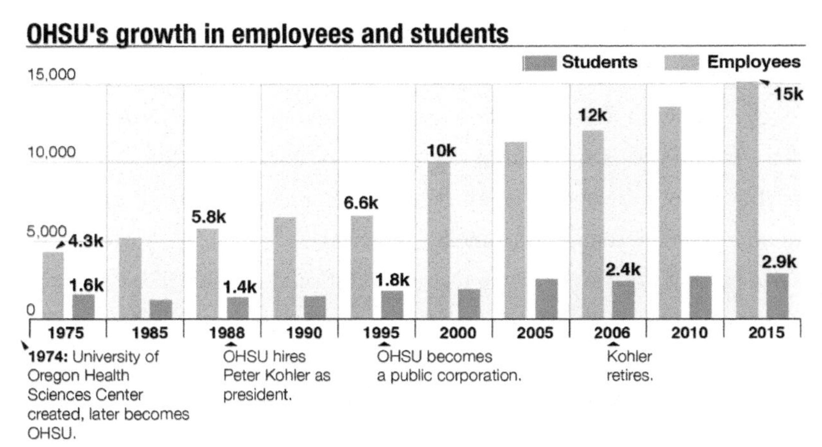

Today in the research labs, geneticist Dr. Markus Grompe and his research team savor the fruits of a more corporate institution. Grompe directs OHSU's Oregon Stem Cell Center and the Pape Family Pediatric Research Institute and works in one of the finest laboratories in the world on the seventh floor of the Hildegard Lamfrom Biomedical Research Building. On one spring day in 2014, Grompe gives a quick tour of his busy laboratory, where researchers and graduate students work at long, spacious black tables. Stretching above the work benches are shelves crammed with boxes, bottles, petri dishes, test tubes, pipettes, jars, cell cultures, machines, and computers. Some dishes hold gels used to sequence DNA and reveal the precise order of the four nucleobases—adenine, guanine, cytosine, and thymine—that form base pairs for the double-helix of a DNA molecule. At one table, a graduate student in a blue T-shirt and white rubber gloves carefully releases a pipette of clear liquid into several small test tubes. The student is adding genes to the genetic code of a virus. Or as Grompe says, "He's building a virus."[62]

Nearby, in a clean, cold, tissue culture room, another student works at a long table enclosed by glass and covered by a fume hood that blows away filtered air to keep everything sterile. She is manipulating cells growing in gel cultures stored nearby in refrigerated incubators. The labs on this floor have at least fifteen hooded tables in seven rooms. The research team has at its fingertips high-powered microscopes, centrifuges, computers capable of doing the billions of calculations required in DNA analysis, and even more specialized equipment. A black box with a camera inside can photograph the faint luminescence radiating from mice tumors genetically altered with glowworm genes. Another machine slices ultra-thin tissue samples for staining and microscope analysis. And a flow cytometer sorts and counts cells tagged with fluorescence color. Paralleling the labs are specially designed, extra wide corridors wired with abundant electrical outlets for refrigerators and liquid nitrogen tanks to preserve cell cultures.

In addition to supporting research, the laboratory has a practical side in producing monoclonal antibodies that it sells to other researchers for marking living cells. "This operation," says Grompe, "is more like a company."[63]

On the research front, his team is working on three quests: to convert gall-bladder cells into insulin producers, to find cells that can help heal diseased or damaged livers, and to discover medicine to cure Fanconi anemia, the rare and deadly genetic blood disorder that leads to bone marrow failure and high susceptibility to cancer. These are among more than 4,000 research projects under way at any given time at OHSU, leading to hundreds of inventions a year, some of which give rise to new businesses.

Now among the top twenty-seven academic health centers in the nation in terms of NIH research grants—and twenty-eight among the 2,450 institutions that receive NIH grants—OHSU has produced a long list of medical breakthroughs.[64] Recently, for example, its scientists conducted the world's first clinical trials on gene therapies that may prevent some types of blindness, discovered a neural stem cell that offers new hope for thwarting certain fatal brain diseases, and converted human skin cells into embryonic stem cells.

Every morning at about 5:30 a.m., Robert Searles—research assistant professor in the division of bioinformation and computational biology, which is to say, DNA analysis—parks at Portland's South Waterfront and rides the tram to the Kohler pavilion 500 feet above. He steps into the hospital wing on the ninth floor, a level connected to a series of hallways and sky bridges that would allow him to reach most campus buildings without going outside. Searles, though, walks through OHSU Hospital and out onto SW Sam Jackson Road, past the Hatfield Research Center and the Biomedical Information Communication Center on his left. And on his right, he passes Baird Hall, the administration building, and Mackenzie Hall, the medical school. He takes a right turn at the OHSU Auditorium, which includes the university's archives. He walks behind the medical school into Richard T. Jones Hall and rides an elevator up to the fifth floor and his office in Room 5327A, which is adjacent to his recently remodeled laboratory. The lab is stocked with more than $1 million worth of equipment, including the $700,000 Illumina HiSeq 2000 Sequencing System. The computerized machine, which looks something like two portable refrigerators pushed together, is capable of ordering 180 million base pairs of DNA an hour, or the entire 3.6 billion base pairs of DNA for each of four human genomes simultaneously in twelve days. Searles, a biochemist, directs this operation, which he calls the Massively Parallel

Sequencing Shared Resource. He also is associate director of the OHSU Integrated Genomics Laboratory. His lab handles gene sequencing for other researchers throughout the university as well as for clients elsewhere in the country and world.[65]

DOCTOR AND STUDENT

Not far from Searles' laboratory, in the emergency room built at street level on the seventh floor of the Mark Hatfield Research Center, teaching resident Dr. Jason Oost works with third-year medical student Moon Yoon one spring afternoon in 2014. Both are in scrubs. The emergency room serves both the OHSU and Doernbecher Children's hospitals. The doctor and medical student discuss a patient in his sixties who has recently been through chemotherapy for epiglottis cancer and has come to them with pain in his left leg. Oost, young with a trim beard and short red hair, examined the patient. Then so did Yoon, whose thick black hair falls nearly to his bushy eyebrows and black-rimmed glasses. Now they sit at a row of computers in the heart of the emergency room, each with a stethoscope slung over his neck, and discuss how to treat their patient.

"He got a water blister and it popped during chemo," Yoon says. "It got infected, first, and it has been difficult to control since then. He developed a left foot abscess during chemo which is presented here as increased left leg pain. There's poor perfusion [flow of blood] to his lower extremities."

Oost quizzes Yoon. Did the patient have a DVT, deep vein thrombosis, a blood clot in a deep vein of his leg? Did he complain of shortness of breath? What does Yoon want to do?

The medical student says he'll get the patient's pain under control, talk to vascular and chemo doctors, and order tests, including a chest X-ray and ultrasound. The medical teacher and student conclude that in addition to the foot abscess, their patient has constricted blood flow to his legs that needs to be checked. They probably will admit him to the hospital for a variety of tests, primarily an angiogram, which is an X-ray using dyes to capture images of blood flow.

Yoon is learning under a new curriculum developed by OHSU and a handful of other top medical schools that marks the biggest change in physician training in a century. Under the new approach, students spend less time in the classroom and more on hands-on interaction with patients. In 2014, a class of 139 students, picked from a record 5,755 applicants, was working with patients within weeks after arriving on campus. Students learn how to work in teams and to assess the social and economic conditions affecting their patients' health. They learn in the new Collaborative Life Sciences Building, which includes a 20,000-square-foot simulation center with twenty clinic rooms and eight mock hospital stages. Professors can observe and converse with students in each of the exam rooms from a director's suite filled with television screens. The students confront simulated health care crises with dummy patients or actors and can view their bedside manner on videotapes. The innovative curriculum is proficiency-based, which allows students to advance at their own paces and potentially complete their training in three years.[66]

LABOR AND DELIVERY

Six floors above the emergency room and a little ways north in what is known as the C-Wing of OHSU Hospital, Tamara and Kevin Wedin of nearby Vancouver, Washington, relax on a sunny morning in the summer of 2014 with their baby boy, Daniel, who has not yet completed his first day on Earth.

The Wedins are in a postpartum suite in the recently expanded Mother-Baby Unit, where big block letters on the wall say "Welcome Mothers, Babies & Families." The spacious suite, with wide windows looking out over OHSU's Physicians Pavilion, has just about everything mother and child could want: a large adjustable bed, a clear plastic bassinet cradled in a wooden base with drawers and wheels, a television, Wi-Fi, vital sign monitors—and quiet. Tamara, thirty-nine, a college student, relaxes peacefully in her bed with baby in arms as Kevin, forty, a Home Depot manager, sits in a comfortable chair nearby. They came to the hospital four days earlier, when Tamara thought that her water may have broken, and went into the maternity triage area where there are small rooms with beds and monitors to determine whether a woman is ready to deliver.

As it turned out, Tamara's water had not broken. But at more than thirty-nine weeks, she was about due and her cervix was slightly dilated, so she and Kevin decided to proceed with an induced delivery. They moved into one of the hospital's spacious private suites in the Family Birth Center on the twelfth floor. The suite includes an attached private bathroom with a jetted tub, private shower, and a sterile bassinet for the newborn. The room also is equipped with computers, fetal heart monitors, and ultrasound equipment. If Tamara wanted to deliver her baby in water, the hospital would bring in a small heated tub. Down the hall on the same floor are surgery suites should she need a cesarean delivery. Also nearby on the same floor is a neonatal unit should the baby need specialized care.

A birth team that included a midwife and nurses cared for Tamara as she was given medicine Thursday evening to induce labor. But little happened for the next twenty-four hours. Or the twenty-four after that. By late Saturday, Tamara was still having only occasional mild cramps. Her medical team suggested it may be time to take the baby by cesarean. Tamara and Kevin had just begun discussing whether to proceed with the operation when Tamara was silenced by severe cramps. Baby Daniel was on his way. He arrived twelve hours later, at 2:00 p.m. Sunday. The midwife immediately placed the baby on Tamara's chest, a modern skin-to-skin practice that stimulates nursing and bonding.

Daniel arrived in Room 12. The Wedins had requested that room because a year earlier, that is where their baby, Marina, died. Doctors had been prepared to take Marina by cesarean, too, because she had some life-threatening congenital disorders. Just as they were about to operate,

Marina's heart rate plunged. That and other vital signs made it clear to doctors and to the Wedins that Marina was not going to make it. So instead of going into surgery, Tamara and Kevin asked their medical team to turn on the ultrasound machine. The parents laid their hands on Tamara's abdomen and watched the ultrasound screen over the next few minutes as their unborn daughter's life slipped away.

Then the labor and delivery staff "circled the wagons around us," says Tamara. "The nurse, the midwives, everybody down there, circled around us like family and gave us space and love. . . . Every single nurse did something over and above her shift duties for us. . . . We were listened to, and we were respected, and we were honored, and that made it possible for us to leave the hospital after a trauma feeling loved."

That level of care brought the Wedins back to OHSU to deliver Daniel, though as military veterans they had plenty of other choices.

"We got pregnant with this little guy three months after Marina died, and we said, 'Well great. We get to go see our people again,'" Tamara says.[67]

The Wedins' experience, once unthinkable at OHSU, is now typical. The hospital offers a variety of childbirth services and delivers about 2,400 babies a year. It is one of the few providers in Oregon who help women who have previously undergone cesarean sections deliver their babies vaginally, and it has the highest success rate in the country for these mothers. About 30 percent of the hospital's births are by cesarean section, which is lower than the national average even though 18 percent of its mothers have high-risk pregnancies, far above the average 6 percent to 8 percent.[68]

A similar expansion in scope, quality, and specialty care has unfolded throughout OHSU's hospitals and out-patients services on Pill Hill and in its clinics in rural and medically underserved areas across Oregon, Southwest Washington and Boise, Idaho. The university offers varying specialty services—nephrology, radiation oncology, psychiatry via electronic telemedicine connections, pediatric cardiology, and much more—in twenty-nine towns and cities outside Portland. For example, the university operates clinics in Bend in Central Oregon, Coos Bay and Lincoln City on the coast, Hermiston in the Columbia Gorge, Enterprise and LaGrande in Eastern Oregon and Klamath Falls and Medford in the state's south.

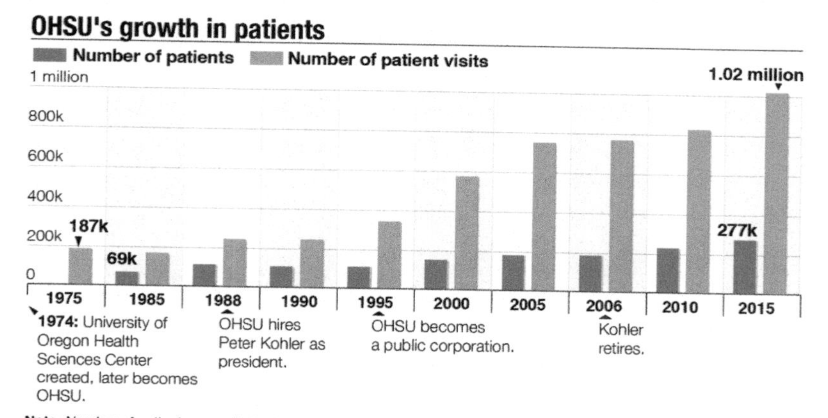

OHSU's expansive health care network, its hospital's spacious labor and delivery wing, Grompe's research labs, Searles' gene sequencing operation, the modern emergency room where Yoon learns medicine by practicing it, and the Collaborative Life Sciences Building did not exist at OHSU two decades ago. And they may have never become part of OHSU had it failed to become a public corporation.

President Joe Robertson told employees in a town hall meeting that becoming a public corporation gave OHSU the structure, the "relative autonomy cemented in public purpose," and the "best enabling legislation of any academic health center in the country," to become a disruptive force.

"We are not the Ivory Tower of academia of old," he said. "We are not your grandfather's university. We are an agent of change."[69]

Mike Thorne, the Pendleton rancher, questions whether OHSU could have survived without becoming a public corporation. As a state senator, he saw its financial problems before its transformation when it was a health center most people tried to avoid. He eventually served on OHSU's first governing board and now sees doctors there himself.

"You feel good about going there," he says. "It just stands out as such a success story for all the right reasons. It is gratifying to be around to see it."[70]

Notes

1 Andy Dworkin, "OHSU Cracks Time's Top 10," *The Oregonian,* Dec. 26, 2007, p. D4.

2 Ted Sickinger, "Get Back to Business, OHSU Chief Urges," *The Oregonian,* June 29, 2007, p. B01. Sickinger wrote, "Robertson's strategic plan is coming together as OHSU generates solid growth at its newly expanded hospital, enjoys an upswing in philanthropic support and investment returns, and sees a bump in funding from the Legislature after more than a decade of eroding state support."

3 Ted Sickinger, "Losses put OHSU at Crossroads," *The Oregonian,* Oct. 30, 2007, p. A01.

4 Ibid.

5 Ashbel S. Green, "High Court Lifts Limit on OHSU Liability," *The Oregonian,* Dec. 29, 2007, p. A01.

6 Sickinger, "Losses put OHSU at Crossroads," p. A01.

7 Ted Sickinger, "Downturn Cripples OHSU Budget," *The Oregonian,* Dec. 2, 2008, business section.

8 Ted Sickinger, "Executives at OHSU take 20 Percent Cut in Pay," *The Oregonian,* Dec. 19, 2008, business section, and (by the same author) "Triage for OHSU's Finances," *The Oregonian,* July 19, 2009, business section.

9 American Hospital Association, "The Economic Crisis: The Toll on the Patients and Communities Hospitals Serve," PowerPoint presentation, April 27, 2009, pp. 5, 6. Online at: http://www.aha.org/content/00-10/090427econcrisisreport.pdf.

10 Sickinger, "Triage for OHSU's Finances".

11 Ibid.

12 Ellion Njus, "OHSU Board Raises Tuition," *The Oregonian,* July 1, 2010, local news section.

13 Joseph Robertson, MD, interview, Aug. 20, 2015, his Baird Hall office, OHSU campus.

14 Bill Graves, "OHSU, PSU Head In Same Direction," *The Oregonian,* Oct. 29, 2010, local news section.

15 Nick Budnick, "$125 Million Gift for OHSU," *The Oregonian,* Sept. 18, 2012, local news section.

16 Andrew Theen, "Knight's $1 Billion Challenge to OHSU," *The Oregonian*, Sept. 22, 2013.

17 "Nike Co-Founder, OHSU Raise $1 Billion for Cancer Research", *Good Morning America*, ABC News.com, http://abcnews.go.com/GMA/video/nike-founder-ohsu-raise-1b-cancer-research-32019274.

18 Andy Giegerich (digital managing editor), "Knight Cancer Challenge hits $1B Goal in Record Time," *Portland Business Journal*, http://www.bizjournals.com/portland/morning_call/2015/06/knight-cancer-challenge-hits-1b-goal-in-record.html.

19 Nick Budnick, "Pursuit of Big Grants Stirs Up OHSU Faculty," *The Oregonian*, March 4, 2014, p. A05.

20 Lynn Loriaux, MD (former chair of the Department of Medicine at OHSU), interview, March 20, 2014, his office on the OHSU campus.

21 Ibid.

22 Betsy Hammond, "In Mega Building, Learning Grows," *The Oregonian*, June 26, 2014, p. A04.

23 Elliot Njus, "The Bridge that Ties it all Together," *The Oregonian*, Sept. 13, 2015, p. A12.

24 Nancy Rommelmann, "Is South Waterfront Portland's Next Great Neighborhood?" *Portland Monthly*, April 27, 2015, http://www.pdxmonthly.com/articles/2015/4/27/is-the-south-waterfront-about-to-become-great-may-2015.

25 Portland Development Commission, "North Macadam URA: Completed Projects," http://www.pdc.us/our-work/urban-renewal-areas/north-macadam/completed-projects.aspx.

26 Brad Schmidt, "City Makes a Deal on Zidell Property," *The Oregonian*, June 7, 2015, p. B01.

27 Lawrence Furnstahl (executive vice president and chief financial officer for OHSU), interview, Oct. 22, 2015, his office on campus.

28 Robertson, interview.

29 *US News and World Report*, Best Medical School rankings for 2016 can be found online at http://grad-schools.usnews.rankingsandreviews.com/best-graduate-schools/top-medical-schools.

30 Carly Minsky, "The World's Best Small Universities 2016," *Times Higher Education* World University Rankings, Jan. 25, 2016, https://www.timeshighereducation.com/student/news/worlds-best-small-universities-2016.

31 Robertson, interview.

32 Ibid.

33 Ibid.

34 Ibid.

35 Ibid.

36 Barbara Archer, interview, Aug. 11, 2015.

37 Barbara Archer, interview, May 7, 2014.

38 Archer, interview, 2015.

39 Archer, interview, 2014.

40 Barbara Archer, "Transformation in Public Organizations" (dissertation presented to the faculty of the School of Policy, Planning and Development, University of Southern California, Dec. 2002), p. 233.

41 Ibid., pp. 242–243.

42 Michael Warren Redding, "Autonomy Policy in U.S. Public Education: A comparative case study of Oregon and Virginia" (doctoral dissertation in higher education management presented to the faculties of the University of Pennsylvania, 2009), pp. 208–14.

43 Ibid., p. 92.

44 Ibid., p. 99.

45 Ibid., p. 214.

46 Ibid., p. 93.

47 John Kitzhaber, MD, interview, Feb. 12, 2016, downtown Portland, Oregon.

48 Ibid.

49 "ACA Continues to Cover Oregonians," (bar chart) OHSU Board of Directors meeting agenda, April 7, 2016, p. 6, https://www.ohsu.edu/xd/about/vision/upload/Complete-set-for-website-20160407.pdf.

50 Redding, "Autonomy Policy in U.S. Public Education," p. 93.

51 Furnstahl, interview.

52 Caryn Ruch (OHSU communications manager), email responding to the author's request on June 23, 2016.

53 Gillian Flaccus, "Six Portland health providers give $21.5M for homeless housing," Associated Press, Sept. 23, 2016, *US News*, http://www.usnews.com/news/news/articles/2016-09-23/6-portland-health-providers-give-215m-for-homeless-housing.

54 Dana L. Director, "The Impacts of Change in Governance on Faculty and Staff at Higher Education Institutions: A Case Study of OHSU" (dissertation, Portland State University), 2013.

55 Ibid., Appendix G, pp. 271–276.

56 Dana L. Director, interview, April 9, 2014, her office at Baird Hall, OHSU campus.

57 Director, *The Impacts of Change in Governance on Faculty and Staff at Higher Education Institutions: A Case Study of OHSU*, pp. 114–117.

58 Ibid., p. 157.

59 J. Peter Bentley, PhD, interview by Linda Weimer, Dec. 10, 1998, interview no. 55 12/10, 1998, transcript, OHSU Oral History Project, pp. 15–17.

60 Joseph Bloom, MD, interview, March 11, 2014, Portland, Oregon.

61 Grover Bagby, MD, interview, April 14, 2014, Heathman Hotel in downtown Portland, Oregon.

62 Markus Grompe, MD, interview, April 16, 2014, Biomedical Research Building, OHSU.

63 Ibid.

64 Blue Ridge Institute for Medical Research ranks OHSU in 2015 as 27th among 138 medical schools in terms of funding from the National Institutes of Health, and it ranks OHSU 28th among all 2,450 universities and institutions that receive NIH money: http://www.brimr.org/NIH_Awards/2015/NIH_Awards_2015.htm.

65 Robert P. Searles, interview, April 24, 2014, Richard Jones Hall, OHSU

66 Andrew Theen, "OHSU Reimagines Med School Curriculum," *The Oregonian*, March 19, 2016, p. A1.

67 Tamara and Kevin Wedin, interview, Aug. 18, 2014, in the labor and delivery suites in OHSU Hospital.

68 These statistics were provided by OHSU's labor and delivery unit for the months of May 2015 through April of 2016.

69 Joseph Robertson, MD, speech for a university town hall, Feb. 17, 2016.

70 Mike Thorne, interview, July 16, 2014, River's Edge Hotel, Portland, Oregon.

Epilogue

A Model for Transformation?

OHSU's conversion to a public corporation presents an intriguing, and even attractive, case study for other stalled—or struggling—public institutions to consider. The question, as with any case study, is the extent to which OHSU's methods and remarkable results can be generalized to other public colleges, universities, and academic health centers. Did OHSU's success stem from the unique mix of people and politics of its time or does it offer a model that can be followed and replicated?

GAINING INDEPENDENCE FOR OREGON'S PUBLICS

As state funding continued to decline for all of Oregon's universities, several of them began looking at following, at least in some measure, OHSU's example by separating from the state bureaucracy—with two different approaches that yielded very different results.

On November 18, 2009, Dave Frohnmayer, former president of the University of Oregon, proposed in a paper written at the request of Chancellor George Pernsteiner that Oregon convert its three largest universities—UO, Oregon State, and Portland State—into public corporations so they would have their own boards and more freedom to raise money and manage their operations. Otherwise, he wrote, the university system would continue to starve financially, which threatens to destroy the state's economic future and render it a "stagnant backwater."[1]

Richard Lariviere, a Sanskrit scholar who became president of UO in 2009, agreed. He could see, as Kohler did at OHSU, that the university could never become great without more freedom and other sources of money. State support was on the decline.

So he asked the state to back $800 million in bonds for UO in lieu of state funding. UO would raise another $800 million and build a $1.6 billion endowment that would allow it to grow without having to keep raising tuition an average 7 percent a year. The state would have no future obligation to UO beyond paying off the bonds.[2]

At the same time, the state board again was exploring the prospects of making the whole seven-campus university system independent of the state and its regulations. The board told Lariviere it liked his creative ideas and would consider them after the legislature passed the OUS reforms, which would give all the universities more independence. Selling both plans at the same time could be confusing and scuttle them both, the board said.[3]

But Lariviere pushed his plan anyway, even wrote about it in a guest column for the *Wall Street Journal*. When the 2011 Legislature convened, lobbyists for the UO Foundation and for the Oregon University System battled for separate bills. Neither passed.

Lariviere continued to push his plan for the 2012 Legislature. He also defied his superiors in other ways. In the difficult economy, Governor Kitzhaber had asked all seven universities to keep increases under 6 percent. He said Lariviere and the other presidents assured the chancellor they would. But then Lariviere raised salaries for more than 1,100 UO faculty and administrators to the tune of nearly $5 million, defying Kitzhaber and others.[4] Lariviere said in an email that he "never agreed to any salary guidelines before I granted the staff raises," and state funds were not used for the increases. The guidelines came after he granted the raises, he said. The UO faculty had had no salary increase in four years, and under Kitzhaber's guidelines, they would have had to endure frozen salaries for three more years, Lariviere said.[5]

While Lariviere had captured the imagination of the UO community, he had estranged the governor and his boss, the state board. He had proposed to govern UO with an independent board and to build a sustainable financial plan. He found a way to raise pay for nearly a third of faculty and administrators. Fall enrollment hit 24,447 students, a record. Incoming freshman were the smartest ever. But on December 3, 2011, the state board voted to fire him. His brash, forceful style appealed to the UO community, but it alienated everyone else and doomed his mission.[6]

"Richard was his own worst enemy," Kitzhaber said. "He was charismatic, and he was interesting. . . . I was totally in support of his vision. . . . He is a great guy, and I'm really sorry he left."[7]

PUBLIC UNIVERSITIES FOLLOW OHSU

Undeterred by Lariviere's failed attempt to win independence for the University of Oregon, the state's universities continued to seek OHSU's status—and this time, followed more of its approach. The State Board of Higher Education and Chancellor George Pernsteiner followed Kohler's example by patiently, quietly lobbying the legislature for more autonomy. The university system worked with Kitzhaber's office and lawmakers in crafting a thoughtful case for making the universities more independent, and in 2013 the legislature gave all seven state universities *some* of the freedom OHSU has. They now have their own governing boards. They can issue their own revenue bonds and contract for their own legal, purchasing, and other services.[8]

But they also have limits on their power that do not apply to OHSU, said Jay Kenton, an administrator for more than three decades in the Oregon higher education system, most recently as interim president of Eastern Oregon University.[9] Unlike OHSU, they all are under the umbrella of Oregon's fourteen-member Higher Education Coordinating Commission, which replaced the State Board of Higher Education as overseer of the state's community colleges and universities. Many of the universities still share services for information technology, payroll, financial statements and other functions. Their staffs receive public retirement and health benefits. Service Employee International Union, which represents all of the universities' classified workers, engages in collective bargaining for a single labor agreement with all seven campuses.

One big limit on the universities' powers restricts their authority to raise tuition. They cannot raise tuition above 3 percent without first notifying the coordinating commission and legislature. The limit reflects fears expressed by student leaders that if the state gave its universities more independence, they would be inclined to raise tuition—just as had happened at OHSU.

It is true that the university on Pill Hill has raised tuition substantially over the two decades since it became a public corporation. Tuition for a medical student from Oregon during that period climbed from about $13,400 to $39,196: a 191 percent increase. Add fees, and OHSU's sticker price for a first-year resident medical student was $44,809 in 2015, the third-highest among the nation's public medical schools, lower only than tuition and fees at the University of Virginia and Oakland University William Beaumont School of Medicine in Rochester, Minnesota.[10] But OHSU's tuition ranked high from the time it became a public corporation. In the 1996–97 school year, for example, OHSU's tuition and fees was sixth highest among public medical schools.[11] And while tuition has grown dramatically since, it has not grown any faster at OHSU than at other public medical schools and universities. In fact, public medical schools on average raised their tuition 232 percent over the last two decades, outpacing OHSU's 191 percent growth.[12] Similarly, tuition and fees climbed an average 221 percent for US public universities during this period, and by 193 percent at the University of Oregon. Oregon's public universities on average saw tuition and fees rise 171 percent since 1995, only a slightly smaller increase than OHSU's. So while tuition and fees are high at OHSU, they have actually climbed a little slower than those at most other public universities and academic health centers across the country.[13]

Other consequences of the increased autonomy given to Oregon's public universities have been mixed, Kenton said. Administering local boards creates new costs for the universities, but having the boards' oversight brings them more attention, more opportunities for philanthropy, more advocacy, and more accountability.

Portland State University has seen positive changes as a result of having its own board and more autonomy, said President Wim Wiewel. More independence has allowed the universities to lobby the legislature, which they could not do before, and the presidents of the seven universities concluded they could do that best by doing it together. They succeeded in winning $700 million from the state for 2015–16 rather than the $670 million the legislative leadership had recommended. That translated into $10 million more a year for PSU, which is "real money," Wiewel said.

"That alone was worth the price of admission" to becoming more independent, he said. "The somewhat ironic result is we are collaborating with the other universities better, and therefore, we have more political power than we ever had under the umbrella of the state board."[14]

PSU also has benefited from a more equitable distribution of state money among the seven universities. And having its own board has given the university more clout, Wiewel said.

"It is not about any particular thing a board member says or does that makes it useful," he said. "It is just that the political world begins to see you as an independent organization that has to be listened to and has to be reckoned with."[15]

PSU also proposed for the November 2016 ballot a metro area payroll tax to raise $25 million to $50 million for student scholarships, something it could not have done under the old State Board of Higher Education. PSU later withdrew the proposal after the Portland Business Alliance, opposed to the tax, promised that the business community would help raise $25 million a year for the university by 2019. And the university's donations climbed dramatically, from $12 million in 2010 to $48 million in 2015, but Wiewel thinks that has more to do with changes in management and strategy than in being more independent.[16]

Despite these positive developments, PSU still remains under the oversight of the Higher Education Coordinating Commission, which has been gaining more authority from the legislature. PSU and the other six state universities must have their requests for state money and capital budgets approved by the commission, which also distributes their money. The commission also must evaluate them against various performance measures such as graduation rates. PSU still must participate in shared services with the other universities including risk management, the Public Employee Retirement System benefits, joint union bargaining, and use of the state treasury. PSU does not have the autonomy OHSU enjoys nor does it have OHSU's money-making capacity as a health care organization, Wiewel said.

Robertson agrees Oregon's universities are not really public corporations with governance structures comparable to OHSU. "They have more autonomy than before," he said, "but it's not an apples to apples comparison."[17]

Oregon's universities, which receive the fourth-lowest level of state support in the nation, are exploring ways to raise more money with their new freedom. They have recruited out-of-state and international students, who pay about three times the tuition of resident students. They have built new dorms to attract students, ramped up campaigns for donors, and pursued entrepreneurial enterprises such as research partnerships with private companies or the creation of company spin-offs. But while Oregon universities are changing, Archer does not see them transforming. They have not made the clear break from the state and functions of the past as OHSU did, she said, and are still governed more by state policies.[18]

TRANSFORMATION ACROSS THE COUNTRY

Although Oregon's large public universities were able to gain only limited autonomy in that same state in which OHSU claimed its independence, there is a more successful example across the country that suggests the move to a public corporation should be possible for any public higher education institution—even a small liberal arts college. One example is St. Mary's College of Maryland, which converted from a state to a hybrid public-private institution, a public honors college.[19] As in Oregon, Maryland was going through a fiscal crisis in 1991 that led the governor to challenge the state's universities and colleges "to explore creative new strategies for financing higher education."[20] The 1,500-student liberal arts college in St. Mary's City, Maryland's first capitol, had its own governing board, which decided to accept the challenge.

The college agreed in 1992 to cap its operating budget request to the state to the amount it received in 1993, and to increase that amount only by the state's inflationary price index. In exchange for this fixed lump-sum support from the state, the college was given more freedom to raise money from non-state sources and to purchase, hire and conduct other functions independent of state agency regulations. Unlike OHSU however, the college at the time was getting half of its money from the state. That dropped to less than a third by 2014.[21]

Like Kohler at OHSU, St. Mary's College President Ted Lewis carefully and patiently sold the autonomy plan to his faculty, staff, students, and alumni and to the legislature.

"St. Mary's College had been so effective with its relations during the years leading up to the new status bill that there was remarkably easy sailing," writes Robert Berdahl, emeritus professor at the University of Maryland and an expert on higher education governance and policy.[22]

The legislation passed with only two opposing votes, one in the Senate and one in the House of Delegates. The legislation unleashed St. Mary's from state regulations, but in exchange the college agreed to maintain its public mission to serve a diverse population of students and not become an upper-middle-class white enclave.[23]

The college thrived under its new structure and freedom. It increased its faculty size, diversity, and quality, restored faculty tenure and improved its student–faculty ratio. It doubled its tuition from $2,500 to $5,000, but used much of its increased income to provide financial aid to students from low-income families. Both the diversity and the SAT college entrance exam scores of its students increased.[24] The college made substantial savings by controlling its own purchases. In building forty townhouses for residential students, the college was able to move quickly, hiring and beginning construction in six months. That would have been impossible as a state agency. Its independence allowed it to take advantage of a tight construction market and lower debt service costs in a favorable bond market, saving $2.3 million on a $4.7 million capital construction project.[25] An accreditation team in 1995, just three years after its conversion to a more autonomous institution, concluded: "St. Mary's has become a public liberal arts college of very high quality—and a nationally recognized model in public higher education."[26] The college has continued to shine. In 2009–10, St. Mary's had the second highest number of student Fulbright winners of any public liberal arts college in the nation.[27] The college has a 10:1 student–faculty ratio and 81 percent graduate rate, which is exceptionally high for a public institution. *U.S. News & World Report* in 2016 ranked it ninety-third among the nation's liberal arts colleges.[28]

Berdahl notes that President Lewis had an "obvious impact" and "crucial role" in St. Mary's transformation during his thirteen years in office. With Lewis at St. Mary's helm, all four forces that Barbara Archer described as necessary for transformational change came to bear on St. Mary's College in 1992. The school faced economic pressures to change, had supportive policies, and had a strong leader who led the institution through a clear break from its principal authority—the state.

Many Maryland leaders concluded that St. Mary's was able to make its remarkable change only because it was so small, Berdahl writes. "The

St. Mary's College model in its entirety then, perhaps is not feasible for all public universities. Yet within this plan, others may find certain pieces to borrow, a direction to take," wrote the president.[29] Inspired by St. Mary's success, eight of the University of Maryland's eleven campuses created local boards. The University of Maryland at Baltimore, which includes the medical school, considered withdrawing from the university system, Berdahl writes, and creating a not-for-profit corporation as its hospital had done thirteen years earlier. In making this deliberation, the university cited "a precedent from Oregon where a public medical campus had been privatized."[30] Although David J. Ramsay, president of the University of Maryland at Baltimore, had brought a team to visit OHSU shortly after it became a public corporation, the university ultimately chose to remain part of the state system.

OHSU INC. AS MODEL

Despite the University of Maryland deciding not to follow in its footsteps, and the limited success of its in-state public peers, OHSU's move to become a public corporation has impressed academic health centers across the country with its transformation, Robertson said.

"We are the envy of every public academic health center across the country with regard to the type of administrative structure we have," he said. "There may be a better structure yet to be devised, but I think it is as good or better than that of any that has been devised to date."[31]

Both Kohler and Robertson have written papers for their academic health center colleagues on how OHSU healed itself by becoming a public corporation. Yet none so far has followed OHSU's path in explicitly seeking legislative approval to become a more independent public corporation. OHSU's conversion to a public corporation is not even mentioned in *The Transformation of Academic Health Centers,* a book published in 2015 with twenty-five chapters written by academic medical center leaders.

Robertson and others said it may be that none has followed OHSU because of the enormous political hurtle they must leap to win so much autonomy. "It takes a legislature that is rather bold to grant the degrees of freedom that we were given," Robertson said.[32]

However, OHSU's transformation does have implications for academic health centers, said Dr. Steven A. Wartman, president and chief executive officer of the Association of Academic Health Centers based in Washington, DC. The academic medical community views the Oregon medical center "as a superb institution that has done some creative and interesting things in terms of its reorganization, its structures, its physical development," he said.[33]

Most academic health centers have not felt a compelling need to change until recently, note some academic health center leaders in *The Transformation of Academic Health Centers.*

"And, in the past, there was not a pressing need to rethink the way we finance and execute our mission; there was little financial incentive to operate differently," they write. "Today's economic exigencies are motivating us to break from tradition and experiment with new ways of delivering health care, conducting research and educating leaders."[34]

So the time may be ripe for other academic health centers to take a closer look at OHSU's story, though it is hard to say how its model might apply as each differs so much in size, structure, and focus. The public corporation model probably makes the most sense for a small number of public academic health centers that are not attached to undergraduate universities, such as the University of California at San Francisco Medical Center, said Lawrence Furnstahl, OHSU's chief financial officer.[35] Today, academic health centers face forces much like those that drove OHSU to transform. The federal Affordable Care Act, or Obamacare, is again advocating various forms of managed care, including integrated accountable care organizations, in which a group of providers receive a bundled payment, rather than fees for services, to manage the health of a group of enrolled patients. As the population ages, with Baby Boomers retiring, academic health centers will be relying more heavily on patients under Medicaid and Medicare, which reimburse providers at about 70 percent to 80 percent of the private insurers. That will mean thinner margins in hospital and clinical operations to subsidize research and education. Research also poses challenges. The NIH has lost roughly one-fifth of its federal funding in real dollars since its peak in 2003.[36] Academic health centers typically estimate they have to subsidize about 15 percent of their research funding. But a group of academic health center administrators launched a study of research costs at thirty-eight medical schools and found they actually subsidize 25 percent to 40 percent of their research spending.[37] The administrators write in their report:

> Academic health center leaders remain especially concerned that the erosion of research funding by the National Institutes of Health poses a serious threat to the long-term financial viability of the academic health center model. Not only is direct funding of research under attack, but as the clinical margin shrinks, academic health centers will be less able to transfer funds from clinical enterprises to cover the "hidden costs" of research.[38]

The long-term trend of declining state support adds to the squeeze on academic health centers. Withering state funding was the chief driver for OHSU to transform, not only because it needed more flexibility to compete in health care, but also because it made no sense to give the state regulatory authority over an institution it was no longer supporting. More public academic health centers may be reaching that conclusion. Less state money combined with declines in Medicare, shifts to bundled health care fees, a flat NIH budget, and rising costs are driving academic health centers to consider dramatic change, maybe even transformational change, says Wartman.

"We are in a disruptive environment," he said. "Disruptive in terms of economics, politics, science, technology, the Internet, patient empowerment—about 20 forces disrupting business as usual."[39]

RESPONDING TO DISRUPTION

Furnstahl said academic health centers have been wrestling with change and predicting "the coming collapse" for the last three decades.[40] Still, academic health centers in recent years have explored innovations in every sector of their operations, most aimed at cutting costs and increasing revenue, in a race to stay solvent. With downward pressure on federal, state, and commercial insurance payments, the private Vanderbilt University Medical Center in Nashville sharpened its administration to adjust to a $200 million loss in revenue in 2014 and 2015. The chancellor put a single person in charge of the medical school and its entire diverse health system, which sees $3.5 billion in annual revenue. The university aggressively retired debt and identified $100 million in cost savings through workforce reductions.[41]

Academic health centers also have looked for more business opportunities, forging partnerships with biotech companies and launching new companies. Johns Hopkins University, for example, collaborated with the private MedImmune, a Maryland firm, in seeking better treatments for rheumatoid arthritis and prostate cancer. The university's research also spawned eight start-up companies in 2014.[42]

Some medical schools have designed new curriculums that can move students more swiftly to completion. Among them, OHSU's new medical school structure is individualized and proficiency-based to allow some students to move faster than others, each at his or her own pace. Schools have also trimmed pre-clinical basic science training, and forty schools offered combined undergraduate-MD programs that reduce total training time to six or seven years.[43]

Academic health centers, including OHSU, also have merged with other health systems in recent years to gain efficiencies through economies of scale. Many other hospitals and health systems have also consolidated for the same reason, creating huge health organizations in competition with academic health centers. Between 2007 and 2012 there were 432 merger and acquisition deals involving 835 hospitals.

"The ongoing consolidation within the health marketplace, especially in the United States, raises serious concerns about the ability of individual academic health centers to compete with far larger national or international health systems," Wartman writes.[44]

The Mount Sinai Health System, an academic health center, merged with the Continuum Health System, producing a Manhattan system of 3,571 licensed beds, 138 operating rooms, and 35,000 employees. New York Hospital-Presbyterian Hospital System includes eleven hospitals in New York's five boroughs along with nineteen other hospitals in the tristate area. These two mergers left the New York University academic health center competing with two mega-systems in Manhattan. Similarly, OHSU also is trying to leverage its resources and capacity, more through partnerships than mergers.

"You need more scale to be successful in this business," Furnstahl said.[45]

In a 2014 member survey by the Association of Academic Health Centers, 41 percent of academic health centers said they were engaged in major expansions of their hospitals or physician networks, a third had launched major cost cuts, one in three opened a new health professions school or branch campus, and 31 percent changed their governance structures.[46] Reorganizing, consolidating, merging, cutting jobs, and streamlining programs are all common and understandable responses by organizations to financial threats.

But these are changes, not transformation.

TIME TO TRANSFORM?

As their book's title suggests, the authors of *The Transformation of Academic Health Centers* argue more radical change may be necessary to keep the nation's medical universities healthy.

"We have a dire need to reengineer our organizations—to transform them in fundamental ways in order preserve our ability to accomplish our public purpose as organizations leading society toward a healthier future," writes Dr. Daniel Rahn, chancellor of the University of Arkansas for Medical Sciences. "This is a time of disruptive, transformational change in every aspect of the academic health center mission."[47]

To truly transform, these complex institutions need to look beyond incremental changes in their business practices and must change their cultures in ways that fit their circumstances and visions. OHSU's story offers a vivid example of what this type of transformation looks like. As Barbara Archer suggests, such transformation may be rare because it requires so much. It demands the right political climate, the support of state policymakers, staff, and the public, and a leadership team willing to make a clear break with authority and with its past. As Kohler said on the day Governor Kitzhaber signed Senate Bill 2 to make OHSU a public corporation, no one should underestimate how hard this is to accomplish.

"It is not the status quo," he said. "It is not the path of least resistance. It is dramatic change."[48]

And when it happens, it can create a work of wonder like OHSU today, said Mark Dodson, the Portland lawyer and state board chair who led efforts to hire Kohler.

"When we were looking for the new president, we had big dreams," he said. "But I don't think we had envisioned anything like this, anything like this at all. I really wanted to think big. I just wasn't capable of thinking this big."[49]

Notes

1 Bill Graves, "Frohnmayer Pitches Idea of Corporate Oregon Universities," *The Oregonian,* Nov. 19, 2009, Metro section.

2 Bill Graves, "Lariviere Put UO First, to a Fault," *The Sunday Oregonian,* Dec. 4, 2011, p. A1.

3 Ibid.

4 Ibid.

5 Richard Lariviere, president and chief executive officer for The Field Museum in Chicago and former president of the University of Oregon, email response to author's questions, May 7, 2016.

6 Graves, "Lariviere Put UO First," p. A1.

7 Governor John Kitzhaber, interview, Feb. 12, 2016: "Richard was his own worst enemy," Kitzhaber said. "He was charismatic, and he was interesting. . . . I was totally in support of his vision. . . . He is a great guy, and I'm really sorry he left."

8 "On Higher Ed, an Incomplete," editorial, *The Oregonian*, July 6, 2013, editorial section. Also see S.B. 270, 77th Legis. Assemb. (Oregon, 2013), https://olis.leg.state.or.us/liz/2013R1/Downloads/MeasureDocument/SB270/Enrolled.

9 Jay Kenton (former vice president of finance for the Oregon University System), interview, Sept. 8, 2015.

10 American Association of Medical Colleges, "Public Medical Schools – Tuition and Fees First-Year Medical Students 2014–15," Tuition and Student Fees Reports, https://services.aamc.org/tsfreports/select.cfm?year_of_study=2015.

11 American Association of Medical Colleges, "Public Medical Schools – Tuition and Fees First-Year Medical Students 1996–97," Tuition and Student Fees Reports, https://services.aamc.org/tsfreports/report.cfm?order_by=tot_res_fee_sort&year_of_study=1997&select_control=PUB.

12 *Digest of Education Statistics 2014*, National Center of Education Statistics, U.S. Department of Education, Table 330:10, online at: http://nces.ed.gov/pubs2016/2016006.pdf; The College Board, "Annual Survey of Colleges," and medical school tuition chart by American Association of Medical Colleges.

13 Ibid.

14 Wim Wiewel (president of Portland State University), interview, Sept. 23, 2015, his PSU office.

15 Ibid.

16 Ibid.

17 Joseph Robertson, MD, interview, Aug. 20, 2015, his Baird Hall office, OHSU campus.

18 Barbara Archer, interview, Aug. 11, 2015.

19 Robert O. Berdahl, "Balancing Self-Interest and Accountability: St. Mary's College of Maryland," in *Seeking Excellence Through Independence: Liberating Colleges and Universities from Excessive Regulation*, ed. Terrence J. MacTaggart & Associates (San Francisco: Jossey-Bass Inc. Publishers, 1998), pp. 59–83.

20 Ibid., p. 65.

21 "FY2015 Operating Budget Testimony," St. Mary's College of Maryland, http://www.smcm.edu/fy2015-operating-budget-testimony/.

22 Berdahl, "Balancing Self-Interest and Accountability," p. 69.

23 Ibid., p. 73.

24 Ibid., p. 73.

25 Ibid., p. 76.

26 Ibid., p.71.

27 Southern Maryland Higher Education Center, "SMCM Awarded Highest Number of Fulbright Scholars in Md.," Oct. 23, 2009, http://somd.com/news/headlines/2009/10669.shtml.

28 "St Mary's College of Maryland," 2016 best college rankings, U.S. News & World Report, http://colleges.usnews.rankingsandreviews.com/best-colleges/st-marys-college-2095.

29 Ibid., pp. 80–81.

30 Ibid., p.81.

31 Robertson, interview.

32 Ibid.

33 Steven A. Wartman, MD (president and chief executive officer of the Association of Academic Health Centers), interview, March 23, 2015.

34 Paul B. Rothman, Edward D. Miller, Landon S. King, and Ellen F. Gibson, "The Changing Ivory Tower: Balancing Mission and Business," in *The Transformation of Academic Health Centers*, ed. Steven A. Wartman, MD, Association of Academic Health Centers (San Diego: Academic Press, 2015), p. 10.

35 Lawrence Furnstahl, interview, Oct. 22, 2015, his office on campus.

36 Rothman et al., "The Changing Ivory Tower," pp. 3–10.

37 Association of Academic Health Centers, "AAHC Benchmarks & Metrics Initiative, Financial Data Project Steering Committee Report", April 2013, pp. 2, 18.

38 Ibid., p. 17.

39 Wartman, interview.

40 Furnstahl, interview.

41 Jeffrey R. Balser, MD, and William W. Stead, MD, "How Academic Health Centers are Transforming in Leadership, Administration and Management: A Case Study," in *The Transformation of Academic Health Centers*, ed. Steven A. Wartman, MD, Association of Academic Health Centers (San Diego: Academic Press, 2015), pp. 23–28.

42 Rothman et al, "The Changing Ivory Tower," pp. 8, 9.

43 Ibid., p. 9.

44 Steven A. Wartman, MS, "Academic Health Center Transformation: Future Shock or Future Success," *The Transformation of Academic Health Centers*, ed. Steven A. Wartman, Association of Academic Health Centers, (San Diego: Academic Press, 2015), p. 253.

45 Furnstahl, interview.

46 Wartman, "Academic Health Center Transformation," p. 253.

47 Daniel W. Rahn, MD, chancellor of the University of Arkansas for Medical Sciences, "Foreword," *The Transformation of Academic Health Centers*, ed. Steven A. Wartman, Association of Academic Health Centers, (San Diego: Academic Press, 2015), pp. xvi–xvii.

48 Peter Kohler, *Talking Points for Bill Signing Ceremony*, May 24, 1995, OHSU

archives.

49 Mark Dodson, interview, Feb. 23, 2016, Multnomah Athletic Club, Portland, Oregon.

Key Players in OHSU's Transformation

THE PRESIDENT AND HIS TEAM

Janet Billups

Janet Billups became OHSU's first attorney when Kohler hired her in 1992, made her part of his leadership team, and gave her the monumental challenge of drafting Senate Bill 2, the legislative and legal framework for OHSU's conversion to a public corporation. She had been working since 1987 for the Oregon Attorney General's Office as the department's assistant attorney general for OHSU and Portland State University. After joining Kohler's team, Billups nearly single-handedly wrote Senate Bill 2, which would define OHSU's powers and obligations as a public corporation, and she helped sell it in the 1995 Legislature.[1]

Billups was a fourth-generation native Oregonian. Ancestors on her mother's side traveled to the state on the Oregon Trail. Her mother died shortly after she was born on July 12, 1952, in Los Angeles. Her father was too young to care for her so she was adopted by family friends there. They later took her to Crescent City, California, and finally to southern Oregon, where she completed high school. She attended a small Seventh-day Adventist college in Walla Walla, Washington, and completed law school at Lewis & Clark Law School in Portland. She passed the Oregon bar exam in 1980, and worked as a law clerk and later as a trial lawyer for Multnomah

County, which includes Portland, under one of the state's legendary trial lawyers, John Leahy. She stayed with the county eight years. Then Leahy retired, and she decided that was a good time to move on to join the state Department of Justice as an assistant attorney general.[2]

After OHSU became a public corporation in 1995, Billups gradually assembled a legal team for the university, including medical malpractice, contract, and employment lawyers. In 1999, after she adopted her daughter, she reduced her own hours, and Steve Stadum, a Portland real estate lawyer, took over as General Counsel for her office. Billups later moved back into the General Counsel position. By 2009, she was overseeing seven in-house and multiple outside lawyers, a position she holds today. She is the only member of Kohler's core leadership team still working at OHSU.[3]

Lois Davis

Lois Davis, former chief of staff for Congressman Ron Wyden (Democrat from Oregon), served as OHSU's chief lobbyist in its public and legislative campaign to convert OHSU to a public corporation. She later served as its vice president for public affairs and marketing, in charge of telling OHSU's story to the people of Oregon.[4]

Davis was born December 5, 1954, in Caldwell, Idaho, the fifth of eight children, and grew up on a farm in the small town of Council in central Idaho, near McCall. She attended Northwest Nazarene University in Nampa, Idaho, became interested in journalism, and transferred her junior year to the University of Oregon. There she earned a degree in journalism and worked as a reporter at the nearby newspaper in Springfield. She went on to law school at Willamette University in Salem. While there, she married Jim Davis in 1978 and became involved in his friend Ron Wyden's first campaign for Congress. After Wyden won, she became his press secretary and later chief of staff.[5]

Davis and her husband and daughter moved back to Oregon in late 1986 when she joined OHSU as a lobbyist. She gave birth to her son, Matt, in OHSU's cramped, outdated labor and delivery wing in September of 1988. After Kohler arrived that year, he made Davis his chief lobbyist in Salem and part of his core leadership team. Following the university's conversion to a public corporation, Davis became vice president for public affairs and marketing. She oversaw the university's promotion and lobbying duties while serving as its chief spokesperson for news events.[6]

She left OHSU three years after Kohler did, in August of 2009, to become chief of staff and vice president for public affairs for Portland State University, where she still works. She loved OHSU, she said, but it had arrived, had reached a state of healthy stability, and it was time for a new challenge.[7]

Timothy Goldfarb

Timothy Goldfarb joined OHSU in early 1984 as an associate administrator of University Hospital and eventually became part of Kohler's leadership team in charge of all of the university's hospitals and clinics. Goldfarb was comfortable in hospitals because he had grown up in one. Shortly after he was born in Jerome, Arizona, in 1949, his father came down with polio and was put into an iron lung to help him breathe. His father spent sixteen years in the iron lung, mostly in hospitals in Cottonwood, which is near Jerome, and in Prescott and Phoenix, before he died of pneumonia, and those hospitals are where Goldfarb spent much of his youth. Since earning his master's in health services administration in 1978, Goldfarb has continued to live much of his adult life in hospitals.[8]

In the summer of 1983, Goldfarb and his wife, Laura, left their jobs in Arizona to work in Oregon, where Goldfarb landed a job as an associate administrator for OHSU's hospital and his wife, a midwife, found work in Woodburn south of Portland. He became friends with Walker, who arrived at OHSU shortly after he did.

Though he expected problems, Goldfarb was shocked by the dysfunction and disrepair at OHSU, especially in contrast to the new, smooth-functioning hospital he left behind in Arizona.[9]

After joining Kohler's administrative team, Goldfarb helped campaign for legislation to make OHSU a public corporation. Kohler later made Goldfarb director of OHSU hospitals and health care systems, and Goldfarb orchestrated the university's expanding clinics and hospital operations.

He became the first member of Kohler's core leadership team to leave OHSU. He departed in 2001 and moved on to more hospitals—this time in Gainesville, Florida, where he became chief executive officer of Shands HealthCare, a health care system affiliated with the University of Florida Health Science Center. That put Goldfarb in charge of a primary teaching hospital, two children's hospitals, a cancer hospital, two specialty hospitals, two home care agencies, and other outpatient services. He retired in 2015.[10] But in August of 2016, OHSU President Joseph Robertson brought him back for five months to fill in at his old job as head of OHSU hospitals and clinics while the university searched for someone to take the post permanently. The Goldfarbs' three daughters all continue to work at OHSU.

Lesley Hallick

Lesley Hallick joined OHSU in 1977 as a molecular biology professor and researcher and became Kohler's vice president of academic affairs, later titled provost, in 1989. As head of OHSU's academic affairs, she oversaw all academic programs at OHSU and took charge of Oregon Regional Primate Research Center after it merged with OHSU in 1998. She also was interim director of the Biomedical Information Communication Center after it opened in 1991. She helped persuade faculty and legislators to support the bill allowing OHSU to convert to a public corporation. Once the bill passed, she helped lead an effort to integrate the hospital and the university's financial and computer systems. Kohler's predecessor, Leonard Laster, often called on Hallick for advice and to head committees and campus initiatives. She appealed to him with her insights, charm, and extraordinary interpersonal and diplomatic skills.[11]

Hallick was born February 4, 1946, in Springfield, Massachusetts; she grew up in Orange, California, the daughter of a World War II fighter pilot, and earned her bachelor's in biochemistry at Pomona College in Claremont, becoming the first person in her family to earn a college degree. She earned her doctorate in molecular biology at the University of Wisconsin, married and had a daughter, and then took a postdoctoral fellowship at the University of California at Berkeley, where she studied the structures of virus DNA and RNA. Hallick taught and launched research that would lead her later to explore virology, simian AIDS retroviruses, and DNA tumor viruses during her twelve years as a faculty member in microbiology at OHSU.[12]

Hallick left OHSU in 2009 to become president of Pacific University.

Peter Kohler

Dr. Peter O. Kohler, an endocrinologist, led Oregon Health & Science University through its conversion to a public corporation in 1995 and its subsequent rise to a nationally prominent academic health center. OHSU is the only institution he presided over, but he held leadership positions through most of his career.

During his eighteen years as president, Kohler led OHSU through a period of unprecedented growth in quality and in clinical and research capacity. Under his leadership, OHSU won $200 million in bonds from the legislature and raised more than $300 million more to expand on Marquam Hill and on Portland's South Waterfront. That expansion helped him attract some of the nation's top researchers and raise the institution's national profile. While Kohler was president, OHSU doubled its building space to more than six million square feet, grew its research awards sevenfold to $294 million, and doubled its employees from 5,800 to 12,000.[13] When he left in 2006, OHSU had reached his goal of ranking twentieth among the nation's academic health centers in terms of its National Institutes of Health (NIH) research grants.[14]

Kohler was born July 18, 1938, in Brooklyn, New York, grew up in southwestern Virginia, and earned an English degree at the University of Virginia and his medical degree at Duke University, where he met his wife, Judy. He served as a clinical associate for two years at the NIH in Bethesda, Maryland, and stayed at NIH for six more years, eventually becoming head of endocrine service for his unit. He and his wife had four children by the time they moved in 1973 to Houston, where Kohler headed the endocrinology division at Baylor College of Medicine and received a prestigious Howard Hughes Medical Institute Investigator award. He went on to be chair of medicine at the University of Arkansas and dean of the medical school at the University of Texas medical center in San Antonio before joining OHSU as president in 1988. He was elected in 1994 to the Institute of Medicine of the National Academy of Sciences.[15]

After leaving OHSU, Kohler returned to Arkansas to serve as vice chancellor at the University of Arkansas for Medical Sciences, where he led efforts to establish satellite medical programs in northwest Arkansas. He worked with local health care providers to establish a campus with rotations for students in medicine, pharmacy and other health professions from the university's Little Rock campus. Currently based in Fayetteville, Arkansas, he leads a major effort to reduce obesity and diabetes among a large migrant population from the Marshall Islands.

Kohler also continues to keep an office at OHSU. He makes regular visits there, often in connection with meetings as a member of the board of directors at Pacific University, a small, private liberal arts university in nearby Forest Grove.

James Walker

The good-humored Jim Walker was working at the University of New Mexico Hospital, enjoying his life as one of the nation's youngest hospital chief financial officers, when he was invited in the fall of 1983 to join OHSU as chief financial officer. Though others warned Walker not to take the job, he accepted the new position. Walker set out to improve University Hospital, which was like a county teaching hospital, serving largely indigent patients. When Kohler arrived at OHSU in 1988, he soon made Walker part of his core leadership team and vice president for finance and administration for the entire academic health center. Walker helped sell Oregon leaders on making OHSU a public corporation. After the change, he led the university through a difficult transition. Among other things, he soon discovered many of his management workers could not handle the rapid shift from a state to corporate culture and was forced to replace them. The university went through "radical change in a very short time," he said.[16]

Walker was born April 10, 1948, in New York City and grew up on Long Island, New York, in a hamlet called Wantagh. He attended Western Kentucky University for two years before joining the US Air Force and marrying his high school sweetheart, Ginny Rowland. After leaving the military, he enrolled at and graduated from California Polytechnic University. He and his wife had two daughters by the time he joined OHSU in February of 1984.[17]

Walker's responsibilities widened over his years at OHSU until he was putting in sixty-hour weeks overseeing not only the university's finances, but its administrative operations, including finance, risk management, purchasing, and labor negotiations. During labor negotiations with the Oregon Nurses Association, he collapsed and went through an emergency appendectomy. He told Kohler "this is my wake up call," and he retired in 2003.[18]

But within months, he went to work for Lewis & Clark College in Portland to help it deal with a financial and political disaster. He stayed for two years. In 2009, OHSU President Joe Robertson called Walker back for nine months to help him deal with the forces of the Great Recession. He helped stabilize OHSU's shaky finances, and then again retired to St. Simons Island in Georgia. Recently, still retired, he was preparing to move back to Albuquerque, New Mexico, completing the circle of his adult life.[19]

STATE OF OREGON AND OHSU LEADERS

Lewis William (Bill) Bluemle

When the State Board of Higher Education consolidated the University of Oregon dental and nursing schools with its medical school and hospital into the academic health center that would become OHSU, it hired Dr. Lewis William Bluemle Jr. as its first president. The university lured Bluemle from his job as president of State University of New York's Upstate Medical Center in Syracuse.[20]

He was a tall, distinguished, and innovative nephrologist with a charming demeanor and sharp mind. He used an electric motor from his phonograph to develop a blood pump for the first clinically applicable artificial kidney program at the University of Pennsylvania.

Shortly upon his arrival at OHSU, he dealt with a crisis: the Joint Commission on Accreditation of Hospitals withdrew University Hospital's accreditation for failing to address shortcomings identified three or four years earlier. Bluemle helped organize the university as an academic health center independent of the University of Oregon. But he found Oregon too parochial and left after less than three years to become president of the private Thomas Jefferson University in Philadelphia, Pennsylvania.[21]

"He didn't like the legislature," recalled Donald Kassebaum, whom Bluemle hired to head the hospital. "He didn't like the mindset. He thought that the faculty was weak and the chairs were weak, and he was right."[22]

Fred Buckman

Fred Buckman, former president and chief executive officer of PacificCorp, served on the Public Corporation Advisory Committee that recommended OHSU become a public corporation. The six-foot-four-inch, low-key executive testified before legislators in favor of Senate Bill 2, the legislation that made OHSU a public corporation, and recommended the institution's president be a member of the OHSU board of directors. Governor Kitzhaber appointed him to the first OHSU board in 1995, and the board elected him chairman. He led OHSU through its early years as a public corporation, including the long and controversial struggle to build an aerial tram connecting the university's Marquam Hill campus to its burgeoning campus on Portland's South Waterfront. He was on the board during its 1999 annual retreat when it decided to seek $200 million in bonds from the Oregon Legislature for its Oregon Opportunity initiative to expand the academic health center's research capacity.[23]

Buckman grew up the oldest of six sons of an insurance adjuster and homemaker in Kalamazoo, Michigan. He graduated early from high school and, at sixteen, enrolled in the University of Michigan. He graduated with a science engineering degree and went on to the Massachusetts Institute of Technology to earn a doctorate in nuclear engineering in 1970 and to Harvard University for a master's in business administration. He married Marion Kasey in 1970.

After leaving MIT, he worked as a nuclear reactor engineer for Consumer Power of Jackson, Michigan, the state's largest electric and gas utility.[24] He was named CEO and president of PacifiCorp in 1994, a position he held four years. He later worked as an executive for a variety of energy companies, including president and CEO of Shaw Group Inc.; managing partner of Brookfield Asset Management Inc.; chairman and CEO of Trans-Elect Development Inc., which he founded in 1999; and president and CEO of Powerlink Transmission Company, a position he still holds. He and his wife live in Vancouver, Washington, and have two children and three grandsons.[25]

Mark Dodson

Mark Dodson, a Portland attorney and president of Northwest Natural Gas, headed the search that led to the hiring of Peter Kohler as president of OHSU in 1988. At the time of the search, Dodson was chair of both the State Board of Higher Education and the board's search committee and pushed hard for the selection of Kohler over other candidates. He was skeptical of the proposal to make OHSU a public corporation. "Do you know what you are doing here?" he asked Kohler. "Is this really the right thing?" But he came to see how it freed OHSU to dramatically expand and improve. He served as the first OHSU board's unofficial secretary and remained heavily involved in OHSU's early years as a public corporation.[26]

Dodson grew up and completed high school in Beaverton, Oregon, a suburb west of Portland, graduated from Harvard University, and attended a Baptist seminary for a year. But the seminary "didn't take," he said, and Dodson became the first male in three generations in his family to choose not to become a Baptist minister. Instead, he went to work doing research on street people in Berkeley, California. While there, he earned a law degree at the University of California at Berkeley. He married in 1968, and moved in 1973 to practice law in Portland, where he and his wife, Ruth Ann Dodson, raised two children. He served in the general counsel office of the US Department of Transportation in 1979 and later as special counsel to the Federal Aviation Administration. He worked for the Ater Wynne law firm for seventeen years before joining Northwest Natural Gas Company in 1997 as senior vice president of public affairs and general counsel. He served as chief executive officer and president of the company from 2003 to 2008.[27]

He was active in public life and provided advice and counsel to government and elected officials. He served on the transition committees for three governors, including his friend Governor Goldschmidt. He has retired, but continues to be active in several industry and business associations including the Northwest Natural Gas board of directors.[28]

Brian Druker

Dr. Brian Druker became one of OHSU's most renowned researchers after he discovered the compound that was later named Gleevec, a simple life-saving pill for people with chronic myelogenous leukemia (CML). In 1992, Druker was a young researcher at the Dana-Farber Cancer Institute in Boston exploring an enzyme involved with CML, a rare but deadly disease in which the bone marrow produces too many white blood cells.[29] After six years at the cancer center as an instructor, he was looking for a move. Dr. Grover Bagby, a top researcher at OHSU, was launching a new Oregon Cancer Center and recruited Druker, who arrived in July of 1993. Within his first six weeks at OHSU, Druker was closing in on a drug that ultimately was going to revolutionize the way the medical world thinks about fighting cancer.[30]

It took five years to get the compound into clinical trials, where it proved to be remarkably effective. By January of 1999, patients trying the drug, called Gleevec, were seeing normal blood counts. Druker and his research team were eradicating cancer with a daily pill and without chemotherapy or radiation therapy or surgery. Today, tens of thousands of CML patients are alive because they take Gleevec daily.[31] Druker gained international recognition with his discovery and "cast a halo over the whole" of OHSU, says Davis, the communications director.[32]

OHSU's cancer center grew into the Knight Cancer Institute, and Druker replaced Bagby as director. In 2014, the center received a $500 million fund-raising challenge from Phil and Penny Knight. OHSU met the challenge, collecting $500 million in less than two years, and will raise an additional $200 million. The money will pay for two buildings and more researchers, who will focus on finding ways to detect cancer in its earliest and most treatable stage.[33]

Druker was born in 1955, and earned a degree in chemistry and his MD at the University of California at San Diego. He completed his internship and residency at Washington University School of Medicine in St. Louis, and then became a fellow, instructor, and researcher at the Dana-Farber Cancer Institute of Harvard Medical School. After a previous marriage, he married Alexandra Hardy, a journalist, and they have three children.[34]

In 2002, Druker was selected for the prestigious position as investigator for the Howard Hughes Medical Institute. He was elected to the American Association of Physicians in 2006 and the National Academy of Sciences in 2007. He's received numerous awards, including the Lasker-DeBakey Clinical Medical Research Award and the Hamdan Award for Medical Research Excellence.[35]

Neil Goldschmidt

Neil Goldschmidt, an energetic, six-foot-one-inch political icon in Oregon, was involved with OHSU from the time he became Portland mayor in 1973, a job he kept through 1979.[36] As one-term governor from 1987 through 1991, he went to bat for OHSU's University Hospital when it had money problems.[37]

After leaving office, he started a law and consulting firm, and in 1994, chaired the Public Corporation Advisory Committee, created by Kohler to explore whether OHSU should become a public corporation or pursue some other change in governance. The committee recommended OHSU become a public corporation, and Goldschmidt testified in favor of the change before legislative committees.

He was appointed to OHSU's first board of directors in 1995 and served through 1999. During his final board retreat in late 1999, he recommended OHSU increase its Big Ask to the Legislature for Oregon Opportunity money from $100 to $200 million, which it did. After leaving the OHSU board, he continued to be involved in the university. He is credited with coming up with the idea of the Portland aerial tram to connect the university's Marquam Hill campus to the South Waterfront. He also urged the Schnitzer family, which was his client, to donate nearly twenty acres on the waterfront to OHSU, and the family did so in 2004. The gift, worth about $35 million, was the largest to date in the university's history and would be used to create a Schnitzer campus for the dental and medical schools. Goldschmidt also represented other owners and developers involved in the South Waterfront.[38]

Goldschmidt, a Democrat, was born in 1940 in Eugene, Oregon. He graduated from the University of Oregon, where he was student body president, and earned a law degree from the University of California at Berkeley in 1967. In 1965, he married Margaret Wood, with whom he had two children. He and Wood divorced in 1990 and, in 1994, he married Diana Snowden, a senior vice president at PacifiCorp.[39] Two years before becoming the nation's youngest mayor in 1973, Goldschmidt was elected as a Portland city commissioner at age thirty. He served as US Secretary of Education under President Jimmy Carter from 1979 to 1981.[40]

Governor Ted Kulongoski appointed him to the State Board of Higher Education in 2003, but he resigned the following spring after *Willamette Week*, an independent newspaper in Portland, revealed that Goldschmidt had a sexual relationship with a fourteen-year-old girl for an extended period during his first term as Portland's mayor.[41] He was not prosecuted for what constituted third degree rape because the statute of limitations had expired. Goldschmidt admitted to the relationship, resigned from several prominent organizations, and dropped out of public life.[42]

Mark Hatfield

US Senator Mark Hatfield contributed to OHSU's expansion throughout a career that made him one of the most influential politicians in Oregon history. As a representative in the Oregon Legislature, he helped find state funds to allow the dental school for the University of Oregon in 1956 to move out of its forty-year-old building in Northeast Portland into a $2.2 million ten-floor building on the OHSU Marquam Hill campus. As a state senator on the Senate Health Committee in 1955, Hatfield carried the bill to the Senate floor that would create a teaching hospital, University Hospital, for what was then the University of Oregon Medical School.

Hatfield worked closely with most of OHSU's leaders, including Dr. David W. Baird, dean of the medical school;[43] President Leonard Laster; and President Peter Kohler. As chair of the US Senate Appropriations

Committee from 1981 to 1987, Hatfield was able to funnel more than $90 million of federal support into construction projects at OHSU such as the Vollum Institute for Advanced Biomedical Research.[44] In 1998, the university honored Hatfield by opening its fourteen-story Hatfield Research Center.[45] After he left the US Senate in 1997, Hatfield served on the OHSU Board of Directors from February of 2000 to May of 2008.

Hatfield, who died August 7, 2011 at the age of eighty-nine, spent most of his life as an Oregon political leader. After graduating from Willamette University in Salem, he served in the US Navy as a landing craft officer in the World War II battles of Iwo Jima and Okinawa. Through his career, he opposed arms proliferation and used his influence instead to improve health care and research. After the war, he earned a master's degree in political science at Stanford University and entered politics as a Republican state representative for four years and member of the Oregon Senate for three more years. He went on to serve a term as Oregon Secretary of State, two terms as governor, and thirty years as a US senator.[46]

John Kitzhaber

John Kitzhaber, a former emergency physician and former Democratic state legislator elected to four terms as governor, attended OHSU's medical school and supported its transformation to a public corporation. Kitzhaber was governor when OHSU introduced Senate Bill 2 in the Legislature. He testified in support of it and signed it into law on May 24, 1995.[47]

He was chief architect of the Oregon Health Plan, which dramatically expanded Oregon's Medicaid population and helped push OHSU to become a public corporation. He also appointed OHSU's first board of directors. He stepped in as governor to urge the Attorney General's Office to grant OHSU a lease on its property so it would have solid standing to borrow money on Wall Street. He helped in a campaign to win voter approval for Measure 11, which allowed OHSU to save money by issuing general obligation rather than revenue bonds. He signed the Oregon Opportunity legislation into law on August 8, 2001, giving OHSU $200 million in state bonds that was paired with $300 million in private donations to support the university's dramatic research expansion. He supported legislation that gave the state's other seven public universities some of the independence OHSU achieved in becoming a public corporation. While supporting OHSU's dramatic transformation and growth over the two decades after it became more independent, he expressed concern that the academic health center was losing its commitment to its public mission of providing health care for the poor.[48] In 2003, after serving his second term as governor, he established the Center for Evidence Based Policy at OHSU.[49]

Kitzhaber, who commonly dressed in his signature blue jeans and cowboy boots, has been one of Oregon's most influential leaders as a legislator and the state's longest-serving governor. He was born in Colfax, Washington, in 1947. He graduated from Dartmouth College before earning his MD from OHSU, and worked as an emergency physician. He was elected to the Oregon House in 1978 and to the Oregon Senate in 1980, where he served three terms and was Senate president from 1985 to 1993. He was elected governor in 1994, served two terms, and then was elected again in 2011.[50] He led broad and systemic reforms in health and education, including an education reform act and the Oregon Health Plan in the early 1990s and the restructuring of the state's education governance system during his third term.

He married Rosemary Linehan in 1971 and they divorced three years later. He married Sharon LaCroix in 1995, and they had one son and divorced in 2003.[51] His current fiancée, Cylvia Hayes, started an environmental consultancy, and became a central figure in his political life. Almost immediately after Kitzhaber took office for his fourth term as governor in 2015, he became embroiled in a controversy over Hayes' work as a consultant for the state and questions about whether she was unethically or criminally advising him about green energy while consulting on the issue.[52] Under pressure from political leaders, both Democrats and Republicans, Kitzhaber resigned, though maintained he had "not broken any laws or taken any actions that were dishonest or dishonorable in their intent or outcomes."[53]

He continues to work as a consultant on health care issues and has indicated he would like to return to public life, telling one newspaper, "I've got runway ahead and gas in the tank."[54]

Phil Knight

Phil Knight, co-founder of Nike Inc., Oregon's largest corporation, has been OHSU's largest donor as well as a leading philanthropist for other enterprises and universities in the state. Knight, and his wife, Penny, pledged in the fall of 2008 to give OHSU $100 million over seven years for its cancer institute, the largest gift in the institution's history.[55] The university subsequently named the institute after him. Three years later, the Knights donated $125 million to establish the OHSU Cardiovascular Institute.[56] Then in 2013, Knight stunned OHSU leaders and guests gathered in the downtown Portland hotel to raise money for the university's Knight Cancer Institute. He and his wife promised to give $500 million to the institute if the university could come up with a match within two years, which it did. Knight said he had confidence that the institute, led by the groundbreaking researcher Dr. Brian Druker, would put a stop to a disease that touches all people. "We are more convinced than ever that cancer will meet its match at OHSU," he said, "and we are proud to play a role in this history in the making."[57]

Knight was born February 24, 1938, in Portland, and graduated from the University of Oregon with a journalism degree and from the Stanford University Graduate School of Business. He was a middle-distance runner at UO, capable of running a mile in four minutes and ten seconds. After a stint in the US Army, he became a US shoe distributer for the Japanese company Tiger. He became a partner in 1964 with his former UO track coach, Bill Bowerman, and they later co-founded Nike, which has grown into a multinational corporation, employing 44,000 people worldwide. The company, headquartered in Beaverton, is one of the world's largest suppliers of athletic shoes and apparel. Knight met Penelope "Penny" Parks in Portland, and they married in 1968.[58]

Knight invested in Will Vinton Studios, an animation company, in 1998 and subsequently purchased the company and renamed it Laika. He resigned as CEO of Nike in 2004, but retained his position as chair of the board until June of 2016. Knight has won many honors for his contributions to businesses, universities, and sports, including his induction into the Oregon Sports Hall of Fame in 2000 and the Naismith Memorial Basketball Hall of Fame in 2012. He was also elected to the 2015 American Academy of Arts and Sciences membership class.[59] His memoir, *Shoe Dog,* was published by Scribner in 2016 and quickly soared onto the *New York Times* bestseller list.[60]

Ted Kulongoski

Ted Kulongoski—former Oregon attorney general, Supreme Court justice, and governor—opposed OHSU's proposal to become a public corporation. He said he saw the conversion of Oregon's State Accident Insurance Fund into a public corporation in the 1980s lead to improprieties and functional problems, and he wasn't in favor of the model. OHSU probably could have been as successful over the last two decades as part of the state and its university system without becoming a public corporation, he said. At Governor Kitzhaber's request, Kulongoski did not publicly oppose OHSU's public corporation quest.[61]

Some OHSU administrators said Kulongoski's opposition to OHSU's public corporation structure appeared to be behind the Attorney General Office's reluctance to give the university a lease from the state on its campus land. But Kulongoski said he was not involved with the lease negotiations. He implied in comments to the State Board of Higher Education on November 17, 1995, however, that the lease posed dangers for the board and state. "Ultimately," he said, "from my perspective, somebody in the State of Oregon is going to be held responsible if there is a default."[62]

Kulongoski, whose full name is Theodore Ralph Kulongoski, was born November 5, 1940, in St. Louis, Missouri. Following his father's death when Kulongoski was four, he grew up in a parochial boys' home. He served in the US Marines, earned undergraduate and law degrees from the University of Missouri and, in 1970, went to work as a labor lawyer in Eugene. He is married to Mary Oberst, an attorney who has edited Oregon historical publications and been active in historical preservation.[63]

Kulongoski, a Democrat, was elected to the Oregon House in 1974 and to the Senate in 1978. Governor Goldschmidt appointed him state insurance commissioner in 1987, and he was elected state attorney general in 1992. He served on the Oregon Supreme Court from 1997 to 2001 and was then elected to two terms as governor from 2003 to 2011. He became a member of the faculty of the Mark O. Hatfield School of Governance at Portland State University after his governorship ended, and he was also chosen to review sentencing guidelines as a member of the Oregon Commission on Public Safety.[64]

Leonard Laster

Dr. Leonard Laster, a handsome, confident gastroenterologist from the East Coast, became OHSU's second president in 1978. He dragged OHSU out of its slumber, expanded its research capacity by building the Vollum Institute, and launched a number of other expansion projects.

He was a brilliant physician and researcher, born and raised in New York City and admitted to Harvard College in 1944 at age fourteen. He graduated from medical school in 1950 at age twenty-one. As a young doctor he joined the Public Health Service and became a researcher at the National Institutes of Health (NIH) when the agency was in its infancy. He stayed twenty-three years during NIH's golden age as it ushered in the modern era of medicine and later produced nine Nobel laureates.[65]

He moved on to become dean of the medical school at State University of New York Downstate Medical Center, and then was recruited to become president of the University of Oregon Health Sciences Center in 1978. His nine-year term at OHSU was marked by both conflict and significant growth, especially in research. He soon discovered that OHSU didn't find much respect within state government and was "not the favored child" in the state higher education system.[66]

He worked with US Senator Mark Hatfield from Oregon to launch a variety of building projects at OHSU, and Tektronix founder Howard Vollum helped him build the eight-story Vollum Institute for Advanced Biomedical Research in 1987, putting Oregon on the national map for biomedical research. OHSU's high-tech Biomedical Information Communication Center, the School of Nursing building, the Center for Research on Occupational and Environmental Toxicology, and the 660-foot-long bridge from University Hospital to the Veteran's Affairs Medical Center were all started by Laster with Hatfield's help. None was completed, though, before he left in 1987 to take his new job at the University of Massachusetts Medical Center. He later retired in Massachusetts.

Laster had conflicts with his administrators and faculty at OHSU, but he worked long hours, railed against mediocrity, and pushed his staff to strive for excellence. He was surprised when some faculty opposed the Vollum Institute as a waste of money. "That was a very, very difficult time—and a shock," said Laster. "I thought I was doing something that would get people starry-eyed."[67]

Barbara Roberts

Barbara Roberts, a former Democratic legislator and Oregon Secretary of State, served one term as Oregon's first female governor from 1991 through 1994 during a period when OHSU was seeking legislative approval to become a public corporation. She was elected governor the same day voters approved Measure 5, the property tax limitation law that pushed OHSU to seek a fundamental change in its governance structure.

Roberts initially asked Kohler and his leadership team to back off pressing for public corporation status because she didn't want their campaign to overshadow her push for tax reform, which included a proposed sales tax. After voters rejected her tax plan in 1993, she stepped up to support OHSU's public corporation proposal. In her 1995–97 budget plan, she pledged support for making OHSU a public corporation, though not for a proposal to give more autonomy to the entire university system. She included an influential budget note urging the 1995 Legislature to consider making OHSU a public corporation. With Roberts' blessing, Kohler and his team in early 1994 launched their public campaign for the law.[68]

Born as Barbara Hughey on December 21, 1936, in Corvallis, Oregon, Roberts spent a portion of her youth in Los Angeles before her family returned to Oregon. By the time she graduated from Sheridan High School in 1955, she'd already been married a year to classmate Neal Sanders. The couple moved to Texas, had two children, and then returned to Oregon. One of the children was autistic, which would eventually lead Roberts into political action. After she graduated from Portland State University in 1964, she began lobbying the legislature for special needs children and served on the boards of Parkrose School District and Mount Hood Community College. She and Sanders divorced in 1972, and two years later, she married Frank Roberts, a state legislator. In 1981, Barbara Roberts, too, was serving in the legislature as a member of the Oregon House of Representatives. She went on to be elected Oregon Secretary of State in 1981 and, five years later, governor. She only served one term as governor, during which her husband died.[69]

After leaving office, she served as director of the Harvard Program for Senior Executives in State and Local Government at Harvard University's School of Governance, associate director of leadership development at Portland State University's Hatfield School of Government's Executive

Leadership Institute, and from 2011 to 2013 as a member of the council of Metro, the Portland area's regional government.[70]

Joseph Robertson

Dr. Joseph (Joe) Robertson Jr., an ophthalmologist, rose from dean of the OHSU School of Medicine to replace departing President Kohler in the fall of 2006. He has presided over the academic health center since.

During his decade as president, Robertson has led OHSU through continuous expansion in keeping with Kohler's vision. He steered the university through a rough patch during the Great Recession, from which the institution quickly recovered. He adopted a strategy used often by Kohler of looking for partners who could help share the cost and increase the value of OHSU investments.[71] He and Portland State University President Wim Wiewel in October of 2010 struck a strategic alliance, pledging to conduct joint research, share faculty, and create a collaborative School of Public Health.[72] In the fall of 2015, OHSU joined Salem Health, which includes Salem hospital, to form a $2.5 billion-a-year integrated health system throughout the northern part of the Willamette Valley, where most of Oregon's residents are concentrated. It also signed a similar agreement to bring Tuality Health Alliance in suburban Portland into the network. Like Kohler, Robertson supports OHSU's rural health network and has helped expand medical education in Eugene and Springfield through partnerships with the University of Oregon and the PeaceHealth System. He said the university is building a statewide health care system.[73]

During his tenure, the university has dramatically expanded its campus on Portland's South Waterfront and attracted unprecedented private donations. In September of 2011, Bob and Charlee Moore, owners of Bob's Red Mill Natural Foods, donated $25 million to OHSU to establish the Bob and Charlee Moore Institute for Nutrition and Wellness at OHSU.

A year later, Nike cofounder Phil Knight and his wife, Penny, donated $125 million to establish the OHSU Cardiovascular Institute. Two years later, they pledged another $500 million for the Knight Cancer Institute if the university could come up with a match within two years, which it did. OHSU would not be able to attract such generous donations and would be half its size today, says Robertson, if it had not become a public corporation, "a foundational change" instrumental in its success.[74]

Robertson was born and raised in rural Indiana, the only child of a flour miller. He earned a degree in neuroscience at Yale University in 1974, and attended medical school at the Indiana University School of Medicine, where he met and married Dr. Margaret Hewitt, in 1976. He completed his residency in ophthalmology at OHSU, and, in 1997, earned a master's degree in business administration from the University of Oregon. In 1999, he and Hewitt, who had two children, divorced. He has remarried.[75]

The president has spent almost his whole career at OHSU. Robertson, who is skilled in performing micro-surgery on the retina, also served as chairman of the Department of Ophthalmology, director of the Casey Eye Institute, and dean of the School of Medicine. He currently serves on the Oregon Health Policy Board, which oversees the Oregon Health Authority.[76]

Steve Stadum

Steve Stadum, an attorney and legal expert on real estate, worked for OHSU in various administrative positions for seventeen years. He was a managing partner at Portland's Ater Wynne law firm when he agreed to help OHSU's Chief Counsel Janet Billups negotiate with the state in 1995 for a lease of OHSU campus property. Stadum commissioned a title search on all of OHSU's property to ensure there were no covenants or disputes that could complicate a lease. After several months of negotiations with the Attorney General's Office and the State Board of Higher Education, OHSU finally secured a fifty-year lease, allowing it to borrow money on Wall Street. Four years later, Stadum joined OHSU as general counsel and in 1999 persuaded legislators to give OHSU a perpetual ninety-nine-year revolving lease on the land.[77]

Stadum helped execute OHSU's expansion on Portland's South Waterfront. In 2004, he was named OHSU's chief administrative officer, overseeing all central administrative functions other than finance.[78] He was later promoted to OHSU executive vice president.

In 2010, Stadum announced he was going to leave OHSU, but President Joe Robertson enticed him to stay with the position of chief operating officer of the OHSU Knight Cancer Institute. In the summer of 2016, Stadum finally left to be executive vice president and chief operating officer for the Fred Hutchinson Cancer Research Center in Seattle.[79]

Stadum credited OHSU's conversion to a public corporation for its extraordinary expansion during the years he worked there. Without that change, he said, "we would have never had a board, we would have never been able to issue debt, and we would not have ever been able to take risks, be entrepreneurial and opportunistic."[80]

Mike Thorne

Mike Thorne, a Pendleton rancher, had left the Oregon Senate by the time President Kohler and his team pushed to make OHSU a public corporation in the Oregon Legislature. But he remained a strong ally, and when he was in the Senate, he helped Kohler move the Office of Rural Health from the State Department of Human Resources to OHSU's control and establish Area Health Education Centers across Oregon. In fact, even before Kohler was hired, Thorne promised to help him expand OHSU services into rural Oregon.[81] The plain-speaking rancher said he admired Kohler's efforts to use the public corporation model to let OHSU work out its own problems rather than turn to the state for money. OHSU showed, he said, that "if people get focused and are willing to commit themselves, you can solve things."[82] Over the years, Kohler sometimes visited Thorne in Pendleton. In 1995, Thorne served on the public corporation advisory board that recommended OHSU convert to a public corporation.

Michael Thorne was born September 25, 1940, in Pendleton, where he "grew up in the saddle on his family's wheat and cattle ranch." He graduated in 1961 from Washington State University, where on a blind date he met his wife, Jill, who was from Olympia, Washington. He worked as a wheat farmer, rancher, and real estate broker. He served as a Democratic state senator from 1973 to 1991, and chaired the Legislature's Ways and Means Committee. Jill organized his campaigns, served as an aide to Governor Goldschmidt, and was chair of the Oregon Trail Sesquicentennial.[83]

In 1991 Thorne became director of the Port of Portland for ten years, followed by three years in Seattle as CEO of the Washington State Ferries. He said he wished he had tried to convert the bureaucratic-laden ferry system into a public corporation.[84] In addition, Thorne is a former member for Benjamin Franklin Federal Savings and Loan Association and Willamette Industries, and a former chairman of a state task force that reviewed Oregon's land-use system.[85]

In 2009, the Thornes returned to their ranch in Pendleton.

Eugene Timms

Senator Eugene (Gene) Timms, a friendly Republican from the eastern Oregon town of Burns, was chief sponsor of Senate Bill 2, the legislation that enabled OHSU to become a public corporation. No one did more to influence the bill's success. As cochair of the Joint Ways and Means Committee, Timms played a key role in ushering the bill through the Oregon Legislature in 1995. The avuncular legislator, well liked by his community and by both Republicans and Democrats, made sure the bill got on the Senate Education Committee's agenda and to a vote by the full Senate. He testified in favor of the bill in committee and on the Senate floor.[86]

He also was concerned about the chronic shortage of health providers in rural Oregon and saw OHSU as an ally in addressing the problem. He worked with Kohler, almost from the day the OHSU president arrived, to move the Office of Rural Health from the State Department of Human

Resources to OHSU's control and to establish Area Health Education Centers across Oregon.[87]

Timms was born May 16, 1932 in Burns and raised there. He graduated from Burns Union High in 1950, earned a bachelor's degree in business at Willamette University, and married Edna Evans in 1953. He served a stint in the military before returning to Burns and his family's business, Alpine Creamery. Timms was active in his community and served in the state Senate twenty-two years. He died in 2014 at the age of eighty-one.[88]

Notes

1 Janet Billups, interview by author, April 2, 2014 in her OHSU office.

2 Ibid.

3 Janet Billups, interview by author, Oct. 6, 2014 in her OHSU office.

4 Lois Davis, interview by author, June 16, 2014 in her Portland State University office.

5 Ibid.

6 Lois Davis, interviews by author, Oct. 3, 2014 and March 9, 2015 in her Portland State University office.

7 Ibid.

8 Timothy Goldfarb, telephone interview, Oct. 2, 2014.

9 Ibid.

10 Timothy Goldfarb, interview by author, Sept. 7, 2015 at his home in Washington County, Oregon.

11 Lesley Hallick, interviews by author on May 27, 2014, Oct. 1, 2014, and Feb. 18, 2015; Lesley Hallick, interview by Charles Morrissey, Sept. 10, 2001, OHSU Oral History Project, OHSU Archives.

12 Ibid.

13 "OHSU and Oregon: Looking to Tomorrow," A Report to the 2007 Oregon Legislative Assembly, chart on "Growth and Change at OHSU—1975–2006," p. 5.

14 Blue Ridge Institute for Medical Research, "2006 rankings for medical schools and their departments," http://www.brimr.org/NIH_Awards/2006/NIH_Awards_2006.htm. Also, Kate Brown (secretary of state), "State Funds Resulted in Expanded Research at Oregon Health & Science University," Secretary of State Audit Report, 2010.

15 Peter O. Kohler, MD, interviews by author, May 17, 2004 and Dec. 5, 2014; Peter Kohler, MD, interview by Charles Morrissey, April 21, 1998, OHSU Oral History

Project, OHSU Archives.

16 Jim Walker, telephone interviews on June 16, 2014, Sept. 29, 2014, and Feb. 25, 2015.

17 Ibid.

18 Ibid.

19 Ibid.

20 Lewis W. Bluemle, Jr., interview by Joan S. Ash, May 22, 1998, OHSU Oral History Project, OHSU Archives.

21 Ibid.

22 Donald G. Kassebaum, MD, interview by Joan S. Ash, Nov. 7, 1997, OHSU Oral History Project, OHSU Archives.

23 Fred Buckman, interview by author, Dec. 10, 2014, in Beaverton.

24 Bill MacKenzie, "Buckman relaxed but ready," *The Oregonian*, June 30, 1996, p. R32.

25 Buckman, interview.

26 Mark Dodson, interview by author, Feb. 23, 2016 at Multnomah Athletic Club, Portland.

27 Ibid.

28 Ibid.

29 Brian Druker, MD, interview by Edward Keenan, Nov. 30, 2011, for the OHSU Oral History Project, OHSU Archives.

30 Brian Druker, MD, interview by author, Feb. 11, 2015, in Druker's OHSU office.

31 Davis, interview, June 16, 2014.

32 Ibid.

33 Andrew Theen, "Knight's $1 Billion Challenge to OHSU," *The Oregonian*, Sept. 22, 2013.

34 "Brian Druker," *Wikipedia*, https://en.wikipedia.org/wiki/Brian_Druker; also see-Andy Dworkin, "Persistence of vision," *The Oregonian*, June 29, 2003.

35 "Druker," *Wikipedia*.

36 Gail Kinsey Hill, "Where's Neil?" *The Oregonian*, March 31, 1996, p. A01.

37 Timothy Goldfarb, interview, Oct. 2, 2014.

38 Neil Goldschmidt, interview by author, June 15, 2015, in his Portland home.

39 Hill, "Where's Neil?"

40 "Neil Goldschmidt," *Wikipedia*, https://en.wikipedia.org/wiki/Neil_Goldschmidt.

41 Nigel Jaquiss, "The 30-Year Secret," *Willamette Week*, May 11, 2004, http://www.wweek.com/news/2004/05/11/the-30-year-secret/.

42 *Wikipedia*; Jaquiss.

43 Mark O. Hatfield, interview by Joan S. Ash, Oct. 22, 1998, interview no. 51 10/22, 1998, transcript, OHSU Oral History Project.

44 Bill Graves, "Federal Largess Benefits OHSU," *The Oregonian*, Aug. 5, 1990, p. D01.

45 Oz Hopkins Koglin, "OHSU will Renew Spirit of Research," *The Oregonian*, Feb. 15, 1998.

46 Jeff Mapes, "Mark O. Hatfield, Oregon's first statesman, dies Sunday at 89," *The Ore-*

gonian, Aug. 7, 2011, http://www.oregonlive.com/politics/index.ssf/2011/08/mark_o_hatfield_oregons_first.html.

47 John Kitzhaber, MD, interviewed by author, Feb. 12, 2016, in downtown Portland.

48 Ibid.

49 "John Kitzhaber, MD," *Wikipedia*, https://en.wikipedia.org/wiki/John_Kitzhaber.

50 Ibid.

51 Ibid.

52 Lee Van Der Voo and Kirk Johnson, "Gov. John Kitzhaber of Oregon resigns amid crisis," *The New York Times*, Feb. 13, 2015, http://www.nytimes.com/2015/02/14/us/kitzhaber-resigns-as-governor-of-oregon.html?_r=0.

53 Ibid.

54 Denis C. Theriault, "John Kitzhaber, with Facebook video and interview, returns to public eye," *The Oregonian*, http://www.oregonlive.com/politics/index.ssf/2016/03/john_kitzhaber_with_facebook_v.html.

55 "Knights to give $100 million to OHSU Cancer Institute," OHSU press release, Oct. 28, 2008, http://www.ohsu.edu/xd/about/news_events/news/2008/cancergift102908.cfm.

56 "Historic gift from Phil and Penny Knight establishes institute for cardiovascular research and care at OHSU," OHSU press release, Sept. 17, 2012, http://www.ohsu.edu/xd/about/news_events/news/2012/cardiology-gift.cfm.

57 Andrew Theen, "Knight's $1 Billion Challenge to OHSU," *The Oregonian*, Sept. 22, 2013.

58 "Phil Knight," *Wikipedia*, https://en.wikipedia.org/wiki/Phil_Knight.

59 Ibid.

60 "New York Times Best Sellers, Hardcover Nonfiction," http://www.nytimes.com/books/best-sellers/2016/05/22/hardcover-nonfiction/.

61 Ted Kulongoski, telephone interview by author, July 18, 2016.

62 Oregon State Board of Higher Education minutes, Meeting No. 647, Nov. 17, 1995, pp. 494, 496.

63 "Ted Kulongoski," *Wikipedia*, https://en.wikipedia.org/wiki/Ted_Kulongoski.

64 Ibid.

65 Leonard Laster, interview by Joan S. Ash, March 5, 1999, interview no. 64 3/5 1999, transcript, OHSU Oral History Project.

66 Ibid.

67 Ibid.

68 Barbara Roberts, telephone interview by author, April 15, 2016.

69 "Barbara Roberts," *Wikipedia*, https://en.wikipedia.org/wiki/Barbara_Roberts.

70 Ibid.

71 Joseph Robertson, MD, interview by author, Aug. 20, 2015, in his OHSU office.

72 Bill Graves, "OHSU, PSU Head In Same Direction," *The Oregonian*, Oct. 29, 2010, local news section.

73 Robertson, interview.

74 Ibid.
75 "Joseph Robertson (OHSU)," *Wikipedia*, https://en.wikipedia.org/wiki/Joseph_Robertson_(OHSU) .
76 Ibid.
77 Stave Stadum, interview by author, Dec. 11, 2014, in OHSU Hospital.
78 "OHSU Names Chief Administrative Officer," OHSU press release, May 26, 2004, http://www.ohsu.edu/xd/about/news_events/news/2004/05-26-ohsu-names-chief-adminis.cfm.
79 "Fred Hutch names new chief operating officer," Fred Hutchinson Cancer Research Center press release, April .29, 2016, https://www.fredhutch.org/en/news/center-news/2016/04/steve-stadum-fred-hutch-coo.html.
80 Stadum, interview.
81 Michael G. Thorne, interviewed by author, July 16, 2014, at the River's Edge Hotel & Spa in Portland.
82 Ibid.
83 Richard Cockle, "Back home in Pendleton, Mike and Jill Thorne still roping in leadership roles, *The Oregonian* Sept. 26, 2009, http://www.oregonlive.com/news/index.ssf/2009/09/back_home_in_pendleton_mike_an.html.
84 Thorne, interview.
85 Cockle; Michael G. Thorne, Oregon State University Board of Trustees member biography, http://leadership.oregonstate.edu/trustees/mike-thorne.
86 Davis, interview, June 16, 2014.
87 Kohler interviews.
88 Eugene "Gene" Timms, obituary, *Blue Mountain Eagle*, April 29, 2014, http://www.bluemountaineagle.com/Obituaries/20140429/eugene-gene-timms.

Timeline

1867

Less than a quarter century after the opening of the Oregon Trail and eight years after Oregon joined the union, Willamette University in Salem welcomes its first medical students to its campus.[1]

1877

Willamette University's medical program relocates to Portland.

1880

The Oregon–Washington Railroad and Navigation Company buys 360 acres of land, sight unseen, with plans to build a railroad depot and terminal, unaware the land is atop Marquam Hill, too steep for trains.

1887

The University of Oregon charters a state medical school in Portland at the request of eight physicians, including four who broke away from the Willamette University program—Simeon E. Josephi, Kenneth A.J. Mackenzie, H.C. Wilson, and George M. Welles. The University of Oregon Medical School enrolls its first class of seven students in the fall. The school occupies two rooms of a former two-story grocery store at NW Twenty-Third Avenue and Marshall Street in Portland.

1898

The Oregon College of Dentistry is founded in Portland.

1899

The Tacoma College of Dental Surgery moves to Portland. The following year it merges with the Oregon College of Dentistry to become the North Pacific Dental College, later renamed the North Pacific College of Oregon.

1913

Willamette University and the University of Oregon merge programs to form the University of Oregon Medical School.

1914

The present 116-acre Marquam Hill campus gets its start with a 20-acre tract donated by the Oregon–Washington Railroad and Navigation Company, and an 88-acre tract donated by the family of C.S. Jackson, former publisher of the *Oregon Journal.*

The statewide Child Development Rehabilitation Center Service Program is established, initially in the School of Medicine to provide diagnostic, treatment, and rehabilitation services for children with disabilities.

1919

The University of Oregon Medical School moves from downtown Portland into a new building at its present location on Marquam Hill in southwest Portland. The medical school's first building, Mackenzie Hall, was named after Kenneth A.J. Mackenzie MD, the school's second dean, who was also the railroad's surgeon.

The University of Oregon in Eugene begins offering courses in nursing.

1920

The Portland School of Social Work begins offering courses in public health nursing.

1923

Multnomah County Hospital opens on the Marquam Hill campus and contracts with the medical school to provide services to indigent patients.

1926

The University of Oregon establishes a five-year program leading to a degree in nursing. The following year a nursing dormitory is built on campus, named Emma Jones Hall after the nursing pioneer and superintendent of Multnomah County Hospital until 1944.

Doernbecher Memorial Hospital for Children is built on the Marquam Hill campus and becomes the first full-service children's hospital in the Pacific Northwest. The hospital was financed primarily by a donation from a charitable trust managed by the heirs of Frank Silas Doernbecher, a prominent Portland businessman who established Portland's leading furniture factory.

1928

The University of Oregon Medical School takes over operation of Doernbecher Children's Hospital.

1931

The outpatient clinic building is constructed and opens on Marquam Hill, allowing medical and nursing students and residents to gain practical experience.

1932

The Department of Nursing begins.

1938

The medical school adds a library and auditorium building, a three-story laboratory wing to Mackenzie Hall and an eighty-bed University State Tuberculosis Hospital, later converted to the Campus Services Building.

1943

Dr. David W. Baird is named dean of the University of Oregon Medical School.

1945

The University of Oregon Dental School begins.

1949

A new building opens for a basic science department and administrative offices, later named after David W. Baird, former dean of the medical school.

1952

A four-story east wing is added to Emma Jones Hall.

1954

The Child Development and Rehabilitation Center facility is built on Marquam Hill.

1956

The Medical School Hospital is built on Marquam Hill. The University of Oregon Dental School moves from Northeast Oregon Street to its present location on Marquam Hill.

1958

Dr. Albert Starr launches an open-heart surgery program at OHSU and produces the world's first successful heart valve replacement.

1960

The Department of Nursing Education becomes the University of Oregon School of Nursing in Portland and part of the Oregon State System of Higher Education.

1971

A new, eight-story, Basic Science Building, later named Richard T. Jones Hall for Basic Medical Sciences, opens as OHSU's example of Brutalism architecture.

1973

University Hospital is created through the merger of Multnomah County Hospital, Medical School Hospital and the outpatient clinics.

1974

University of Oregon Health Sciences Center is formed as an independent institution under the direction of the Oregon State System of Higher Education. The schools, hospitals, and all of the university's programs are brought together under one umbrella to create this new center, which becomes Oregon's only academic health center and one of 125 in the nation.

The Oregon State Board of Higher Education hires Dr. Lewis William (Bill) Bluemle, president of State University of New York's Upstate Medical Center in Syracuse, to be the Oregon medical center's first president.

1977

Lesley Hallick arrives at OHSU to be a professor and researcher, leaving the University of California at Berkeley, where she studied the structures of virus DNA and RNA.

1978

Leonard Laster, a gastroenterologist and dean of the medical school at State University of New York Downstate Medical Center, is hired to become OHSU's second president.

1981

The institution is renamed Oregon Health Sciences University.

1983

A $20 million Shriners Hospital for Children opens on Marquam Hill with thirty-nine beds and 80,610 square feet.

1984

Timothy Goldfarb leaves his job as senior associate administrator of the new hospital at the University of Arizona's medical center in Tucson to join OHSU as associate director of the University Hospital.

James Walker leaves the University of New Mexico Hospital to work as OHSU's chief financial officer.

1985

Legislators propose House Bill 2596, calling for a task force to study closing OHSU's hospital and, thereby, threatening the entire academic health center. The bill does not survive.

1986

Lois Davis leaves post as chief of staff for US Representative Ron Wyden, a Democrat from Oregon, to become government relations director for OHSU.

1987

Construction is completed on the Vollum Institute for Advanced Biomedical Research building. The institute is dedicated to the study of the brain and nervous system at the molecular level.

OHSU is designated one of two Level 1 trauma care centers in Oregon.

Leonard Laster leaves to become president of the University of Massachusetts Medical Center.

Janet Billups arrives as the Oregon Attorney General's Office representative at OHSU.

1988

Dr. Peter O. Kohler, an endocrinologist, leaves his post as dean of the medical school at the University of Texas medical center in San Antonio to become OHSU's third president.

New Veterans Affairs Medical Center opens on Marquam Hill.

1989

The Center for Ethics in Health Care is created to promote interdisciplinary study of ethical issues in health care.

The State Office of Rural Health becomes part of OHSU to help rural areas better address their unique health care needs.

The Area Health Education Centers program is established to promote better access to adequate health care and to facilitate medical student primary care clerkships.

1990

Dotter Interventional Institute is established at OHSU to carry on the work of the pioneer of interventional radiology.

Oregon voters approve Measure 5, a property tax limitation law that puts a squeeze on state funding for higher education.

1991

Casey Eye Institute opens on Marquam Hill.

Construction is completed for the Biomedical Information Communication Center, which provides library, audiovisual, and teleconferencing services; public computer services; and health informatics.

President Peter Kohler appoints a task force of business leaders, legislators, and representatives from OHSU to consider reorganizational options, including merging with the Oregon Health Division, becoming fully private, or transforming into a public corporation. The task force recommends it become a public corporation.

1992

The Center for Research on Occupational and Environmental Toxicology building opens. CROET is one of the first facilities in the world to combine the use of molecular and cell biology to study the adverse effects of chemicals on the body and, in particular, the nervous system.

The Veterans Affairs Medical Center bridge opens. The 660-foot-long suspended pedestrian enclosed skybridge is the longest in North America.

The Oregon Cancer Center is established with a grant from the National Cancer Institute of the National Institutes of Health, and Dr. Grover Bagby is appointed as its director.

The School of Nursing building opens.

1993

The School of Nursing begins coordinating a statewide integrated nursing education system that includes programs at OHSU, Eastern Oregon University, Southern Oregon University and the Oregon Institute of Technology.

Oregon Health Policy Institute, an interdisciplinary center of OHSU, Portland State University, and Oregon State University is created as a resource center for collecting, analyzing, and disseminating health policy information.

Physicians Pavilion opens on Marquam Hill to provide modern outpatient services.

Dr. Brian Druker, researcher who discovered the compound that became Gleevec, a virtual cure for chronic myelogenous leukemia, is hired by OHSU.

1994

The Oregon Regional Primate Research Center joins OHSU as an affiliate research institute.

OHSU Foundation and the Oregon Medical Research Foundation, owner of the Oregon Regional Primate Center, merge.

President Peter Kohler creates the Public Corporation Advisory Committee, chaired by former Governor Neil Goldschmidt, which urges state leaders to allow OHSU to become a public corporation.

Oregon Health Plan, led by Senate President John Kitzhaber, receives funding for implementation.

Governor Barbara Roberts endorses OHSU's public corporation proposal and gives President Peter Kohler and his team a green light to campaign for it.

1995

OHSU becomes a public corporation and independent of the Oregon State System of Higher Education and of state government regulations. Governance of OHSU changes from the State Board of Higher Education to the OHSU Board of Directors, whose members are nominated by the governor and approved by the Oregon Senate. The new board begins meeting in July.

Two floors for labor and delivery are added to the C-Wing of University Hospital, nine years after the project began.

The American Federation of State, County and Municipal Employees Local 328 go on strike for four days, the first labor strike in the medical school's history.

After more than four months of tense negotiations with the Attorney General's Office and the State Board of Higher Education, OHSU secures a fifty-year lease of its campus property. Four years later the lease is extended to ninety-nine years.

1996

OHSU issues a $215 million bond package backed solely by its good faith and credit as a public corporation.

University Hospital is renamed OHSU Hospital.

The first of OHSU's primary care neighborhood clinics opens in southwest Portland.

1997

Planning begins for the Center for Women's Health, and an interim director is named. The center offers a place where women's concerns can be addressed in a comprehensive, comforting, and supportive manner. The center uses a collaborative model that encourages women to actively participate in their care.

Portland Mayor Vera Katz appoints a twenty-five-member steering committee to study development of land on the city's South Waterfront.

1998

The Mark O. Hatfield Research Center is dedicated. The center houses a variety of basic and clinical research programs that have the potential to spark new therapies. It includes such programs as the Clinical Research Center, the Oregon Hearing Research Center, Doernbecher Children's Hospital Pediatric Research Laboratories, the Bone and Mineral Unit's osteoporosis studies, the Oregon Stroke Center, and the Oregon Cancer Center.

Doernbecher Children's Hospital's new state-of-the-art pediatric medical complex is opened. Built with private funding and bond revenues, Doernbecher provides the widest range of health care services for children in the region.

The Neurological Sciences Institute leaves Legacy Good Samaritan Medical Center in Portland and joins the university as its fifth research unit. NSI researchers conduct research to advance understanding of the brain and neurological disorders.

The Oregon Regional Primate Research Center becomes an OHSU research unit.

1999

During its annual retreat at Skamania Lodge in the Columbia Gorge, OHSU board agrees to pursue its Big Ask. The board will ask the legislature for $200 million in bond money financed by tobacco lawsuit settlement money.

Portland city staff and consultants produce the first draft of a development plan on Portland's South Waterfront.

2000

President Peter Kohler and his leadership team launch a campaign for $200 million in bonds from the legislature, arguing that it will help Oregon get a foothold in the burgeoning biotechnology business. OHSU board officially supports the plan, which is named Oregon Opportunity and also calls for raising $300 million in donations.

2001

The Oregon Legislature approves Senate Bill 832, also called the Oregon Opportunity Act, allowing the state to use its tobacco settlement money to finance $200 million in bonds for OHSU's research expansion. Governor Kitzhaber signs the bill on August 8, 2001.

The Vaccine and Gene Therapy Institute and Neurological Sciences Institute buildings open on OHSU's West Campus in Hillsboro.

OHSU's name changes to Oregon Health & Science University as Governor Kitzhaber signs legislation expanding OHSU's mission and paving the way for merger with Oregon Graduate Institute of Science and Technology. The merger took place July 1, 2001.

OHSU Board of Directors expands from seven to ten members.

Oregon Cancer Center changes its name to OHSU Cancer Institute.

Oregon Nurses Association union at OHSU goes on strike, which lasts nearly two months before a settlement.

Timothy Goldfarb, director of OHSU hospitals and the health care system, departs to work as chief executive officer of Shands HealthCare in Gainesville, Florida.

2002

Oregon Regional Primate Research Center changes its name to Oregon National Primate Research Center.

President Kohler's staff completes a thirty-year Marquam Hill Plan, guiding development on the hill and on the South Waterfront. Marquam Hill is designated a "plan district" by the Portland City council. Portland Planning Bureau releases proposed zoning and design guidelines for South Waterfront.

Portland City Council approves construction of a tram from South Waterfront to OHSU.

OHSU uses Oregon Opportunity money to create the Oregon Rural Practice-based Research Network.

2003

OHSU breaks ground for its first building in the South Waterfront District.

OHSU breaks ground for a new research building on Marquam Hill campus.

James Walker, vice president for finance and administration, retires from OHSU, and shortly thereafter goes to work as finance director for Lewis & Clark College.

2004

The Schnitzer Investment Corporation donates nearly twenty acres of riverfront property in South Waterfront to OHSU.

2006

Hildegard Lamfrom Biomedical Research Building opens on Marquam Hill.

Peter O. Kohler Pavilion opens as a state-of-the-art patient care facility on Marquam Hill.

The Center for Health & Healing, one of Oregon's greenest buildings and winner of the LEED (Leadership in Energy and Environmental Design) Platinum award, opens on the South Waterfront by the Willamette River.

The Portland Aerial Tram begins operating between OHSU's Marquam Hill Campus and South Waterfront.

Oregon Graduate Institute School of Science and Engineering and the Neurological Sciences Institute are dismantled. Some of their researchers join other OHSU departments, others leave.

OHSU ranks twentieth among nation's academic health centers in terms of research money from National Institutes of Health, reaching President Peter Kohler's central longtime goal.

Peter Kohler retires from OHSU, passing the torch on September 14 to OHSU's fourth president, Dr. Joseph Robertson Jr. Kohler goes to Arkansas to serve as vice chancellor at the University of Arkansas for Medical Sciences.

2008

A gift of $100 million from Nike cofounder Phil Knight and his wife, Penny, helps evolve the OHSU Cancer Institute to the OHSU Knight Cancer Institute.

2009

Lois Davis, vice president for public affairs and marketing, leaves OHSU to become vice president for public affairs for Portland State University.

Lesley Hallick, OHSU provost and vice president for academic affairs, leaves to become president of Pacific University in Forest Grove, Oregon.

2010

OHSU and Portland State University agree to a strategic alliance that includes joint research, shared faculty and a collaborative School of Public Health.

2011

The OHSU/OUS Collaborative Life Sciences Building and Skourtes Tower groundbreaking takes place on the Schnitzer Campus.

A gift of $25 million establishes the Bob and Charlee Moore Institute for Nutrition and Wellness at OHSU.

2012

A gift of $125 million from Phil and Penny Knight creates the OHSU Knight Cardiovascular Institute.

OHSU celebrates its 125th anniversary.

2013

Legislature approves bill giving Oregon's seven state universities more independence and authority to have their own governing boards.

2014

The OHSU/OUS Collaborative Life Sciences Building and Skourtes Tower opens on the Schnitzer Campus in Portland's South Waterfront District.

2015

OHSU sets fundraising record by meeting the challenge of Phil and Penny Knight and matching their pledge of $500 million.

OHSU joins Salem Health and Tuality Health Alliance to form a $2.5 billion-a-year integrated health system throughout Oregon's northern Willamette Valley.

2016

OHSU breaks ground on Portland's South Waterfront for the 320,000-square-foot Knight Cancer Institute research building, which will house up to 600 researchers and administrators.

OHSU also starts construction on the South Waterfront for the Center for Health & Healing South, a twenty-four-story building that includes a health care center, a guest house, and other mixed uses.

Notes

1 This timeline includes information from a historical timeline on the OHSU website: "History," About OHSU, http://www.ohsu.edu/xd/about/facts/history.cfm.

Index

Bold references are brief biographical profiles; *italic* references are images

CPSIA information can be obtained
at www.ICGtesting.com
Printed in the USA
BVOW05*1921100417
480865BV00005B/6/P

9 781945 398988